JANIE SPELTON WEINBERG, R.N., M.S.

Nursing Faculty
Thomas Jefferson University
Philadelphia, Pennsylvania

with contributions by

SHEILA GROSSMAN, R.N., M.S.

The University of Connecticut
Storrs, Connecticut

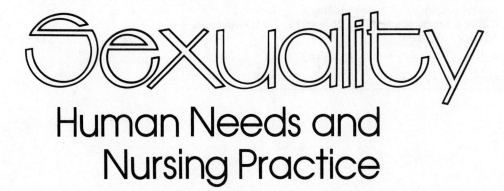

Sexuality
Human Needs and
Nursing Practice

1982
W. B. SAUNDERS COMPANY
Philadelphia   London   Toronto   Mexico City   Rio de Janeiro   Sydney   Tokyo

W. B. Saunders Company: West Washington Square
Philadelphia, PA   19105

1 St. Anne's Road
Eastbourne, East Sussex BN21 3UN, England

1 Goldthorne Avenue
Toronto, Ontario M8Z 5T9, Canada

Apartado 26370 — Cedro 512
Mexico 4, D.F., Mexico

Rua Coronel Cabrita, 8
Sao Cristovao Caixa Postal 21176
Rio de Janeiro, Brazil

9 Waltham Street
Artarmon, N.S.W. 2064, Australia

Ichibancho, Central Bldg., 22-1 Ichibancho
Chiyoda-Ku, Tokyo 102, Japan

Library of Congress Cataloging in Publication Data

Weinberg, Janie S.

Sexuality, human needs and nursing practice.

1. Sex (Psychology)   2. Sex (Biology)   3. Sex.
4. Sick — Sexual behavior.   5. Nursing.   I. Grossman,
Sheila.   II. Title.

BF692.W33   613.9   81–48671

ISBN 0–7216–9152–8   AACR2

Sexuality: Human Needs and Nursing Practice   ISBN   0-7216-9152-8

© 1982 by W. B. Saunders Company. Copyright under the Uniform Copyright Convention.
Simultaneously published in Canada.   All rights reserved.   This book is protected by copyright.
No part of it may be reproduced, stored in a retrieval system, or transmitted in any form or by any
means, electronic, mechanical, photocopying, recording, or otherwise, without written permission
from the publisher.   Made in the United States of America.   Press of W. B. Saunders Company.
Library of Congress catalog card number 81-48671.

Last digit is the print number: 9   8   7   6   5   4   3   2   1

To Sandy

PREFACE

Although there has been a significant increase in the number of texts available on the topic of human sexuality, few have been written specifically for nurses. Of those that have, nursing interventions are rarely included in each chapter. The nurse is the appropriate professional to collect sexual histories and to formulate care plans that include sexuality as an integral part of client care. Nurses spend a great deal of time with clients, and have the opportunity to establish a rapport with them that is often impossible for other health care workers to provide. Nurses are well trained in the social sciences, including communications, sociology, psychology, and human development, as well as in the medical sciences, including anatomy, physiology, and the study of disease and health states. The nurse is often the only member of the health care team who views the client as a whole individual. Partially as a result of this social science approach, the field of nursing has stressed holistic care— care of the entire person. Sexual health care is a vital aspect of this total care to which nurses have committed themselves.

This text is intended for both students and practicing nurses. It is presented as an overview of human sexuality, specifically as it relates to nursing practice. Sexuality throughout the life cycle is presented in depth, with special attention to nursing interventions appropriate at each level of the life cycle. Each chapter includes discussion of the nurse's feelings and attitudes and of roles for the nurse. This individual approach to nursing in each topic area is a unique feature of this text. Commonly encountered situations are discussed, as are appropriate actions for the nurse. Such examples serve to clarify theory and its application. Clarification is essential in order for nurses to function effectively in sexual health care delivery.

The issues of contraception, abortion, homosexuality, and rape will be covered in Unit III of this text, with specific nursing topics addressed. Finally, sexuality will be discussed in terms of illness.

Anatomy and physiology of sexuality is not covered in depth here. The biological aspects of sexuality and human sexual functioning are adequately covered in other texts and other sectors of the nursing curriculum. Readers wishing further information on the biological, physiological, and mechanical aspects of sexual behavior are advised to consult the references at the end of each chapter. Sources that deal with these complex topics have been included.

Nursing is in a unique position to provide for the sexual health care needs of clients. This care is appropriate to the goals of health promotion and primary prevention in nursing. It allows nurses to function as advocates for clients, and enables them to meet the growing demand for informed, responsible client care. It is with the purpose of helping to prepare nurses to fulfill this challenging new role that this text has been written.

JANIE S. WEINBERG

CONTENTS

UNIT I

Nursing and Sexuality

1

PERSPECTIVES ON NURSING AND HUMAN SEXUALITY

1. Each individual has the right to his or her own beliefs and convictions.
2. All people are sexual, regardless of personal, cultural, or health variables.
3. An individual or family unit, although sexually independent, is very much affected by the sexual milieu of the community and society.
4. The sexual self evolves as an integral component of the total physiological, psychological, and sociological development of the individual. The evolution is an ongoing process, extending from the moment of conception until the moment of death.
5. The reproductive system is not the sole physiological component of sexuality. The physiology of sexuality is expressed in the physiology of the whole body.
6. Puberty, conception, pregnancy, and menopause are all both physiological and psychological events that affect aspects of sexuality.
7. A person's state of health or illness will necessarily affect that person's sexuality, biologically, psychologically, and sociologically.
8. The physical sexual response cycle affects each body system, and therefore has the potential to affect symptoms of some illness.
9. Therapeutic modalities, including hospitalization, may affect the sexuality of the client and his or her family. The effect may be viewed positively or negatively.
10. The nursing process is the means through which the nurse provides sexual health care.
11. Professionals must be familiar with current knowledge about sexuality and sexual behavior.
12. A necessary prerequisite to helping others is the ability to talk openly and nonjudgmentally about sex.

PERSPECTIVE 1

Each individual has the right to his or her own beliefs and convictions.

All people are affected by their background, their culture, and their specific situation. Each of us develops a sense of values and beliefs as a part of growing up. For some, these values are unchanging throughout life; for others, much of life is spent in a re-examination and redefinition of these values. It is highly unlikely that any two people, regardless of their backgrounds, will hold exactly the same beliefs and attitudes.

For some individuals, including some nurses, encountering people with different values and beliefs is a highly emotional and threatening experience. To encounter beliefs sharply different from one's own requires that the individual either re-examine long-held beliefs in order to determine if they are still appropriate or retreat from the individual with the "different" and therefore "bad" beliefs. Either of these alternatives can be difficult.

It is in the encounters in which nurses must deal with people of different orientations (sexual or otherwise) that discussions of nonjudgmental behavior often occur. Nurses are admonished to set aside their own beliefs and attitudes in order to meet the patient at his or her level, and deal with the patient's problem. In situations in which values held by the patient differ from the nurse's but are not vitally important to the nurse, critical, objective evaluation and treatment of the client is easily accomplished. In situations in which values of great importance to the nurse are challenged, nonjudgmental treatment becomes a much more difficult task. If an individual strongly disagrees with the orientation of the nurse, whether through behaviors displayed or by verbal statements, the nurse will react at some level to this disagreement. Statements that challenge the values of the nurse *will* be responded to.

The way in which nurses respond to patients with sharply different views on topics of importance to them is highly significant. Ideally, nurses will be able to recognize their own biases in order to minimize their effect on interactions with patients. Nurses need not change their own attitudes on issues in order to deal with patients, nor is it necessary for nurses to persuade patients to change their views to conform to the nurse's. Nurses must recognize the inherent right of all people to hold values and beliefs that may differ from their own. This is not an easy task. Recognition of one's own value system is a difficult procedure to undertake and must be repeated frequently. Having understood their own biases, nurses may recognize previous nontherapeutic behaviors that were utilized as a reaction to patients with different values. Recognition of this negative behavior can be painful for the nurses whose interests lie in helping patients. Value clarification is a necessary first step, however, if nurses are to be able to truly respect the individuality of their patients. It is only through a thorough understanding of the self that a true respect for others can develop. Given this respect, nurses will be able to internalize the rights of others to hold their own beliefs and convictions.

PERSPECTIVE 2

All people are sexual, regardless of personal, cultural, or health variables.

In order for nurses to adequately deal with their patients as sexual people, they must recognize that they too are sexual, subject to the same types of feelings, insecurities, fears, joys, and pleasures as the rest of society. It is not appropriate for nurses to attempt to deny their sexuality in order to be more "objective" about their clients' concerns. In trying for such objectivity, nurses run the risk of losing their own warmth and understanding. More importantly, it is virtually impossible for any individual to be anything but sexual. The expression of sexuality may differ, according to background, sexual preferences, and health status, but the individual is sexual nevertheless.

Once nurses have recognized and internalized the reality of their own sexuality, they can be more open to the sexuality and the sexual health needs of their clients. The tendency to think of young adults as the only members of our culture who are sexual is a common one. All patients encountered in the health care delivery system, from the youngest infant to the oldest patient, are sexual. The identification of self as male or female, which begins at birth, is a sexual process. One need only watch a six-month-old infant handling his or her genitals to see that the baby is indeed sexual. The pleasure at examining objects with the mouth is another obvious indication of the sexual interest demonstrated at this early age. The natural curiosity of children about sexual activity, sex roles, and behavior indicates their interest in sexual matters. In short, all people at all stages and situations in life are sexual. To ignore this aspect in planning care for patients within and outside of the hospital is to deny and invalidate a part of the patient that cannot and should not be ignored.

Critically ill patients, dying patients, disoriented patients, paralyzed patients, patients in nursing homes, and any other patients who are encountered by nurses are sexual. Even in cases in which the nurse's tendency is to ignore the sexual needs of clients, the sexual needs do exist. Sexual needs encompass more than the needs for sexual intercourse. The need for privacy for bathing and dressing, for example, is a sexual need. All people are sexual, regardless of personal, cultural, or health variables.

PERSPECTIVE 3

An individual or family unit, although sexually independent, is very much affected by the sexual milieu of the community and society.

In examining the sources for sexual attitudes held by people in our culture today, Frieze (1978) identified three major areas from which our beliefs about sexuality arise: religion, Freud, and research in human sexuality. A brief overview of historical religious attitudes and recent scientific research in human sexuality is given in Chapter 3; however, the influences from these three areas are interwoven into all chapters. Some of our understanding of the psychological and physical aspects of human sexual development has undergone tremendous change because of scientific research. At times, when society tries to deal with issues that involve sexuality, the influences of religion and research come into conflict. The issues surrounding sexuality engender strong emotions, heated public debates, committed political movements, and nearly unsolvable legal questions.

When does life begin? Is abortion a crime or a private matter between a woman and her doctor? Can minors receive contraceptive information without parental knowledge? Is homosexuality a sin or an acceptable alternative lifestyle? How are the rights of individuals to decide on their own sexual behavior balanced with society's need for order and conformity? All one needs to do is to look around at our social institutions to realize the tremendous range of values and beliefs about sexuality in our society. On the one hand, religious groups with strong traditional standards about sexuality are growing in membership and political influence; on the other hand is the reality that

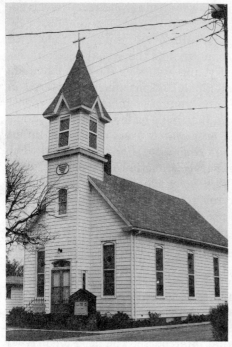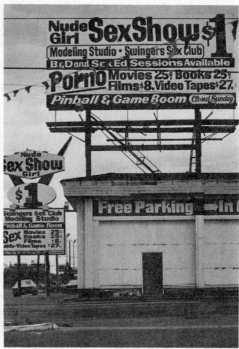

Photographs by L. Newman

Attitudes toward sexuality vary greatly in our society. In every large city, blatant commercial exploitation of human sexual needs can be found. These establishments offend many people, but their existence and their profitability indicate that they do serve some people's needs. On the other hand, strong religious influences support traditional values that sexual activity has a spiritual aspect and is moral and permissible only between married men and women.

sexually explicit television programs, books, magazines, movies, and even cassettes for home video players are widely accepted and profitable. What some groups view as "disgusting and immoral filth" others see as legitimate artistic expression or as profitable commercial ventures.

Obviously, what is considered acceptable public or private sexual behavior varies greatly among communities and cultural groups. It is precisely for this reason that the nurse, who interacts with people from all classes and backgrounds, must be aware of the influences that have shaped the beliefs and attitudes about sexuality in society today.

PERSPECTIVE 4

The sexual self evolves as an integral component of the total physiological, psychological, and sociological development of the individual. This evolution is an ongoing process, extending from the moment of conception until the moment of death.

Physiological development of the sexual self begins at the moment of conception, when the chromosomes determining the sex of the fetus are combined. In most cases, individuals with the XX combination of sex chromosomes become females, and those with the XY combination become males.

Hormones further affect the biological sex of the fetus in utero. As individuals develop hormones, they are further differentiated as males or females.

During adolescence, the individual's sexual self is bombarded by a variety of stimuli, all of which impinge on the sexual self. The hormones that determine the secondary sexual characteristics lead to both physical changes and psychological swings. The very appearance of the secondary sexual characteristics (the development of breasts in the female, facial hair in the male, and so on) has a profound effect on the individual. The individual can no longer identify himself or herself as a boy or a girl. The definition must now be as a young man or woman. This change is dramatic and requires the individual to redefine the self-concept. The redefinition can be a difficult one, for it entails an acceptance of the inevitability of adulthood and adult responsibilities. Another factor in this change in self-concept is the effect of the added hormone levels on the sexual desires of the adolescent. Suddenly, the adolescent may experience sexual feelings to a far greater degree than in the past. These feelings are confusing and somewhat frightening for even the well-prepared adolescent. Again choices must be made about behavior, attitudes, and beliefs. The adolescent must develop his or her own value system, separate from that of the parents. The value system includes more than the expression of sexual behavior. Indeed, the individual must begin to make the type of decisions that will ultimately determine his or her course through life.

The psychological adaptation to the sexual self continues throughout life. The decisions made in adolescence are not irrevocable. As the adolescent passes into young adulthood, new decisions and roles must be tried and incorporated into the self-concept. Forming a lasting relationship may be a part of the development of the young adult. The decision of whether or not to have children is another challenge to the identification of the individual as a sexual person. Middle age is a period of further changes in both lifestyle and physiological functioning that requires redefinition of the sexual self. Finally, in old age, the individual must again define himself or herself in terms of sexual functioning, life aspirations, roles as parent, grandparent, retiree, and so on.

The sexual self does not occur in a vacuum. The appropriateness of sexual behavior and expressions, as well as the appropriateness of sex role behavior, is largely determined by the society in which the individual lives. The choices available to the individual may be severely limited in some societies and seemingly unlimited in others. It is difficult to realize that the socially acceptable roles and behaviors for our culture and our Western society are not the same as those for individuals of other cultures. The tendency to view one's own culture and society as the "best" is one that can potentially make for real difficulties for the nurse faced with patients from other cultures. An awareness of the differences is necessary for acceptance of these differences.

In attempting to place the patient in the proper perspective, then, the nurse is faced with examining the individual's physiological status, the psychological status, and the society in which the individual has been living. Examining any of these components separately, or viewing them as static, leads to significant misunderstandings with the patient. The three components, physiological, psychological, and sociological, cannot be separated. The changes that each individual experiences as a part of living must also be realized and dealt with. The sexual self is complex and interactive. It cannot be examined only in its component parts. It must be viewed in the light of its existence—as an evolved set of complex interactions.

PERSPECTIVE 5

The reproductive system is not the sole physiological component of sexuality. The physiology of sexuality is expressed in the physiology of the entire body.

Physiological sex is determined during the embryonic period. Although the actual steps involved in determination of sex and sexual orientation are still widely debated, it is clear that in most cases, at birth the baby possesses all the required systems that determine sex.

Perhaps as a side effect of teaching reproduction as sex education, it is the tendency of most people to equate sexuality only with the reproductive organs. In fact, each body system contributes to the sexual functioning of the individual. This is most readily apparent when an individual experiences any alteration in function of a given system. The effect on the individual's sexuality, if investigated, will invariably show itself. For example, if the individual's endocrine system is compromised, sexual desire may be eliminated or significantly heightened. In the case of a woman in a state of estrogen deprivation, atrophy of the vaginal walls may lead to a decreased sexual desire as a result of pain experienced during intercourse. This pain can be eliminated with the use of estrogen creams or sterile lubricants before intercourse. If, however, the nurse or physician fails to inquire about this potential side effect, the patient may be too embarrassed to report her painful intercourse to the nurse or physician and may instead try to convince herself that sexual activity has ended for her.

In evaluating the sexual response cycle, Masters and Johnson (1966) clearly outlined some of the physiological changes that occur. Each of the body systems was demonstrated to be affected by sexual stimulation.

Another system, often absent in discussions of sexual function, is the psychological system. Disturbances in normal psychological functioning have a significant effect on the individual's sexual functioning. Often, for example, depressed patients report (if asked) a significant decrease in sexual desire.

Investigation of the physiological components of sexuality, therefore, must include all of the body systems. In the physical examination of an individual, sexuality must be included as a topic of investigation in all of the systems, not just the reproductive one.

PERSPECTIVE 6

Puberty, conception, pregnancy, and menopause are all both physiological and psychological events that affect aspects of sexuality.

Puberty is a stressful time for all involved with the individual experiencing it. The "child" is beginning to emerge as an adult. The transformation can be readily seen by all involved, and thus cannot be ignored. The adolescent must make what appear to be momentous and irrevocable decisions about sexual identity, sex role behavior, and sexual expression. Although on later reflection these decisions are seen as fluctuating greatly, the adolescent in the throes of puberty is intent on deciding these issues once and for all. Perhaps the most striking aspect of puberty that has a major effect on the adolescent is the tremendous increase in the desire for physical sexual expression that accompanies the increase in hormonal function. Values must be decided upon. Pubescent males or females must determine what values are acceptable in their own lives. No longer are the values of the parents accepted without question. At this turning point in their lives, most adolescents find themselves questioning everything and every value. Issues of relationships and roles emerge. Premarital sexual activity becomes an interesting possibility, which must be placed somewhere in the value system. Peers and their reported sexual activities have a great impact on the emerging sexuality of the adolescent.

For some, adolescence is the true awakening of sexual feelings. Of course, they have experienced sexual feelings from infancy, but their current feelings are much stronger and more difficult to ignore. It is a turning point in their sexual self-concept.

A second developmental milestone occurs for some individuals with the conception of a child. The pregnancy may be viewed as a joyous event to be celebrated, as a dreadful occurence that must be "dealt with," or somewhere in between. In the past, it has been commonly accepted that all individuals will marry and have children. This view of marriage with children is being challenged in modern times. The growing divorce rate, combined with the greater necessity for both partners to work, has tended to negatively affect the appeal of child-bearing. As a result, more couples are choosing to remain child free, or are having much smaller families. These decisions have a definite impact on the sexuality of the partnership.

In cases in which pregnancy is planned and wanted, the couple, although happy with the pregnancy, must sooner or later experience an alteration in their pattern of sexual expression. Early in pregnancy, the woman may be quite ill with morning sickness or fatigue, and may experience a decrease in sexual desire. Alternately, she may feel increased desire, since she is freed from having to use contraceptives and freed from the worry of becoming pregnant. Of course, the man's reaction to the pregnancy will have an effect on future sexual expression as well. Fear of harming the child may prevent him from enjoying sexual activities that he had previously enjoyed. On the other hand, he too may be thrilled at no longer having to use contraception. Whatever the reaction, both future parents are faced during pregnancy with temporary alterations in their sexual functioning, and a permanent role change once they become parents. New forms of sexual expression may need to be discussed. The importance of body contact and closeness during these times of change cannot be stressed enough. As during puberty, the individuals involved are facing significant role changes that will cause them to re-examine their sexual identities, sex roles, and sexual expression.

Menopause, and generally the age at which menopause occurs (around 50), represents another developmental milestone for both women and men in our culture. For the woman, menopause irrevocably tells her that she no longer can produce children. While for most women, childbearing has ended years before menopause, the physiological reality may lead some to depression. Most susceptible are those whose major self-perceived role has been that of "mother." Perhaps more important than the physiological event is the realization that the woman is aging, as is her partner. Along with aging in our society goes the unfortunate myth of sexlessness. Again, individuals in this age group must re-evaluate their sexual identities and sexual expression. For those who viewed sexual expression (especially intercourse) as intertwined with reproduction, the value of sexual activity in light of the absence of the possibility of reproduction must be re-examined.

The role changes experienced by both men and women in their careers as they age also have an impact on their sexual self-concept and general sense of well being. No longer are they seen as young "up and coming" workers. Instead, they may be seen as "old fashioned" and "outdated." These changing roles lead inevitably to the self-questioning and reassessment of the entire self, including the sexual self. The love and support of a partner can be instrumental in emerging stronger and more confident from this stressful period.

PERSPECTIVE 7

A person's state of health or illness will necessarily affect that person's sexuality, biologically, psychologically, and sociologically.

As discussed in the previous assumptions, an individual's sexuality is determined by his or her biology and psychological makeup and by the society in which he or she lives. It follows then, that any alteration in the normal function of the individual, including physiological and psychological spheres, will have an effect on that person's sexuality.

When patients are ill, the illness itself may lead to changes in their sexuality. The symptoms of the illness may lead to these changes. For example, an individual with compromised cardiovascular functioning may find the exertion required during most sexual activity to be too tiring to endure. In fact, the individual may be advised to refrain from sexual activity altogether in order to avoid overexertion. Although the individual suffering from these symptoms will need teaching and counseling to arrive at a form of sexual expression that is available and appropriate, given the limitations of the symptoms of the illness, the individual nevertheless need not be informed that sexual expression must end. In such a case, however, the illness has a significant effect on that person's sexuality.

In addition to the physical effects of the symptoms of illness, individuals suffer from psychological effects of variations in their health status. For some, just being defined as "ill" may be so debilitating to the self-concept that the individual may withdraw from many of the activities that had previously been an integral part of life. An individual who has recently experienced removal of some or all of the bowel and is left with a colostomy may refuse to engage in sexual activities with his or her partner for fear that lack of control, body odors, or the colostomy itself will be disagreeable to the sexual partner. The potential for a shortened life span may further inhibit this individual's capacity for sexual enjoyment. (It should be noted that in some cases, a diagnosis that includes a shortened life span has been found to increase the sexual desire of the individual.) The individual's self-concept as a sexual person and a sexually desirable person has been adversely affected by what is perceived by the individual to be severely mutilating surgery. Some surgeries that are required are indeed mutilating. Patients who have undergone such procedures will require great support and assistance to regain the self-confidence to resume their sexual activities. In some cases, the forms of sexual expression may need to be altered. In no case, however, must an individual cease to function as a sexual person. Physically handicapped persons in our society are rarely perceived as sexual persons. As a result of this, their sexual needs are often ignored. It is only recently, for example, that patients in rehabilitation units have been given sexual information following spinal cord injuries. Injuries that result in paralysis and lack of function of the genitals have for too long been equated with the death of sexual expression. This long-term disability is not easily placed in either the illness or health category. It is a condition, however, that necessitates intervention in order to assure the patient that a rewarding sexual life can indeed exist, even in the face of physical difficulties.

Illness of any kind will have some effect on the individual's sexuality. Because an individual's sexual self is such an integral part of the person's "self," illness must be seen as a disruption of this self.

PERSPECTIVE 8

The physical sexual response cycle affects each body system, and therefore has the potential to affect symptoms of some illnesses.

Perhaps the most commonly encountered illness in which the sexual response cycle affects the symptoms of illness is found in patients suffering from cardiac abnormalities. Many cardiac patients are encouraged to greatly curb physical activity in order to avoid the increased blood pressure, pulse, and respirations normally associated with the sexual response cycle. Patients who have suffered heart attacks are often very fearful of resuming sexual activity. They feel that the exertion may lead to another heart attack. They may fear that the body cannot withstand the pressure of the weight of another person during intercourse. For many, unless counseling is received, sexual expression stops after a heart attack.

Research indicates that resumption of sexual activity can indeed take place. One rule of thumb is that when an individual who has suffered from a heart attack is able to climb two flights of stairs without difficulty, he or she may resume sexual activity. In order to decrease the strain on the heart, most post–heart attack patients are advised to avoid sexual activity immediately after ingestion of a large meal or alcohol, during extreme cold or hot temperatures, near an anxiety-provoking setting or situation, and immediately prior to or following strenuous physical activity. The changes in the body system experienced during the sexual activity will bring about the symptoms of decreased cardiac efficiency but not to a dangerous level, provided that the individual's recovery has progressed to the aforementioned point.

The individual with any illness should be evaluated in terms of the effect of sexual activity on the symptoms of the illness. In the vast majority of cases, with proper planning and educative efforts, the individual can be restored to an acceptable level of sexual functioning. Some changes in the previous pattern of activity may be required. However, with the understanding of the necessity for changes, and the awareness that the sexuality of the individual is of great importance to the very concept of the self, a positive sexual identity can be preserved.

PERSPECTIVE 9

Therapeutic modalities, including hospitalization, may affect the sexuality of the client and his or her family. This effect may be viewed positively or negatively.

One of the greatest deterrents to the expression of sexual feelings of hospitalized people is the lack of privacy experienced by virtually all patients in the hospital. In addition to making sexual activity with a partner nearly impossible, the hospital situation practically rules out sexual expression. Even worse in denying privacy and the opportunity for sexual expression to patients are nursing homes and other types of long-term care institutions. This lack of privacy, at least in nursing homes, is seen by some as an extension of the denial of elderly persons as sexual beings.

When an individual is hospitalized, depending on the illness, his or her sexual desire may be greatly diminished or entirely absent. However, in other cases, the hospitalization itself may be the only deterrent to sexual expression for that person. In any case, since most individuals in our society are involved in partner relationships regarding sexual expression, the partner of the hospitalized patient is often left without an outlet for sexual expression. He or she may greatly miss the intimacy and sharing of the sexual act, and may wish to recapture this intimacy with the partner even within the hospital. Often it is this lack of sharing that is the motivating factor which leads to partners climbing into bed with patients. In some instances, sexual relations may be attempted. It is not uncommon in cases such as these for the couple to be interrupted by a staff member. The reaction of the individual who has unintentionally interrupted the patient and partner is of great importance. There may be great benefit to be derived for the patient from close contact with a loved one. The embarrassment experienced by all involved in cases where such activity is unintentionally encountered must be dealt with. One way to avoid such embarrassing situations is to provide more carefully for the patient's privacy. For example, nurses should knock and wait for the patient to tell them to enter before entering the room. This will provide an opportunity for both the nurse and the patient to escape a potentially embarrassing situation.

In providing for the privacy needs of patients, all patients must be considered. It would be inappropriate, for example, to have a couple in one bed of a semiprivate room engaging in intercourse while the patient in the next bed was in the room. It would be similarly inappropriate to have the patient without a partner leave the room in order to provide the necessary privacy for the couple. In some cases the nurse may fear for the patient's safety should the patient not respond to a knock at the door. Because of such difficulties, most attempts at privacy for patients are usually ignored. This overreaction is unnecessary and particularly dehumanizing. All individuals require and should be given some privacy.

Hospitalization is not the only modality that affects an individual's sexuality. Many drugs commonly given to patients have a significant effect on the sexual drive or libido of the patient. In most cases, drugs that have an adverse effect on the libido can be changed. In the few cases when this is not possible, the patient should be informed of this effect. The knowledge that the change in libido is related to the prescribed drugs can take a great deal of pressure off of the individual. If this information is not given, the patient may try in vain to explain the changes in feelings. This attempt to justify changes beyond his or her control can contribute greatly to a loss of self-esteem. This entire situation can be avoided by adequate and appropriate anticipatory guidance.

Not all therapies have a negative effect on the individual's sexuality, however. Certainly, some forms of reconstructive surgery, psychotherapy, and other forms of therapy that increase the patient's energy level may be seen as having a very positive influence on the person's sexual functioning. Any

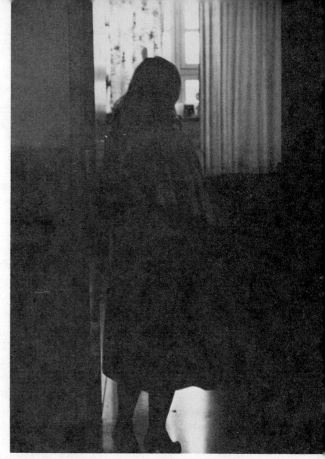

Hospitalization brings worries, fears and loneliness, both for the patient and for the partner who waits. Intimate contact can be a source of great comfort and healing, within the physical limitations of the patient's medical problem. However, when only a thin curtain and an unlocked door protect the couple's privacy, intimacy can be difficult or impossible.

Photograph by Jim Tackett

treatment that results in increased self-esteem is likely to have as a benefit improved sexuality.

PERSPECTIVE 10

The nursing process is the means through which the nurse provides sexual health care.

The steps of the nursing process include assessment, planning, implementation, and evaluation. The data base upon which nursing assessments of sexual care needs are made is the sexual history. The nurse collects these data in order to make an assessment of the patient's sexual health status and of his or her needs for education, counseling, or physical care. Any changes that may affect the patient's sexuality are included in the sexual history. This encompasses a great deal of the patient's life. But the role of the history and the specific information elicited by the nurse is important. It is not necessary or appropriate for a nurse to collect a detailed sexual history (or any detailed history for that matter) without some plan or notion of the use to be served by it. If the nurse does not plan to address potential problem areas uncovered in the history taking, the nurse must examine the value of eliciting such information. For example, the patient admitted to an acute care setting with an illness that will require short-term hospitalization need not be subjected to a complete sexual history; it is likely that issues raised will not be addressed during his or her short stay in the hospital. This is not to say that the sexual information included in a general history should be eliminated for such a patient. This general sexual information is indeed necessary, and can be addressed even in a short-term hospitalization. A complete, detailed history, such as the type presented as a model later is not necessary for such a patient.

The second portion of the assessment stage includes the physical examination. The nurse may or may not actually carry out the examination. Regardless of this, it is essential that the nurse understand the procedures and their purposes, so that the patient can be educated about them.

In planning for the sexual health care of patients, based on the assessment made by the nurse, three major roles for nurses in sexual health care emerge: The nurse as educator, counselor, and therapist. As more nursing programs include human sexuality in their curriculums, graduates of such programs will approach their patients with a firm base of knowledge in the field of sexuality. The role of the nurse as educator is one that can and should be filled by the graduate nurse. Generally, additional training is not necessary, provided that the undergraduate work in human sexuality was appropriate and sufficiently in depth. In the process of eliciting answers to some of the commonly asked questions about sexuality, the nurse is in an excellent position to educate the patient, on the spot and when the information is most likely to be well received and understood. For example, in asking a female patient what she was told about menstruation (as a follow-up question to her age at menarche) the nurse may learn that the woman continues to believe erroneous information passed on to her years ago, and be able to correct these misconceptions. The opportunities for patient education are practically unlimited for the nurse who is knowledgeable in and comfortable with sexual matters. The knowledge that the nurse possesses can frequently serve as a valuable tool to combat sexual fears and to help explain sexual feelings and behaviors for patients. By careful evaluation of the nursing process, nurses can better prepare themselves for their roles as sex educators, counselors, and therapists.

PERSPECTIVE 11

Professionals must be familiar with current knowledge about sexuality and sexual behavior.

Several factors are responsible for the lack of available sexual health care and for the seeming resistance in the health professions to providing this care. First, and perhaps of greatest importance, is the fact that for many individuals who are now involved in health care, sexuality and the sex act were not acceptable topics for discussion in the home. The prohibition continues to be expressed in adult life and does not automatically disappear when an individual becomes a nurse or physician. The student requires desensitization and resensitization in order to be able to discuss sexuality with comfort (Downey, 1976).

A second reason for not giving clients sexual information is that health professionals are inadequately prepared to discuss sexuality. Most nurses and other health professionals have not acquired the knowledge and skill during their formal education that would have enabled them to provide sexual health care to their clients. This lack of knowledge can at least partially explain the feelings of personal discomfort in discussing sexuality reported by Renshaw (1975).

Despite findings in studies of sexuality in nursing curriculums that indicated that sexuality was covered inadequately or not at all, instructor expectations of students regarding their roles in sexual health care were quite high (Woods, 1976). While these expectations are appropriate for most new graduates, it is impossible to realize these potentials without including comprehensive teaching of human sexuality in all phases of the basic nursing curriculum.

The role of sex therapist is one that can be filled only after extensive training in the field of human sexuality. Nurses should be aware of individuals who have been prepared to perform sex therapy, so that they can be sources of referral should the nurse encounter someone in need of this therapy. Sex therapists deal in cases of sexual dysfunction and in cases where more intensive therapy is required. Once again, the line between the sex counselor and the sex therapist is often indistinct.

Regardless of the role being performed by a given nurse in a given situation, interviewing skills are a prerequisite. Communication techniques can be utilized to help increase the patient's comfort level and to help the nurse to collect the necessary data to educate, counsel, or refer a patient to therapy.

The intervention stage of the nursing process includes those interventions that the nurse thinks will be most likely to help achieve the stated goal. In some cases, these interventions will center largely around education and supportive measures. In others, they will be involved in seeking out and following up on referrals. This followup is the responsibility of all nurses. It is imperative that nurses be sure that they are securing the best treatment for the patients they refer. Followup ensures feedback for nurses to adequately assess the referral source.

In the evaluation stage of the nursing process, the nurse determines whether or not the objectives stated in the planning phase have been met. The criteria should be measurable, so that evaluation is possible. For example, it is not possible to evaluate a goal that states that a patient will understand some aspect of sexual functioning. The nurse would need to include some criteria by which the objective would be evaluated. The patient could demonstrate understanding by explaining in his or her own words. Knowledge that the majority of people masturbate can be a great relief and reinforcement that they are "normal." The fact that certain practices are widespread does lead the patient to understand that his or her behavior is within the normal limits generally acceptable in our culture.

In the role of educator, nurses spend a great deal of time correcting misconceptions. Many people have never received formalized information on sexuality, and many continue to function on erroneous and misleading information learned in childhood. Learning correct physiological functions can clarify many misconceptions. Learning of common behaviors can further enhance the individual's sense of self-esteem and "normality." Of course, the nurse does not define "normal" or "abnormal." The educator role need not occur only after the initial assessment has taken place. The teaching can be informal and brief. It is not impossible for some of the educative value to arise from the history taking itself. (The educator role will focus primarily on the presentation of clear, concise material that can be easily understood by the patient.)

The role of counselor is somewhat more involved than that of educator and includes an emphasis on counseling. The roles are not mutually exclusive by any means, and should not be viewed as such. Counseling skills are essential, as is a good understanding of the physiological and psychological bases of sexual function and dysfunction. In simple situations in sex counseling, the graduate nurse should possess the skills necessary for counseling. Much of the role would overlap with the educator role, with only basic counseling skills necessary. For more-in-depth counseling, however, additional training is necessary (AASECT, 1973).

PERSPECTIVE 12

A necessary prerequisite to helping others is the ability to talk openly and nonjudgmentally about sex.

The idea of holistic care in nursing, that of caring for the whole person, has been common in nursing literature for a long time. It is only recently that the nursing profession has realized that it has been considering clients to be asexual, thereby ignoring a significant aspect of the client's life. Sexual health care has become a recognized need of patients that nurses can and should meet (Barnard, 1978; Downey, 1976; Rubin, 1965; Schiller, 1977). The nurse is often the first member of the health team to be approached by the client with questions regarding sexuality. These questions are critical to the client and should not be ignored or left unanswered.

The need for nurses to educate themselves is encountered with relative frequency in the literature dealing with sexuality. It has been determined in an excellent study (Payne, 1976) that, in fact, the more knowledge nurses have of human sexuality, the more favorable will be their attitude toward it, and the more comfortable they will be in professional situations involving sexuality. Here, then, is a major rationale for increasing education in the field of sexuality. By including this concept consistently in nursing curriculums, nurses who are comfortable with sexuality and who will include sexuality issues in their care can be prepared.

If a separate course in sexuality is not available, workshops could be utilized to supplement content. These workshops could serve the additional function of ongoing faculty education in sexuality and sexual health care. Because sexuality varies from culture to culture, students need the chance to clarify questions and to struggle with their impressions from youth, as well as educate themselves regarding values and goals. Workshops and small discussion groups could help to meet this need. Finally, the teachers of these students must develop expertise in sexuality counseling. Teachers who are prepared in this area can serve as role models for the students in both academic and clinical settings (Fitzpatrick, 1977; Hanson, 1978; Pfeiffer, 1968; Walker, 1971).

References

AASECT, 1973.

Bernard, Martha Underwood, Clancy, Barbara, and Krantz, Kermit: *Human Sexuality for Health Professionals.* Philadelphia, W. B. Saunders Co., 1978.

Downey, Greggs W.: "Sexuality in a Health Care Setting." *Modern Health Care*, Vol. 5, May 1976.

Fitzpatrick, Gehnevieve: "Filling the Gap in Education: Sexuality Issues and the Nursing Curriculum." *Nursing Care*, Vol. 10, August, 1977.

Frieze, Irene: "Sexual Roles of Women." *In* Frieze, Irene H., Parsons, Jacquelynne E.,

Johnson, Paula B., Ruble, Diane N., and Zillman, Gail L. (Eds.): *Women and Sex Roles: A Sociological Perspective*. New York, W. W. Norton and Co., 1978.

Hanson, E. Ingavarda: "Sexuality Curriculum and the Nurse." *In* Rosenweig, Norman, and Pearsall, F. Paul (Eds): *Sex Education for the Health Professional: A Curriculum Guide*, New York, Grune and Stratton, 1978.

Masters, William H., and Johnson, Virginia E.: *Human Sexual Response*. Boston, Little, Brown and Co., 1966.

Payne, Tanya: "Sexuality of Nurses: Co-relations of Knowledge, Attitudes and Behavior." *Nursing Research*, Vol. 25, No. 4, July-August, 1976.

Pfieffer, Eric, Verwoerdt, Adrian, and Wang, Hsiohshan: "Sexual Behavior in Aged Women and Men." *Archives of General Psychiatry*, Vol. 19, December 1968.

Renshaw, Meena C.: "Nurses Need Formal Sex Education." *Journal of Nurse Education*, Vol. 14, November 1975.

Rubin, Isadore: *Sexual Life After Sixty:* New York, Basic Books Inc., 1965.

Schiller, Patricia: "The Nurse's Role as Sex Counselor." *Nursing Care*, Vol. 10, July 1977.

Walker, Edith G.: "Study of Sexuality in the Nursing Curriculum." *Nursing Forum*, Vol. 10, No. 1, 1971.

Woods, Nancy, and Mandetta, Anne F.: "Sexuality in the baccalaureate nursing curriculum." *Nursing Forum*, Vol. 15, No. 3, 1976.

THE SEXUAL HISTORY AND PHYSICAL EXAMINATION

In keeping with the nursing process, assessment is the first step the nurse undertakes in the sexual health care of clients. Assessment includes a sexual history and a physical examination. To collect sexual history information, nurses must be comfortable with and knowledgeable about the topics covered in order to perform the "on the spot" teaching that accompanies sexual history taking.

The second step in the assessment of the client is the physical examination. The physical examination cannot be excluded if the health care worker is to get a complete objective as well as subjective data base from which to plan care. The sexual examination includes the female and male pelvic examination. Both afford nurses the opportunity to teach their clients. For example, women may be taught about breast self-examination and male sexuality during the procedure. Often in our society, women are not taught about male sexuality or physiology, and men are not taught about female sexuality or physiology. This lack of information leads to tremendous misconceptions on both sides, which can be reduced by education by nurses in the field of sexual health care. Men should be taught about testicular self-examination and female sexuality during their examinations.

This chapter includes the sexual history, including interviewing techniques, and a sample history outline. The second portion of the chapter describes the physical examination of both the male and the female. Human sexual response will be discussed in Chapter 3.

THE SEXUAL HISTORY—INTERVIEWING

Although many individuals in the health fields believe that sexual health is a necessary component of care, they are reluctant or too embarrassed to collect the necessary baseline data from which to formulate nursing care plans. An appropriate sexual history is a prerequisite for adequate assessment of the client. Taking the sexual history can serve to facilitate the development of an environment in which the client will feel comfortable while discussing sexual health. By including sexual history data with the rest of the medical and social data usually collected, the nurse communicates an acceptance of the importance of sexual health (Green, 1975). In addition to providing an atmosphere that permits clients to discuss their sexual health, the process of eliciting data may be therapeutic in that it permits verbalization of anxieties that the client might not otherwise have volunteered. The nurse can then reassure the patient of the widespread nature of most sexual acts, such as masturbation and oral-genital sex. The patient can then determine that, indeed, the behaviors are acceptable. The potential for education and anticipatory guidance is apparent, given the historical data (Payne, 1976; Roznoy, 1976).

THE INTERVIEW SITUATION

Taking a sexual health history need not be a traumatic situation for either nurse or client. It is appropriate to take the sexual history at the same time that the medical history is taken. Nurses should be aware that it may take more than one session to collect the history data. They should keep in mind that baseline data are always being enlarged, and must not feel pressured to complete every detail of the history at the first meeting.

Interviewing involves many complex skills. In approaching the sexual interview, whether it is concerned with a specific problem, such as illness, or whether it is to obtain the necessary baseline data, skillful nurses utilize all of the communication and interviewing skills at their disposal. Prior to a discussion specific to the sexual history, the interview situation will be discussed, including the interviewer's contribution to the interview and the phases of an interview. A discussion specific to sexual history will then follow.

When approaching the counseling situation, establishment of a trusting and therapeutic relationship is of the utmost importance. Four ingredients that are necessary for the establishment of such a relationship will be discussed here in terms of the nurse and the client. This relationship should not be viewed as one that occurs only in an institutional setting. The nurse is a highly visible individual and may make contact with people in a variety of settings. The four areas to be discussed are as follows (Benjamin, 1969; Lief, 1976; Semmens, 1978):

1. Sensitivity of nurses to their own personal attitudes, values, and feelings.
2. Sensitivity of nurses to the client's attitudes, values, and feelings.
3. Assurance of confidentiality.
4. Developing trust.

Sensitivity of Nurses to Their Own Personal Attitudes

Throughout the nursing literature one encounters the admonition to thoroughly know oneself in order to deal effectively with the problems and lives of others. This maxim is definitely true in the area of sexuality and sexual counseling. Only through an understanding of ourselves can we understand our biases and strengths and be able to control our behavior. By exerting this control we are able to better understand and to appreciate the behavior of others.

What, then, do nurses bring to the interview situation? They bring knowledge and information, professional skills, experience, and all of the resources that they have at their command. In addition, nurses bring themselves to the interview. The unique self of the nurse combines a desire to be of use and a warm regard and liking for others with the background prejudices and shortcomings common to all humans, and the nurse's own internal frame of reference. The importance of the nurse's awareness of self cannot be overemphasized. Clients are very sensitive to the affect or feeling tone of the interviewer. In stressful situations, such as that in which sexuality is discussed, the person being interviewed is even more attuned to the feelings of the interviewer. If the interviewer is struggling with but is unaware of her or his own problems, this uncomfortable feeling will almost always be transmitted to and picked up by the person being interviewed. Clearly, this can greatly interfere in a therapeutic relationship. Interviewers who are comfortable with themselves and the topic are free to concentrate fully on the client, unencumbered by their own working through of feelings. The feeling of comfort with self can contribute greatly to putting the client at ease and to the eventual establishment of trust in the relationship.

In becoming aware of the effect of self on the interview, the nurse must be aware of nonverbal communication. Facial expressions, body gestures, and tone of voice are often more important to the conversation than are the actual words. Consider the following situation: You are to meet an old friend for lunch and you arrive a half hour late, for whatever reason. You apologize, and he tells you that he is not angry that you are late. However, he sits through your interaction tapping his foot, speaking in short, quick sentences, on the edge of his seat, during what would otherwise have been a relaxed and enjoyable meeting. Despite his words, you clearly receive a nonverbal message of anger. These nonverbal aspects must be considered by anyone involved in counseling. The video taping of interviews can be most useful in learning some of the possibly unconscious nonverbal behaviors that an individual may exhibit.

Cultural biases must also be examined by nurses. All of us have grown up in a society that has some very rigid ideas about sexuality. We must become more aware of the effect that our upbringing has had on us, and recognize the biases inherent in each of our experiences. Most nurses come from middle class family systems that may not correspond to the situations of our clients (Green, 1975).

For example, the majority of individuals involved in family planning and contraception have a general bias toward planned families, in terms of both spacing and number of children. It is difficult, then, to accept the client who is pregnant with her ninth baby in 12 years and who refuses contraception because her husband will not allow her to use any form of birth control and will not use any himself. Many cultural biases are evident in this example. Health care professionals who feel strongly that the population problem must be addressed by having smaller families are at risk of becoming quite angry with women they feel are contributing to the population problem. Nurses who are concerned with the quality of care that children receive from their parents may feel that couples in this situation would not be able to adequately meet the needs for love and support of so many children. Health care workers who are concerned with the individual's right to control her own body may feel anger toward clients for not standing up for their rights and insisting that either they use birth control or their partners use some method of contraception, including the possibility of permanent sterilization.

Sensitivity to Client Attitudes, Values, and Feelings

What has not been considered here is the cultural background, beliefs, and values of clients and their family systems. Perhaps fertility is a major source of status within the culture of a particular family, and, as such, is of great value to both of the partners involved. What is important is that the health workers have brought their own biases to the situation and have reacted to them. This reaction will probably be noted by clients, who may not return for the prenatal care they need. It must be stressed that nurses, or any health care workers, will have feelings about clients, particularly those whose values differ from their own. It is not necessary that the nurses change their attitudes. What is required is that they acknowledge prejudices, beliefs, values, and biases and possess the ability to prevent them from interfering with the provision of the best possible care for clients.

Sensitivity of the nurse to the attitudes, values, beliefs, and feelings of clients implies an overall acceptance and respect for them. Clients must be treated as individuals and as equals. By showing a sincere interest in clients and their world, the interviewer demonstrates a respect for them. Honesty is another essential component of the therapeutic relationship. The interviewer should avoid assuming an all-knowing attitude, and should tell a client if he or she does not understand or know the answer to a problem. Together, then, interviewer and client can search for solutions. By excluding external interference as much as possible, the interviewer demonstrates respect for the individual. Privacy for the interview is essential. The nurse demonstrates acceptance of the client by regarding the thoughts and feelings of the client with sincere respect. It is not sufficent to state that the client is "OK." The behavior of the nurse is the crucial element in demonstrating respect. By respecting the feelings and thoughts of the client, the nurse is not bound to agree with or share the values of the client. What the nurse demonstrates by this respect is a recognition of the right of the individual to hold unique values, and the right of the individual to be listened to in a nonjudgmental fashion.

Another way in which nurses can show respect for and acceptance of clients is to allow them to use their own language regarding sexuality. This requires that nurses be familiar and comfortable with this terminology. To expect clients to be able to utilize medical terminology is to expect them to conform their perceptions to the value system of the interviewer. This is not to say that nurses must utilize "street language." Clients and nurses should use mutually understood terminology.

In order to be effective listeners, nurses must strive to understand clients. Understanding has been described by Benjamin (1969) as occurring on three different levels. On the first level, we may be thought to "understand about" another person. This level of understanding emcompasses the understanding that we receive from the perceptions of others. We may read about the individual, or hear others talk to us about the individual, or we may receive some kind of verbal report from another person. This level of understanding is necessarily superficial and may not agree with our later understanding of the individual.

The second level of understanding of a person is the understanding that occurs when we see another person with our own eyes. By using our own perceptual apparatus such as thinking, feeling, knowledge, and skills, we come to understand the individual in terms of ourselves. This second level is obviously much deeper than the first level of understanding, but carries with it the inherent bias and lack of true understanding of how events will and have affected individuals from their own frame of reference.

The final level, which is strived for and may or may not ever actually be attained, is the level at which nurses develop an "understanding with" the other person. This level of understanding requires that nurses put aside their own feelings and try to understand how clients feel from their point of view. The purpose of this high level of understanding is not to agree or disagree with people, but rather to understand how they are feeling. This final level has been called empathy (Lief, 1976) and is thought to be the ultimate sensitivity to clients.

The levels of understanding discussed above can sometimes be confusing. In order to clarify them, an example will be utilized. The situation involves a nurse, Diane, and her patient, Ms. Jones. Ms. Jones is a 30-year-old patient on an obstetrics and gynecology floor. Two days ago she had a complete hysterectomy. At report, Diane learns that Ms. Jones has two children at home, and has what seems to be a happy marriage. Her husband has been in to visit her both days, and although the children were too young to visit, they have managed to sneak into the room to see their mother. In the report, the nurse going off duty tells Diane that Ms. Jones has been very upset, becoming tearful at times. The nurse feels that Ms. Jones is upset at the loss of her uterus, since it means that she can no longer have children. At this point in her understanding with Ms. Jones, Diane is on the first level. She has learned about Ms. Jones from someone else. The other nurse has provided her with factual information and his own perceptions of the problem.

When Diane is seeing each of her patients for the first time on the shift, she walks in and finds Ms. Jones crying. Diane offers to sit with Ms. Jones until she is feeling better, but Ms. Jones tells her that she would rather be alone. Diane respects Ms. Jones's wishes, telling her that she will be back, and perhaps then Ms. Jones will feel like talking. In the interim between their first and second meeting, Diane attempts to pull together her knowledge of other patients she has encountered who have become depressed following a hysterectomy. She notes that Ms. Jones is young for such

a procedure and might indeed be mourning her loss of reproductive capacities. She also considers other possible explanations for Ms. Jones's depression. Ms. Jones may be crying because she is experiencing a great deal of pain, or she may have had an argument with her husband. Diane wonders how she would feel if she had just undergone a hysterectomy. Having proceeded to the second level of understanding, Diane returns to Ms. Jones, who is more composed and seems ready to talk.

In their somewhat superficial opening discussions, Ms. Jones tells Diane (rather sheepishly) about the incident in which her children violated hospital rules to visit her. She tells Diane that it was important for her to see them, since she feared that they would think that she was never coming home to them. Diane takes this opportunity to ask Ms. Jones if she had planned to have any future children. Ms. Jones says "No!" quite emphatically, and adds that at least now she won't have to worry about contraception.

As the discussion continues, Diane asks Ms. Jones what she feels will change (if anything) in her life as a result of the surgery. At this point, Ms. Jones again begins to cry, telling Diane that she is afraid that she will no longer be able to enjoy sexual relations with her husband. When Ms. Jones relates this fear, Diane is able to move into the third level of understanding. She is able to look at Ms. Jones's problem from Ms. Jones's point of view. In addition, of course, Diane can and does provide the information and sexual counseling that Ms. Jones so desperately needs.

The stages of understanding are not separate, distinct stages, but are best viewed as part of a continuum. On the early end of the continuum is the superficial knowledge and understanding of a client, while at the other end is the feeling of empathy.

Assurances of Confidentiality

A highly sensitive and important area that must be covered in any interview situation is the confidentiality of the information. All clients must be advised as to what material will remain between the nurse and the client only, and what material, if any, will be shared with others. Both parties must be clear on this, and must agree before a trusting relationship can be established. Most nurses will encounter and care for clients in conjunction with other health team members. The issue of how much of the information gathered should be shared with the rest of the team can be a confusing one for the nurse. Generally, it is best to "reveal everything that is absolutely necessary, and absolutely nothing that is not" (Benjamin, 1969). Often a client will divulge more information than is necessary or pertinent to the care given by other members of the health team. Again, the nurse must be certain to discuss with the client exactly what will be divulged, to whom, and for what purpose. The client may then take an active role in his or her care by participating in the decision making process.

Developing Trust

Perhaps the most important factor in the development of trust between a client and a nurse is the interest, understanding, and accepting attitude toward the client that is displayed by the nurse. An open and honest attitude is of great importance. The interviewer must be "human" during the relationship. The cold, aloof counselor will find it almost impossible to form a trusting relationship with the client. The difference between the nurse and the client is that the nurse has specific knowledge that the client needs and does not possess. This difference in knowledge and skills does not, or should not, place the client in a subordinate position to the health care professional.

Listening skills are an integral part of the repertoire of a good counselor and are necessary to the development of trust. Good listening requires giving full attention to the client, hearing the way things are being said (including tone, expressions, and gestures), and hearing what is not being said (those things that are hinted, held back, that which is beneath the surface). This therapeutic listening is difficult, especially for the new nurse or counselor, who must learn to listen to the client rather than focusing on what to say next (Benjamin, 1969).

PHASES OF THE INTERVIEW

Most interviews consist of three distinct phases. The first phase involves a statement of the purpose of the interview. The interviewer should state as precisely as possible the purpose for initiating the interview. A statement of the time that is available and the time that is considered adequate should also be a part of this introductory phase. An example of this is, "Mr. Abbott, my name is Ms. Peters. I am the nurse who will be helping you to plan your care during your hospital stay. I would like to spend some time talking with you so that I can get to know you better. In the next hour, I would like to discuss your past history with you and look at some concerns you may have upon entering the hospital."

The second phase of the interview is the content phase. It is characterized by a mutual probing of some matter. It is during this stage that many of the techniques of the interviewer are utilized. Some of the more familiar techniques are silence, restatement, clarification, explanation, and listening.

For some people silence is the most difficult communication technique to employ. Beginning interviewers are often very uncomfortable with silence and may have an overwhelming desire to fill them. Silence may occur during an interview for any of several reasons. The most common cause is a lengthy pause by the interviewee in order to sort out thoughts or feelings. During this time, he or she may be reflecting on what has been said. If the interviewer speaks at this time, the effect may be to break the other person's train of thought and possibly cause general confusion in the person.

Confusion itself may be the cause of periods of silence in the interview. Of course, the interviewer will wish to clarify any confusion that the person being interviewed might have. Generally, if the client is confused, the interviewer will see some sign, such as a perplexed facial expression. Such nonverbal behavior can be very valuable in determining when to allow silence to continue and when to validate that the impression of confusion is in actuality the reason for the silence.

Finally, silence may arise out of some resistance on the part of the client to participate in the interview. Perhaps the timing is poor or sufficient rapport has not yet been established. The client may not feel comfortable enough to discuss what may be seen as a personal matter. The nurse who encounters resistance to a given topic may wish to go back to a less threatening topic until he or she feels that the client is ready to proceed.

Restatement is utilized by the interviewing nurse to let the client hear what she or he has said. The interviewer acts as an echo. This may encourage the client to go on speaking, to examine and look deeper. It also helps to communicate to the client that the interviewer is listening. The nurse does not attempt to interpret what the client has said in restatement.

Clarification usually involves the interviewer making a statement that is very close in meaning to that made by the client, but in a more simplified version, in order to determine whether the interviewer has "gotten the message" intended by the client. It should be noted, however, that the client may need the nurse to clarify what the nurse has said. This need is appropriate and should not be ignored.

Explanation involves the use of descriptive statements that may or may not contain evaluations by the nurse. As a rule, the explanation is neutral in tone, tending to be impersonal and logical. Explanations may be utilized as an orientation to a situation: for an explanation of behavior, for an explanation of causes, or for an explanation of the interviewer's position.

Listening is very important in interviewing and has been discussed earlier. It is not necessary to listen any differently when listening to sexual matters than when listening to any other concern. A genuine interest in the client is necessary, as is an understanding and accepting attitude in the nurse.

The final phase of the interview is the closing. At the end of the interview, both participants should be aware that the interview is coming to an end. As a rule, no new information should be introduced or discussed in the closing portion of the interview. The main concern at this time lies with what has already been discussed. Restatement and summation are often utilized during the closing of an interview. In order to let the client know that the interview is soon to be over, the nurse could say, "Well, our time is just about up. Is there anything you'd like to say before we try to see where we have arrived?"

This tells the client that the interview will soon be over and paves the way for restatement and summation. It also serves the purpose of allowing both participants to feel a sense of closure to the interview.

Summary: Interviewing

The preceding discussion on interviewing has been somewhat lengthy. At this point, a summary of the factors discussed will clarify the general principles that should be utilized in sexual interviewing (Elder, 1973; Lief, 1976; Mims, 1977; Schiller, 1977).

Nurses should remember that a sexual history is a conversation between two people. Counseling techniques are of great importance in a conversation of this type.

Interviewers must be comfortable in discussing sexuality. They must be aware of the fact that clients usually see them as informed authorities and are receptive to their attitudes about sex. This places a great deal of responsibility on nurses. They must possess sufficient knowledge of related medical, psychiatric, psychological, and other behavioral sciences to be able to recognize when referral for more specialized help is needed.

Clients should be allowed to arrive at their own answers when exploring moral issues. It is up to the nurse to provide an atmosphere in which the client can express feelings without fear of rejection from the nurse.

It is the responsibility of the interviewer to provide privacy for the interview and to insure confidentiality. The issue of confidentiality is an important one. The client must be sure that information disclosed will be treated responsibly. He or she should participate in decision making regarding disclosure of information to other health team members.

Good listening skills are essential. Listening is a prerequisite for a trusting relationship. Listening requires giving full attention to what an individual says. The listener must be aware of that which may be beneath the surface in the interaction (Benjamin, 1969). Many new interviewers initially have a great deal of trouble listening because they tend to be thinking of what they will say next while the interviewee is talking. It is imperative that the interviewer listen rather than focusing on her or his own next statement. The silence needed for the interviewer to collect her or his thoughts is time well spent provided that the interviewer can then attend to what the client has said.

Sufficient time should be allowed to cover the discussion topics adequately. If it is not possible to accomplish this in one interview, as is sometimes the case, another interview should be scheduled before the client leaves. If the interviewer has a suspicion that the data required may take more than one interview, the client should be informed of this as early in the interview as possible. In addition, the time available should be stated clearly, so that both the client and the interviewer understand this limitation.

Vocabulary must be clarified during the interview. It is essential that both participants understand how they are using words. The language utilized must reflect an understanding between the two. Nonverbal communication must also be considered. Facial expression, body gestures, and voice tone are important components of communication, and potentially carry greater weight than the spoken word. Interviewers must pay great attention to their own nonverbal communication, as well as to that of the interviewee.

Interviewers must guard against making assumptions about clients that have not been validated. For instance, individuals who report that they are sexually active are not necessarily heterosexual. This type of assumption is easy to make, and is commonly encountered, but can be very detrimental to the establishment of a working relationship. On a more emotional level, nurses should avoid labeling patients. Labeling can be very damaging to the individual, who may carry the label throughout his health care experiences.

Finally, the nurse should *determine in advance, if possible, how much detail to obtain during the interview.* Naturally, at times such plans must be modified, but having some idea of the depth of the interview can enable the nurse to better judge the amount of time needed and the most appropriate setting for the interview.

THE SEXUAL INTERVIEW

A general rule of thumb often encountered in the literature regarding sexual history-taking is the principle of beginning the interview with the topics that are easiest to discuss, and then, without haste, proceeding to those that, in our culture, are more difficult (Green, 1975; Roznoy, 1976; Wahl, 1974). Utilizing a life chronology is a good way to accomplish this. The interviewer can begin the discussion by asking the client how he or she first learned about sexuality during childhood. Using statements of universality can help to decrease anxiety in the client. For example, the nurse may state, "Many people tell me that they had their own ideas about where children came from when they were young. Before anyone spoke to you about this, what were your ideas?" By prefacing direct questions about sexual experience with such universal statements, the nurse can help to create an atmosphere in which the client feels comfortable to reply. It is neither the purpose of nor is it appropriate for the nurse to judge any behavior or information as right or wrong. Once a question has been asked, the nurse should allow time for the client to answer the question fully, or to modify the response.

During the interview, questions are a primary source through which the nurse will be gathering information from the client. An open question is the most likely to elicit detailed information. It allows the client full scope in answering. By asking an open question, a nurse is soliciting the thoughts and feelings of the client. An example of an open question that a nurse might ask during an interview is, "How do you remember feeling when you first learned about menstruation?" A question such as this is far more likely to allow the individual to discuss feelings than is a question that includes the answer, such as "You really felt afraid when you first learned about menstruation, didn't you?" Asking a double question limits both the client and the nurse. For example, the nurse may ask, "Were you happy or sad when you first learned about menstruation and that it would happen to you?" By asking this double question, the interviewer has given the client only two choices—happy or sad. It is entirely possible that the client had mixed feelings. She might not be comfortable enough with the question to answer anything other than one of the two choices. Bombarding is another type of questioning that is almost always confusing and tends to stop discussion rather than encourage it. For example, an inexperienced nurse could ask, "How old were you when you first learned about menstruation? How did it make you feel? Did you find out from your parents or your friends?" Obviously, the client isn't going to know which question to answer first, or whether she should answer all of them or none of them. Bombarding is often a problem for beginning interviewers who may not be comfortable with silences that may follow the initial question. In order to "fill" those silences, the nurse may add another question, compounding the problem of silence. The nurse should strive to utilize open questions whenever possible. In some situations, particularly ones in which an initial history is to be obtained, closed, direct questions are necessary in order to obtain certain concrete facts, such as age of menarche, marital status, etc. Often the data learned by the nurse from the concrete closed information type questions can serve as the basis for the deeper, more open line of questioning that will allow the client to discuss his or her concerns.

On occasion, inexperienced nurses may find that, somehow, despite their best efforts, the interview has not gone well. They may wish to learn the reasons for this. Some of the most common impediments to communication are enumerated:

1. *Interruption.* The interviewer who does not allow the client to finish what he or she is saying is likely to anger clients, and may misinterpret what they were going to say next. In any event, the interview will not go smoothly with a nurse who interrupts.
2. *Advice giving.* This behavior is not appropriate. It is the clients who must ultimately decide what is right or wrong in their specific situations. The role of the nurse is to provide support and guidance.
3. *Moralizing.*
4. *Use of approval and disapproval.* This technique is utilized by some interviewers both consciously and unconsciously. The nurse is not in a position to judge right or wrong, and therefore should neither approve nor disapprove of a client. To use this technique is to take unfair advantage of the power inherent in the counseling relationship, and will lead to the eventual loss of a relationship between equals.
5. *Ridicule.*
6. *Disbelief.* This implies to the client that the nurse feels the client is incapable of accurate perceptions.
7. *Contradiction.*
8. *Denial and rejection.*
9. *Scolding/punishment.*
10. *False encouragement.*
11. *The use of "why" questions.* For many, being asked "why" they have done something or why they think or feel something carries with it the connotation of disapproval or displeasure, even if the nurse doesn't wish it to. Because of this, "why" questions should probably be avoided, whenever possible.

Ethical Issues

In discussing the gathering of history data of any kind from patients, the issue of confidentiality is usually addressed. Assuring the patient that information gathered will not be shared with others if such action is not necessary for the patient's care is a significant step that is essential for the establishment of a trusting relationship. The patient must feel free to disclose intimate information without fear that the information will be used in an irresponsible manner. In the area of sexual information, confidentiality must be combined with a firm sense of what the information will be used for in planning the patient's care. If the nurse is not able to determine what will be done with the sexual information elicited, this data collection tool must be re-evaluated. Each individual's sexuality and sexual history has a tremendous impact on that person and must not be ignored. However, in their zeal to provide the sexual health care that has been omitted for so long, nurses need not overreact to the extent that they collect irrelevant and unusable information.

A very detailed and extensive sexual history adapted from the Marriage Council of Philadelphia's sexual history outline follows. It is appropriate to use such a data collection tool for patients who are seeking sexual therapy. In most cases, however, nurses will not be dealing with such patients, and therefore will need to choose from this outline those areas that are pertinent and appropriate for the patients they usually encounter. For example, nurses who work in gynecological nursing will probably care for women who are about to undergo hysterectomy. In the initial screening, it would be appropriate to the nursing care of the patient to determine what she learned in adolescence about menstruation, since many of the ideas surrounding the beginning of menstruation are related to ideas and beliefs about the ending of menstruation. Also important for a woman about to have a hysterectomy are her feelings about herself as feminine and her general sexual adjustment at the present time. By looking through the sexual history guide, the nurse can identify areas that are appropriate to the specific client and will in this way be laying the foundation for individualized and more personalized care for the patient, based on appropriate data collected in the nursing history. The more complex tool should be used as a guideline and a reference tool to remind the nurse of areas that may have been overlooked previously.

THE SEXUAL HISTORY

As are other assessments, the sexual data base is composed of subjective and objective data. The subjective data, the actual history information obtained, will be discussed at some length here. Objective data include the pelvic and breast examination findings for women and the findings of the genitourinary examination for the male.

In the following pages a somewhat lengthy form will be provided for the taking of a sexual history (Barnard, 1978; Masters, 1970). A thorough history has been included here to give the reader a comprehensive model from which to individualize formats. By the time sexual data are discussed during the initial interview, the nurse will already have learned a great deal about the client. If sufficient rapport has been established, the interview will go smoothly and quickly. It is important that the nurse not repeat questions during the sexual history that have already been answered elsewhere in the history. This may convey to the client that the nurse has not been listening to the previous information that has been discussed.

Recording the history information can be difficult. It is not conducive to discussion for the client to be faced with a nurse who is furiously scribbling notes on all that is being said, or who is trying to fill in the blanks on a history form. If the nurse is unable to recall data after using only brief notes, it may be preferable to utilize a tape recorder for the interview, in order to accurately report the information given, unhindered by the need to take notes. Of course, the client must give permission for this. The nurse and the client should both understand what is to be done with the tape after the history is transcribed, and must be assured of the confidentiality of the information. Although the use of the tape recorder may be threatening to both the client and the nurse at first, both seem able to forget about it as the interview proceeds.

Sexual History

    I. Demographic Data
       A. Client
          1. age
          2. sex
          3. marital status (single, number of times previously married, currently married, separated, divorced, remarried)
       B. Parents
          1. ages
          2. dates of death and ages at death
          3. birthplaces
          4. marital status (married, separated, divorced, remarried)
          5. religion
          6. education
          7. occupation
          8. congeniality
          9. demonstration of affection
          10. feelings towards parents
       C. Siblings (as indicated)
       D. Current Primary Relationship-Partner
          1. age
          2. marital status (number of times previously married; remarried, if divorced)
          3. place of birth
          4. religion
          5. education
          6. occupation
          7. cultural background
       E. Children
          1. ages
          2. sex
          3. strengths
          4. problems
   II. Childhood Sexuality
       A. Family attitudes about sex
          1. degree of parents' openness or reserve about sex
          2. parents' attitudes about nudity and modesty
          3. behavior about nudity and modesty: (a) parents; (b) client
       B. Learning about sex
          1. asking parents about sex: (a) which parent; (b) answers given; (c) at what age; (d) nature of questions; (e) feelings about it
          2. information volunteered by parents: (a) which parent; (b) what information; (c) at what age; (d) feelings about it
          3. explanations by either parent (indicate which parent or parent substitute): (a) sex play; (b) pregnancy; (c) birth; (d) intercourse; (e) masturbation; (f) nocturnal emissions; (g) menstruation; (h) homosexuality; (i) venereal disease; (j) age at time of each explanation; (k) feelings about such learning
       C. Childhood sex activity
          1. first sight of nude body of same sex: (a) age ("how young"); (b) feelings; (c) circumstances

2. of opposite sex: (a) age ("how young"); (b) feelings; (c) circumstances

3. genital self-stimulation: (a) age ("how young"); (b) before adolescence at first occurrence; (c) manner; (d) orgasm? ("how often"); (e) feelings (pleasure, guilt); (e) consequences, if apprehended

4. other solitary sexual activities (bathroom sensual activity regarding urine, feces, odors)

5. first sexual exploration or play (playing doctor) with another child (possible reply may be never): (a) age; (b) sex and age of other child; (c) nature of activity (looking, manual touching, genital touching, vaginal penetration, oral-genital contact, anal contact, other); (d) feelings (pleasure, guilt); (e) consequences, if apprehended (what and by whom)

6. other episodes of sexual exploration or play with other children before adolescence (subcategories as in #5 above)

7. sex activity with other persons: (a) at what ages; (b) ages of other persons; (c) nature of activity; (d) willing or unwilling; (e) force or actual attack involved?; (f) feelings

D. Childhood exposure to intercourse
   1. parents' intercourse: (a) hearing; (b) seeing; (c) feelings
   2. other than parents: (a) hearing; (b) seeing; (c) feelings

E. Childhood sexual theories or myths
   1. thoughts about conception and birth
   2. functions of male and female genitals in sexuality
   3. roles of other body orifices or parts (e.g., umbilicus) in sexuality and reproduction (e.g., oral impregnation, anal intercourse, anal birth, pregnancy by kissing, etc.)

F. Other childhood sexuality

III. Onset of Adolescence
   A. In girls
      1. preparation for menstruation: (a) informant; (b) nature of information; (c) age given; (d) feelings about way in which information was given; (e) about the information itself
      2. age: (a) at first period; (b) when breasts began developing; (c) of appearance of pubic and axillary hair
      3. menstruation: (1) regularity (initial, subsequent, present); (b) frequency; (c) discomfort; (d) medication; (e) duration; (f) Kotex, tampons; (g) feelings about first period; (h) about subsequent periods

   B. In boys
      1. preparation for adolescence: (a) informant; (b) nature of information; (c) age given
      2. age: (a) of appearance of pubic and axillary hair; (b) change of voice; (c) of first orgasm; (d) with or without ejaculation; (e) frequency of orgasm; (f) for how many years?
      3. emotional reactions: (a) to early or delayed onset of adolescence; (b) to first orgasm

   C. Sexual orientation
      1. (a) attracted to opposite sex; (b) feelings
      2. (a) attached to same sex; (b) feelings

IV. Orgastic Experiences
   A. Nocturnal emissions (male) and orgasms during sleep (female)

1. frequency: (a) adolescence; (b) young adult; (c) adult; (d) middle age; (e) old age
2. accompanying dreams

B. Masturbation
1. age when begun
2. ever punished?
3. frequency per week: (a) during teens; (b) during twenties; (c) during thirties, etc.
4. method: (a) usual; (b) others tried; (c) others used
5. current partner's knowledge of past or present masturbation
6. practiced with others: (a) before current relationship; (b) current partner
7. emotional reactions
8. accompanying fantasies

C. Necking and petting ("making out")
1. age when began
2. frequency
3. number of partners
4. types of activity

D. Intercourse (see also section IX on next page)
1. frequency of occurrence
2. number of partners
3. kinds of partners (fiancé(e), lover, friend, prostitute, unselective)
4. contraceptives used: (a) needed? (homosexual relationship)
5. feelings about premarital intercourse: (a) for women; (b) for men; (c) for different ages
6. accompanying fantasies

E. Orgastic frequency (overall)
1. during teens
2. during twenties
3. during thirties
4. during forties, etc.
5. orgasmic difficulties
6. effect of partner or situation on orgasm

V. Feelings About Self as Masculine/Feminine
A. The male client
1. does he feel masculine?
2. popular?
3. sexually adequate?
4. any feelings about being a "sissy"?
5. does he feel accepted by his peers? belong to a group?
6. feelings about: (a) body size (height, weight, etc.); (b) appearance (handsomeness, virility); (c) voice; (d) hair distribution; (e) genitalia (size, circumcision, undescended testicle, virility, potency, ability to respond sexually); (f) cross-dressing (any experience in doing so)
7. wish to change sexual relationships

B. The female client
1. does she feel feminine?
2. popular?
3. sexually adequate?
4. was she ever a "tomboy"?
5. does she feel accepted by her peers? belong to a group?

      6. feelings about: (a) body size (height, weight, etc.); (b) appearance (beauty); (c) breast size, hips; (d) distribution of hair; (e) cross-dressing (any experience in doing so)

      7. wish to change sexual relationships

VI. Sexual Fantasies and Dreams
    A. Nature of sex dreams
    B. Nature of fantasies
      1. during masturbation
      2. during intercourse

VII. Dating
    A. Age ("how young")
      1. first date
      2. first kissing: (a) lips; (b) deep
      3. first petting or "making out": feelings
      4. first "going steady": feelings
    B. Frequency: feelings about frequency of dating

VIII. Engagement
    A. Age: (formal or informal?)
    B. Sex activity during engagement period
      1. with fiancé(e): (a) kissing; (b) petting; (c) intercourse
      2. with others: (a) number of individuals; (b) frequency; (c) nature of activity

IX. Primary Relationship
    A. Vital statistics
      1. date of marriage: (a) if not married length of relationship
      2. age: (a) interviewee; (b) spouse/partner
      3. partner's occupation
      4. is partner present at interview?
      5. previous relationships: (a) interviewee; (b) partner
      6. reason for termination of previous relationships (death, divorce, etc.): (a) interviewee; (b) partner
      7. number, sex, and ages of children from previous relationships: (a) interviewee; (b) partner
    B. Sexual relationship with partner (if not previously covered)
      1. how long knew each other before becoming sexually involved
      2. what attracted client to partner? what is unattractive?
      3. do partners confide in each other? share?
      4. talk about sex life in and out of bed?
      5. relationships with other partners during this primary relationship?
      6. partner's other relationships: (a) feelings
      7. petting: (a) frequency; (b) feelings about it
      8. intercourse: (a) frequency; (b) feelings about it
      9. contraceptives used: (a) needed; (b) kind used, if any
      10. level of commitment to relationship
      11. Are partners satisfied with the relationship?
    C. Wedding trip (honeymoon)
      1. social and geographic particulars: (a) where; (b) duration; (c) generally pleasant or unpleasant?
      2. sexual considerations: (a) frequency of intercourse; (b) was sex pleasant or unpleasant?; (c) was spouse aroused?; (d) was orgasm achieved (occasionally, always, never)?; (e) was spouse consid-

erate?; (f) any complications (impotence, frigidity, pain, diffi-
culty in penetration, "honeymoon" cystitis)
  D. Pregnancies
      1. number
      2. at what ages
      3. results (normal births, cesarean deliveries, miscarriages, abor-
         tions)
      4. effects on sexual adjustment (fear of pregnancy)
      5. number wanted and number unwanted
      6. sex of children wanted or unwanted
 X. Sex After Death of Spouse, Separation, or Divorce
  A. Outlet
      1. orgasms in sleep
      2. masturbation
      3. petting
      4. intercourse
      5. homosexuality
      6. other
  B. Frequency of past or current resort to outlet
  C. Feelings about such experience

OBJECTIVE DATA

A complete physical examination, especially pelvic, Pap, and breast examinations for women and genitourinary examination for men, is indicated after
collection of the sexual history. In addition to ruling out the possibility of
organic dysfunction, the physical examination offers the nurse an excellent
opportunity for teaching the client about sexuality (AASECT, 1978). The
nurse may or may not actually perform these physical examinations, but they
are necessary in order to complete the sexual health assessment.

An appropriate teaching role during the collection of the woman's objective data is the teaching of breast self-examination. If the woman reports
that she does this, the nurse can have the client demonstrate her techniques
in order to validate the methods being used. She may then reinforce the
client's good efforts or may teach the client the appropriate methods of breast
self-examination.

During the examination of the male genitalia, the nurse can teach the
male client the proper technique of checking for testicular tumors. In addition,
the nurse can take the opportunity to inform the male client about symptoms
of urinary infections, and the fact that venereal diseases are becoming more
and more asymptomatic. A discussion of female sexuality may arise during
discussions of contraceptive use with the male client.

The Female Pelvic Examination

Many women report negative feelings about pelvic examinations. Even women
who report that they have never had any uncomfortable or otherwise upsetting
examinations still dread the routine pelvic and Pap smear. Settlage (1975)
has outlined five reasons why women have negative feelings regarding pelvic
examinations. The first of these involves exposure and manipulation of a

person's genitals. Normally, only those with whom the client is very intimate are given access to the genitalia. This exposure is most often in the context of mutual trust and closeness. The lithotomy position contributes to women's discomfort about this exposure, despite any attempts at draping. In addition to the exposure and manipulation of the genitals, most women fear that the examiner will find or validate some pathology.

A second source for the reluctance of women to undergo pelvic examinations is closely related to the first. The pelvic examination is a violation of the body privacy of the client by a person who is at best an awesome, friendly stranger. Regardless of the fact that the stranger is friendly, the privacy is violated.

Many women (and men) express confusion about the covert and overt sexual overtones of the examination. This has been found to be true, regardless of the sex of the examiner or the client. This exploration of an individual's sexual organs can be embarrassing to clients who fear that they will evidence some signs of sexual excitement from the examination. This is particularly true during the examination of the man's prostate. Many men will find to their dismay that their penis becomes erect during the examination.

The fear of physical discomfort from the procedure accounts for a great deal of anxiety about the physical examination. Invariably, people hear from well-meaning friends that their examination was excruciatingly painful and that they hope their friend does not have to go through that pain. In fact, the pelvic examination is not painful when the examiner and the client have established a rapport, and the steps outlined below are followed. The experience of having a speculum inserted and opened in the vagina is subjectively uncomfortable for some women, but with adequate relaxation and reassurance this discomfort can often be reduced to the level of something that feels "different" rather than uncomfortable.

For some women, though, the pelvic examination in the past has been an uncomfortable experience. Some women (and men) may seek a pelvic examination during a time in which they are experiencing some difficulty, such as a vaginal infection in the woman. The irritation from the infection may indeed make the experience of the pelvic examination a negative and painful one. The woman may then fear future examinations, thinking that they will all cause the discomfort she recalls from her past experience.

The nurse should have an idea of the client's past experience with pelvic examinations prior to the actual examination. During the history taking phase of the interaction, the nurse and client have usually established a rapport that can be of great benefit to both during the examination. The client should be informed of the rationale for the pelvic examination in terms of ruling out any pathology and in terms of preventive care and education.

In the past, few nurses performed the actual pelvic examination. This is no longer true, with the increasing number of nurses trained in these expanded skills. Nurse practitioners trained in gynecology and family planning often perform the major sexual health care for healthy female populations. Female patients often state that they prefer to have a nurse examine them for several reasons. First, they feel more comfortable having the examination performed by a woman. Nurse practitioners in gynecology are predominantly female. Women have a better intuitive feeling for the location of the interior pelvic structures than do men, and may be better able to palpate these structures without using a pressure that may be uncomfortable to the client. A second and important reason clients report greater ease with a nurse practitioner is the fact that it is usually the nurse who has gathered the history information. The client has had an opportunity to establish a relationship with the nurse, which readily continues during the pelvic examination. If another individual (even another nurse) enters to perform the examination, the client must then establish rapport with this individual.

If the nurse in a given situation is not performing the pelvic examination, the valuable function as patient advocate during the examination can still be utilized. Since the relationship has probably been established prior to the examination, the nurse can work to make the experience more positive for the client.

Perhaps the most important action that the nurse or the examiner can take to reduce the client's anxiety during the pelvic examination is to provide a running explanation of what is being done and what is about to be done. This should include whether the client is likely to feel any discomfort from a particular activity (such as some discomfort when the ovaries or testicles are palpated) and the reasons for the various parts of the examination (AASECT, 1978). The client should be instructed to tell the examiner if anything that is being done is uncomfortable. The issue of asking the client to report any discomfort brings up the value of the client's nonverbal communications. Some clients, especially those who expect the examination to be painful, will not tell the examiner if something is hurting them. Instead, they may grimace or hold their breath. The examiner should be aware of this and arrange the drape (if one is being used) in such a way that the client's face can be seen during the examination. Elevating the head of the examining table 30 degrees can make this eye contact easier to accomplish for both the client and the examiner (Settlage, 1975).

In beginning the examination, the nurse-examiner can help to begin the examination in a relatively nonthreatening area by palpating the abdomen. Having established this touch with the client, the examiner should keep touching the client throughout the remainder of the examination. For example, the nurse should keep one hand on the client's abdomen and place the other on her breast for the breast examination. (The client will be told that the breast examination will be done prior to moving the hand onto the breast.) In examining the breasts, the nurse can ascertain whether or not the client is aware of the proper methods of breast self-examination, and can either teach the client or reinforce the client's practice. Following the examination and discussion of the breast examination, the nurse can assist the client into the lithotomy position, continuing his or her touch on the client's knee. Finally, as the pelvic examination begins, the nurse can touch first the client's thigh, and then proceed to the external genitalia.

Prior to actually examining the external genitalia in both the female and the male patient, the nurse should note the distribution of hair on the individual's genital region. As discussed in the chapter on sexual development, the distribution of hair gives the examiner valuable information on the hormonal levels of the client, and may give the examiner information on any endocrine problems the client may be experiencing. Following the superficial observation of the external genitalia, checking for any lesions, growths, or abrasions, the examiner begins the examination of the external genitalia.

The clitoral hood (prepuce) should be retracted so that signs of inflammation, lesions, adhesions, and smegma may be noted. At this point, the nurse can educate the client about the fact that the clitoris has no direct means of lubrication, and can become painfully sensitive with direct stimulation (AASECT, 1978; Masters, 1966; Settlage, 1975). Information on the use of lubricants can follow here. The labia minora will then be checked for

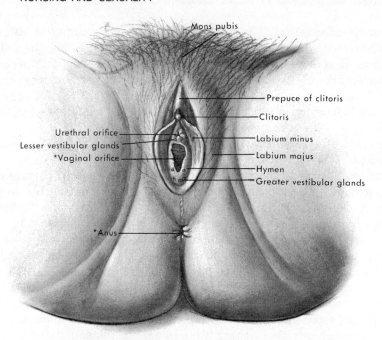

Mons pubis

Prepuce of clitoris

Clitoris

Urethral orifice

Lesser vestibular glands

*Vaginal orifice

Labium minus

Labium majus

Hymen

Greater vestibular glands

*Anus

*The clinical perineum lies between these two openings.

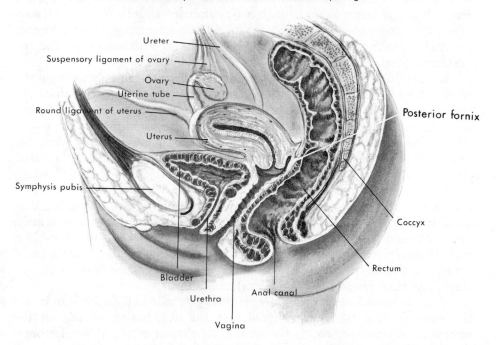

Ureter

Suspensory ligament of ovary

Ovary

Uterine tube

Round ligament of uterus

Uterus

Posterior fornix

Symphysis pubis

Coccyx

Rectum

Bladder

Anal canal

Urethra

Vagina

lesions, adhesions, inflammation, and varicosities. During this portion of the examination, the nurse can discuss the size of the labia with the client, reassuring her that most women have labia that are not exactly the same size, and that this finding is not indicative of any problem. A mirror can be provided to enable the client to look at herself and understand the teaching more clearly.

The perineal body and the introitus are evaluated next. The nurse should be especially careful here to check for signs of abrasion and erythema, which may indicate a chronic vulvitis or vaginitis. Such a chronic condition may cause dyspareunia (pain on intercourse) or may result from painful intercourse. If these findings do exist, the client should be asked if she has had dyspareunia in the past or if she has it now. During this phase of the examination, the nurse can insert one finger into the introitus and evaluate the pubococcygeal muscle. This muscle is important in orgasmic response. The woman can be instructed to squeeze the examiner's finger to determine muscle tone. Also during this time, with one finger in the vagina, the nurse can evaluate the client for signs of vaginismus, for anxiety level, and for an intact hymen. All of these findings will affect the remainder of the examination.

Following the examination of the external genitalia, a speculum examination is usually performed. The speculum should be warmed and be of an appropriate size for the client. Warm water can be useful in helping to lubricate and warm the speculum, and does not interfere with the collection of vaginal and cervical samples for laboratory evaluation. In inserting the speculum, care should be taken to avoid hitting the urinary meatus with the speculum. This is painful to most women, and is easily avoided by inserting the speculum at an angle into the vagina. Also, pressing down on the introitus with the free hand and the speculum aids in increasing the client's comfort during the insertion of the speculum. With the speculum in place, Pap smears, GC cultures, and the collection of samples to check for various types of vaginal infections can be accomplished. In addition to collecting samples, the nurse will examine the vaginal mucosa and the cervix for any signs of inflammation, lesions, growth, or color changes, all of which may affect the client's sexual functioning as well as her health. The use of a plastic speculum is preferred by some in order to more easily visualize the entire vagina. If the traditional metal speculum is used, it should be turned 90 degrees when being removed, so that the entire vagina can be visualized. Care should be taken to avoid the urinary meatus when removing the speculum.

The bimanual examination follows, during which the examiner inserts

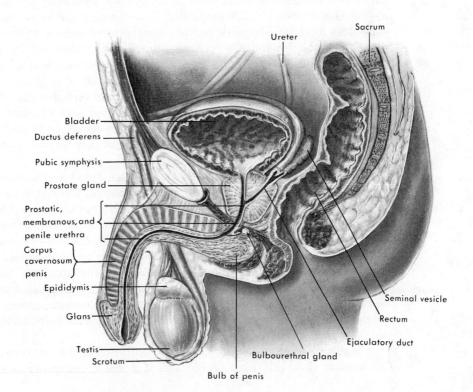

one or two fingers into the vagina and places the other hand on the client's abdomen. The position, shape, and movement of the uterus are evaluated at this time. In addition, the ovaries, tubes, and broad ligaments are palpated. A rectovaginal examination is essential in the complete pelvic examination. It is required in order for the nurse to evaluate the posterior pelvis, the posterior aspect of the uterus, and the posteriorly positioned ovaries, tubes, masses, and uterosacral ligaments. The rectal portion of the examination is most stressful for the client. She may feel an urge to defecate during this procedure, and should be assured that this urge is natural, and that she will not actually have a bowel movement at this time. The nurse should be particularly careful during the examination to remember that the client is probably unaware of the medical terminology that has become commonplace to health care workers. The client must be allowed to utilize her own language, and the nurse must be certain that both she and the client understand what is being said.

After the examination is finished, the client should be helped to a sitting position and given tissues to remove the lubrication utilized during the examination. It is helpful to allow the client to dress in private, assuring her that the nurse will return when the client is dressed. After the client is dressed, any tests taken should be fully explained (including the time needed for the results), as should any findings. The next scheduled examination should also be discussed. Time should be allowed to answer the client's questions. Some reinforcement should be provided at this point in the interview, since many clients are unable to concentrate on information received during what may have been a stressful examination.

The Male Pelvic Examination

The pelvic examination can often be as anxiety producing for the male client as for the female. If the examiner is a female, the male client may be especially anxious. The male pelvic examination begins with the history data and the establishment of a relationship with the client. If the examiner is a female, some discussion of the client's feelings about having a female examiner may be helpful. When the client is in a standing position, the external genitalia are observed, beginning with the hair distribution. If the man is uncircumcised, the foreskin should be retracted and checked for signs of irritation, lesions, and smegma. Proper hygiene should be taught at this point if necessary. The penis should be evaluated for any lesions, growths, discolorations, or painful areas.

The testes should be palpated for varicose veins and atrophy as well as for masses. During the examination of the testes, the nurse can inform the client that most men find that one testicle is higher than the other, and that this is normal. (Approximately 85% of men have the left testis lower than the right.) In the process of palpating the testes, the nurse should check the scrotum for any lesions, inflammation, masses, or tenderness. In addition, testicular self-examination should be explained and taught.

The rectal examination is an integral part of the pelvic examination of the male. The prostate must be palpated to check for size, consistency, shape, tenderness, and so on. In many older men, the prostate is found to be enlarged on examination.

Many men become erect from the stimulation of the prostate. They should be warned that this may occur, and if it does, reassured that this is an involuntary response that does not indicate sexual arousal as a result of the procedure.

The position utilized for the rectal examination in the male client consists of having the client bend over the end of the examining table. This position, like the lithotomy position for the female, can be seen as a very vulnerable one, in which the man is likely to feel uncomfortable. Eye contact during the rectal examination of the male is not possible. However, the running explanations and the eliciting of verbal responses in case the procedure is painful continue to be necessary.

Following examination of the male client, the nurse should allow the client to dress in private, and then should return to discuss the examination and any findings. The nurse is in an excellent position to teach male clients about their sexuality and sexual functions as well as about the sexuality of women. Many men have never received any information about female sexuality. They may be too embarrassed to ask for information, but may readily accept an offer to discuss the similarities and differences in the sexual responses and sexual behaviors of men and women. As always, the nurse must be comfortable with and be knowledgeable about the subjects to be discussed, and must have worked through his or her own feelings about sexual issues such as masturbation, sex for purposes other than procreation, nonmarital sex, and different cultural orientations toward sexuality. When nurses have a thorough understanding of their own biases they will be able to put them into proper perspective and deal more appropriately with the problems of their clients. The role of teaching in relation to the pelvic examination is tremendously important. During the examination, nurses have many opportunities to correct misconceptions held by clients. They can reassure patients that their behaviors are well within the normal limits and that many people experience many of the same fears about sexual functioning.

PLANNING

Once the nurse has collected the subjective and objective data base, a nursing plan may begin. It may be useful to categorize the sexual problems encountered into the following areas:
1. Biological—illness, use of drugs, aging.
2. Behavioral—secondary to guilt, anxiety.
3. Socioenvironmental—interpersonal components that may indicate a partner approach for counseling.

Having categorized the problems, the nurse will give them specific priorities and then proceed to the planning stage. In some cases, the problems will be beyond the scope of training and expertise of the nurse, who must be aware of the limitations of the nurse's role, and be able to recognize when referral is necessary. In referring clients, nurses must be aware not only of the availability of referral but also of the quality of care given by the agency or individual to whom the client will be referred. Some general problems that should be referred are the following (Glover, 1977):
1. Impotence, premature ejaculation, or retarded ejaculation that is unresponsive to treatment.
2. Severe dysfunctions (vaginismus, unusual dyspareunia) that are unresponsive to treatment.
3. Destructive tendencies, such as sticking foreign objects into the genitourinary tract during masturbation (note: this does not include vibrators).

4. Cases of untreated venereal disease or genitourinary infections. Of course, some nurses will be prepared to deal with the aforementioned problems. Discussion of the advanced training necessary to deal with these problems is beyond the scope of this text.

A common fear expressed by nurses is their inability to handle questions that the clients may ask of them during a sexual history or other sexual interviewing situations (Benjamin, 1969; Ujhely, 1976). Nurses who feel confident of their ability to deal effectively with clients who ask personal questions not relating to sexuality sometimes become unsure of what to do when questions are asked about the nurse's sexuality. Nurses must remember that, as in any situation, if another individual is to ask a question or make a demand on them, they are not obligated to answer the question or meet the demand. In fact, not all questions call for answers. Every question, however, demands respectful listening on the part of the nurse. The client must know that the question or demand has been heard. Usually some personal reaction on the part of the nurse is expected.

In some cases it may be feasible and appropriate for the nurse to supply the information requested. Often, clients are not asking just the question stated. Different needs or feelings may be behind such personal questions. Clients may feel that unless they demonstrate an interest in the personal concerns of the staff, the staff will not pay attention to them. Personal questions may be used by clients to direct the conversation away from them. Patients may ask highly personal questions in order to express what little power they feel they have left. Because of their feelings of helplessness, they may assert themselves in a hostile manner in order to keep the nurses away from them. Whatever the reason for the questioning of nurses, they must listen to what is not being asked. If they choose to answer questions asked by clients, these questions should not take over the interview. The discussion should revert to the client as soon as possible following a concise, short response by the nurse.

SUMMARY

This chapter has spent a great deal of time on the sexual interview in general, and on the sexual history. Skilled assessment and planning are essential prerequisites for quality care of all clients. The basics presented here will form the baseline for nursing assessment of the sexual health care needs of clients. Succeeding chapters will present these basic skills in light of the specific issues covered.

References

American Association of Sex Educators, Counselors and Therapists (AASECT): *The Physical Examination in Sex Counseling and Therapy*. Washington, D. C., American Association of Sex Educators, Counselors and Therapists, 1978.

Barnard, Martha Underwood, Clancy, Barbara, and Krantz, Kermet: *Human Sexuality for Health Professionals*. Philadelphia, W. B. Saunders Co., 1978.

Benjamin, Alfred: *The Helping Interview*. Boston, Houghton Mifflin, 1969.

Elder, Mary-Scovill: "The Unmet Challenge . . . Nurse Counseling on Sexuality." *In* Browning, Mary, and Lewis, Edith (Eds.): *Human Sexuality: Nursing Implications*. New York, American Journal of Nursing Co., 1973.

Glover, Benjamin, H.: "Sex Counseling of the Elderly." *Hospital Practice, 12*:101–104, June 1977.

Green, Richard: "Taking a Sexual History." *In* Green, Richard (Ed.): *Human Sexuality: A Health Practitioner's Text*. Baltimore, Williams & Wilkins, 1975.

Lief, Harold, and Berman, Ellen: "Sexual Interviewing of the Individual Patient Through the Life Cycle." *In* Oaks, Wilbur W., Melchiode, Gerald A., and Ficher, Ilda (Eds.): *Sex and the Life Cycle*. New York, Grune and Stratton, 1976.

Masters, William H., and Johnson, Virginia E: *Human Sexual Response*. Boston, Little, Brown and Co., 1966.

Masters, William H., and Johnson, Virginia E.: *Human Sexual Inadequacy*. Boston, Little, Brown and Co., 1970.

Mims, Fern H., and Swenson, Melinda: "Improving Sexual Health Care" *Nursing Care*, Vol. 10, Oct. 1977.

Payne, Tyana: "Sexuality of Nurses: Correlations of Knowledge, Attitudes and Behavior." *Nursing Research, 25*:4, July-Aug. 1976.

Roznoy, Melinda Swenson: "The Young Adult: Taking a Sexual History." *American Journal of Nursing, 76*(8):1279–1282, Aug. 1976.

Schiller, Patricia: "The Nurse's Role as Sex Counselor." *Nursing Care,* Vol. 10, July 1977.

Semmens, James, and Semmens, Jane: "The Sexual History and Physical Examination." *In* Barnard, Martha, Clancy, Barbara, and Krantz, Kermit (Eds.): *Human Sexuality for Health Professionals*. Philadelphia, W. B. Saunders Co., 1978.

Settlage, Diane S. Fordney: "Pelvic Examination of Women." *In* Green, Richard (Ed.): *Human Sexuality: A Health Practitioner's Text*. Baltimore, Williams & Wilkins Co., 1975.

Ujhely, Gertrude B.: "Two Types of Problem Patients and How to Deal with Them: The Patient Who Gets Too Personal." *Nursing 76, 6*:5, May 1976.

Wohl, Charles W.: "The Art of Taking the Sexual History." In *Counseling Sexual Problems in Medical Practice*. Ortho Panel New Jersey: 1974, Ortho Pharmaceutical Corporation.

SEXUALITY: HISTORICAL ATTITUDES AND RESEARCH

One of the perspectives discussed in Chapter 1 was that "An individual or family unit, although sexually independent, is very much affected by the sexual milieu of the community and society."

The sexual milieu of a community or society evolves slowly and changes according to the prevailing attitudes and values of the time. To define the sexual milieu of a given time, the sexual history of that society must be addressed. As mentioned in Chapter 1, Frieze (1978) identified three major areas from which beliefs about sexuality in Western culture arise: religion, Freud, and research in human sexuality. In this chapter, an overview of historical religious attitudes is given, and the research of Kinsey et al. and of Masters and Johnson is presented. The research conclusions of Masters and Johnson about the human sexual response are detailed, and their theories about the kinds and etiologies of sexual dysfunctions in both men and women are given.

The chapter concludes with a discussion of nursing implications of both traditional attitudes and new "myths" that have arisen from research in human sexuality.

HISTORICAL AND RELIGIOUS ATTITUDES

In the following discussion of religion and its effects on sexuality, the use of the word "church" does not specify any religious denomination, but rather a sociological definition (Walum, 1977). "Church," as used here refers to the beliefs and rituals about the sacred that bind people together in a moral community. Since our historical background is largely the Judeo-Christian model, the following discussion has been based on Judeo-Christian concepts.

The view of women as inferior has been long established among the Hebrews. For example, there is an Orthodox Jewish daily prayer that reads, "I thank Thee, O Lord, that Thou has not made me a woman" (Walum, 1977). Traditional Judaism has viewed women largely as possessions, necessary for bearing children. In some of the writings, however, one can find references to the possibility for deep love between "man and wife" (Frieze, 1978). The use of the terms "man and wife" rather than "man and woman" or "husband and wife" clearly indicates the role that was considered important in the Orthodox Jewish Church.

According to Jewish tradition, although women were considered necessary for bearing children, their bodies and body functions have been viewed as essentially unclean and requiring purification following each menstrual period and pregnancy. The ritual involved in purification, called the Mikvah, is a ceremonial bath taken by the woman following menstruation (during which she has been separated from the rest of the group) and delivery of a child. Interestingly women are considered to be "unclean" for a longer period of time following delivery of a female child (two weeks) than following delivery of a male child (one week). With the growth of more liberal sects of Judaism, this view of women has changed somewhat. For example, menstruation no longer requires separation from the family, and most Jewish women no longer have the Mikvah following menstruation. However, the basic ideology still persists.

In Christian tradition, women are seen in one of two major images, either that of Eve or that of Mary. Eve is seen as the first "sinner" and is held ultimately responsibile for the loss of Paradise. She epitomizes the sexual evil of the temptress and seducer of men (Frieze, 1978; Walum, 1977). In the role of temptress, an ancient and often repeated fear is evident. Women are seen as having a basic sexual nature that is a constant threat to the salvation of men, since woman distracted man into thoughts of sex rather than thoughts of God.

Women were thought to possess naturally boundless, albeit usually repressed, sexual appetites for men, who had to be sure not to release this appetite by too often engaging in sexual relations (Parker-Benfield, 1977; Ehrenreich, 1977; Frieze, 1978; Walum, 1977). According to Weidger (1976), the most damning tradition attached to menstruation, and indeed to women in general, reflects the belief that the monthly flow of blood is the curse of God laid upon woman for her sin in Eden.

The second image of women seen in early Christianity is the image of Mary, which combines virginity and motherhood. Mary is not seen as being interested in sex, but in earthly matters and children. She is seen as the epitome of "perfect obedience" (Walum, 1977).

In the Christian tradition, men fare no better in terms of the models they are encouraged to emulate. The first model, that of God the Father, is seen as unattainable, as is the second, God the Virginal Son. Both men and women seem to be faced with impossible models toward which to strive. Women were seen as primarily involved with the rearing and bearing of children. They were not seen as being involved in spiritual matters, since their major concerns revolved around their procreative and nurturing roles on earth. Men, on the other hand, were seen as striving for spiritual purity, having to fight their dangerous sexual urges. Achievement was stressed for men. It is interesting to note that of some 464 saints in the Catholic Church, only 60 are women. All of these saints were either virgins or martyrs. The role models presented to youth of women were symbols of either virginity or death. Men, however, were much more widely represented (396) in all fields. The male saints were bishops, abbots, popes, martyrs, doctors, apostles, etc. The role model for the male saint was either an achievement model or a death role model.

Around the 16th century, Calvinism was the basis for behavior. Unlike earlier Christian attitudes, the Calvinist doctrine of self-denial and postponed gratification was aimed not at a better lot in the next world but at greater rewards in this one. Of all the pleasures seen as needing postponement, sex was the foremost. Sexual activity was seen as a spending of energy that was needed for business. Marriage and the family were idealized as the models of righteousness. Sexual activity was to take place only within marriage, and then only for the purpose of procreation. In this way, the man would have the maximum energy available to spend on his business. The role of the woman during this time was to bear children and to satisfy man's sexual desires (Gordon, 1976). The idea of "motherhood as destiny" arose during this period. Women were seen to exist only for the purpose of procreation. It was through motherhood that women were promised redemption. Around this time there existed an "ideology" of motherhood (Gordon, 1976), which consisted of three main components. The first of these, the biological, included pregnancy, childbirth, and suckling. From this role, the woman became the symbolic universal nourisher, and the giver of love and rules of society to a new generation. The second component, the social one, involved childrearing. This role later became one of such importance that it was considered harmful and dangerous to separate childbearing from childrearing. (This insistence that only the biological mother can adequately rear a child still exists today, especially among the vocal individuals who speak out against day care on this basis.)

The final step in the ideology of motherhood viewed men as incapable of childrearing, since it was defined as "mothering" and as something for which women were destined. Once women were defined solely as mothers, their potentials were also defined. The qualities of feminine motherliness were seen as the essential qualities of all women (Gordon, 1976).

In the late 16th and early 17th centuries, the medical profession was beginning to form. During this time, individuals calling themselves "doctors" began to practice, often employing so-called "heroic" measures such as bleeding and using strong cathartics to cure a variety of illnesses. Women, having been defined as destined to motherhood and childrearing were necessarily excluded from these positions as "doctors." As a response to dangerous and often fatal reactions to treatment, the Popular Health Movement began in the 1830s and 1840s (Ehrenreich, 1977; Marieskind, 1977). Women made up the backbone of this movement, which stressed preventive care. The focus of the popular health movement was that the mind and body were one, and that harmonious balance between the two would lead to personal well-being. The members of the Popular Health Movement promoted such "radical" ideas as frequent bathing, loose fitting clothing for women (the style of the day included whalebone corsets that were often so tight that they actually did damage to the internal organs of the woman!), healthy diets, and temperance. In addition, some of those involved in this movement advocated birth control. For many, given the standard view of women and their destiny, this was too radical to accept. With this radicalism and the rise of the American Medical Association in 1848, the Popular Health Movement seemed to disintegrate. Men were almost exclusively in control of health care (such as it was), with the exception of midwives, who experienced a tremendous amount of pressure to stop their practice. (Midwifery and its evolution will not be covered here, although it is of great interest in the study of the evolution of the medical profession. The reader is encouraged to consult the reference list in this chapter for more information on midwifery.)

During the Victorian era, commencing in the mid 1830s and 1840s, men and women began to be seen not only as different, but actually as opposites. The Calvinist views of reproduction as the basis for sexual activity continued, but were applied to women only. Women were seen as having no sex drive. In fact, it was thought that the drive that motivated women to take part in sexual activities was the maternal instinct. Men, however, were seen as having tremendous sex drives. Sex was seen as dirty, immoral, and undignified, and was removed from respectable discussion (Gordon, 1976). In fact, men were encouraged to visit prostitutes rather than to expose their more genteel wives to their own savage sexual urges. This description of sex as lacking respectability must surely have led to great feelings of guilt among the men of the times on the occasions they did engage in sexual activities with their wives. Learning that sex was dirty and immoral, combined with the learnings that wives were genteel and moral women, would seem to make enjoyable sex between husband and wife impossible.

During this period, there was a continuation of the role of the woman taking place solely in the home. She was expected, because of the moral influence she obtained from her innate capacity for motherliness, to temper the savagery of capitalist competition to which her husband was exposed, and to make the home a "haven" for her husband. It was expected that he could leave the "cutthroat" business world and return to his calm, serene wife and home. In the United States in the years 1865 to 1920, industrialization was taking place, and there developed two quite distinct classes: the working class and the affluent class. In order to discuss the roles of men and women in these classes, they must be examined separately.

During this period of industrialization, one indication of a man's success was an ornamental wife who did not have to work. The wives of these affluent men were considered too weak and delicate for any but the mildest pastimes. The slightest shock was thought to be sufficient to send the frail and somewhat sickly affluent woman to her bed. Of course, during menstruation it was expected that she would remain in bed. In 1871, Dr. W. D. Taylor, a physician, wrote in his book, *A Physician Counsels Women in Health and Disease*, the following concerning the proper behavior for women during menstruation:

We cannot too emphatically urge the importance of regarding these monthly returns as periods of ill health, as days when the ordinary occupations are to be suspended or modified. . . . Long walks, dancing, shopping, riding, and parties should be avoided at this time of the month invariable and under all circumstances. . . . Another reason why every woman should look upon herself as an invalid once a month is that the monthly flow aggravates any existing affection of the womb and rekindles the expiring flames of disease.

From this quote, we see something of a continuation of the early separation of menstruating women from the rest of the family.

This period of "female invalidism" was fashionable for affluent women. However, the reader should not assume that these women did not face real risks in their lives. In 1915, the death rate for women in childbirth was approximately 30 times greater than it is today (Ehrenreich, 1977). In addition, the death rate from infection following delivery was also far greater than today, as there were no antibiotics available at the time. Tuberculosis was also a greater danger. The disease seemed to be more prevalent among young women. Some have proposed that this greater propensity to contract the disease was the result of the hormonal changes accompanying puberty and childbearing. Ehrenreich (1977) suggests that it is the look of the women suffering from this disease that defines the prevailing standards of feminine beauty in our culture. The woman suffering from tuberculosis is pictured as having bright eyes, translucent skin, red lips, and as being very thin.

Working women of this time were seen as innately healthy and robust. In fact, they were not given time off from the factory jobs for pregnancy, for recovery from childbirth, or for their menstrual periods. They were also not subject to the care of the early "physicians," which, with the level of care at the time, may have been a benefit. Although the idea of the strong but poor working class woman was incorrect, it persisted. With the acceptance of the germ theory of disease transmission, the working woman was soon seen as being the carrier of disease, particularly venereal disease. The ghetto, the area in which all of these women lived, was regarded as dangerous because individuals merely passing by were at great risk of suffering from illness as a result of the germs believed to exist primarily in the slum areas. Little is written about the role of the working woman and her role as a childbearer. The necessity of working in order to eat and to feed children seems to have been stronger than the conviction that women were unable to function in the fashion required of the affluent woman.

During the Victorian age, a theory called the "Conservation of Energy" became popular and was considered by many to be a basic physiological law. According to this theory, each human body contained a set quantity of energy. This energy was utilized as needed by one organ or another. The sex organs were regarded as in competition with all other organs for this fixed supply of energy. Because of the emphasis on reproductive functions in women, their reproductive organs were viewed as in almost total command of their limited energy. In fact, the reproductive organs were seen as essentially in charge of the entire woman. Women were encouraged to concentrate their physical energy internally, towards the womb. Women were advised to slow down or cease all other activity at the time of peak energy use, such times being menstruation, pregnancy, and menopause.

A byproduct of the Conservation of Energy theory was the move to restrict women from too much education. Since they needed all of their available energy for their uteruses, it was hypothesized that learning or other use of the brain could lead to atrophy of the uterus. In pregnant women, the use of the brain was thought to lead to malformed children or even spontaneous abortion. The push to exclude women from formal education was given support from learned men in society. The president of the American Medical Association gave a lecture in 1905 endorsing less education for women. In his discussion, this physician clearly sums up the prevailing view of women in light of the Conservation of Energy doctrine.

The causes of physical decay in women are numerous and varied. . . . I can only touch disconnectedly on this one . . . education. . . . Nature has ordained that the vast majority of women shall become wives and mothers, and if they are exhausted mentally (from education) as well as physically, how is it possible to keep the race strong and healthy?

The Conservation of Energy theory was applied to men as well as to women during this period. Men were admonished to avoid masturbation and too frequent intercourse, in order to avoid depletion of their energies by this "base" activity. They were instructed instead to save this energy and put it into the building of capital used for business. This conservation and putting of energies into the workplace for men was consistent with the economic values of the time.

The step from the Conservation of Energy Principle to the so-called "psychology of the ovary" is a small one. The idea that the woman's energy was directed at her internal organs of reproduction led to a general acceptance of the notion that the problems women encountered must also be due to their reproductive organs being in some way dysfunctional or diseased. Gynecological surgery became the treatment of choice for "female disorders." The disorders themselves were varied, ranging from masturbation to domineering characteristics to "not knowing her proper place." The gynecologic surgery that began around the 1860s was practiced primarily on affluent women who could afford the treatment.

One treatment that was successful was the removal of the clitoris as a solution for excessive female masturbation. Clitoridectomy was also performed to check women's mental disorders. It was introduced in 1858 by the English gynecologist Isaac Baker-Brown and was first performed in the United States in the late 1860s. Removing the major site for female sexual stimulation certainly would reduce mastrubatory behavior!

The surgical removal of the ovary, oophorectomy, was invented in 1872 by a physician in Georgia (Barker-Benfield, 1977) and flourished between 1880 and 1910. This procedure largely gave way to the general use of the hysterectomy combined with the oophorectomy. The first successful hysterectomy was performed in 1853 by Dr. L. P. Burnham of Lowell, Massachusetts (Barker-Benfield, 1977).

In all of the various types of female castration, the expected "cure" would return the woman to her more tractable, orderly, "tame" self (Ehrenreich, 1977). The woman was thought to return to her role as dependent, submissive, supportive, smiling, and nurturing following castration (Barker-Benfield, 1977; Ehrenreich, 1977). Indeed, given the risks from surgery at this time, the mere threat of such intervention was probably enough to induce many women to behave according to the notion of what was "correct" for a woman of the time.

The discussion on gynecologic surgery has thus far addressed only the problem of unnecessary castration. The husbands of these women, the physicians, and indeed, probably many of the women themselves felt that the women in question were sick and that such treatment would make them well again. There was probably no malicious intent in any but a small proportion of the cases of female castration. Throughout history, there have been many examples of medical practices that, in the light of current knowledge, were harmful and even barbaric. It must be recognized that the people of this time were acting on what was currently accepted knowledge and thought of the time. It was the function of the restrictive roles of both men and women during this period that led to such operations.

The epitome of the cult of female invalidism is expressed in the disease commonly called hysteria. This was thought to be a disease of the uterus that had no organic base, and that was not susceptible to medical intervention. The literal definition of hysteria is "wandering uterus." The womb was actually thought to either float to various parts of the body or to send out energy to distant body parts that would cause illness. Some manifestations of hysteria included fainting (vapors), loss of voice, loss of appetite, and paralysis (with no organic base). Ehrenreich (1977) has suggested that women themselves used this behavior in order to exert some small amount of control over their husbands and their lives. A husband witnessing his wife having a "fit" may well have been at a psychological disadvantage initially. The wife may have gotten her way about something, but ultimately this role confirmed the prevailing notion of women as irrational, unpredictable, and sick. Hysteria could serve some valuable functions for women, however. It could mean that sex could be avoided. By manipulating the physician into prescribing abstinence, the women could be freed from sexual activity that she may truly have found to be unpleasant, and she could avoid the possibility of pregnancy.

As physicians began to suspect that women were faking their complaints, some became more punitive and radical in their treatments, including the gynecologic surgical procedures discussed above and the advocacy of freezing baths or other treatments intended to "shock" a woman back into her prescribed role. Freud was perhaps the first to suggest that hysteria was a mental disorder rather than a physical one. He did not address the idea of whether or not the woman was faking. Instead, he wrote that hysteria stemmed from the woman's resentments and rebellious feelings. His advocated treatment, psychotherapy, was aimed at helping the woman to accept her role as a woman.

In his writing about women, Freud supported the historical belief in the greater sexual aggressiveness of men and the passivity of women. He wrote that the male sex cell (sperm) was mobile and active, while the female sex cell (ovum) was immobile and passive, awaiting the male sex cell. Freud viewed this as biological confirmation of his own psychological theory (Fortier, 1975; Frieze, 1978).

Freud also postulated that women were sexually inferior to men. He used this inferiority to explain the alleged lower sexual drive of women. Women were viewed as submitting to sex, never actually enjoying or participating in sexual activities. Women were seen as sexually inferior because of their lack of a penis and their sex drive was thought to be aimed at pregnancy not sexual pleasure alone. Masturbation was thought to be a male activity that should be avoided by women.

Freud had a great impact on the ideas of the general public about female orgasm. He postulated that clitoral orgasm was an immature orgasm that would give way to vaginal orgasm as the married woman matured. Despite the fact that it has been proven that the clitoris is the major site of sexual excitement in women, and that the inner two-thirds of the vagina has very few nerve endings, the idea of the superiority of the vaginal over the clitoral orgasm continues today. Actually, both the vagina and the clitoris are involved in female orgasm.

Many feminist writings seem to condemn Freud as lacking knowledge and sensitivity about women. Others hint that he based his theories on too few cases and that he basically did not care for women. In fact, Freud himself admitted that he knew little about women. Some of his work has had positive effects on both men and women in the field of sexuality. Freud was one of the first professional people to support the idea that sexual feelings were normal in women and children as well as in men. He also had some great insights into the negative effects of sexual repression, and he supported the growing belief that sexuality should be encouraged for everyone.

By the early 1900s, the cult of invalidism and hysteria seemed to be on the decrease. Women were rejecting the sick role and were leaving home more (Ehrenreich, 1977). In employment outside of the home, women were expected to take on roles that were appropriate to their class. These roles were essentially extensions of the wife and mother role. Today, these continue to be the major women's professions, such as nursing, teaching of children, social work, and volunteer work.

As the industrial revolution continued, the increasing demand for labor led to more and more single women leaving the home to work in factories. Prior to the end of the 19th century, most women, whether married or single, worked exclusively in the home or as unpaid laborers in family enterprises.

Some of the jobs filled by women in the home were in child care, upkeep of the house, cultivation and preparation of food, and manufacture of many household goods. However, with the advent of the industrial revolution, many of the foods and products were manufactured outside of the home, and thus the woman's role there chiefly involved childrearing and cleaning (Lewis, 1978). This decrease in actual work in the home was another factor motivating women to leave the home and work in the outside world.

In reviewing the roles of women and men through history, even in such a brief fashion as this, certain patterns become evident. Throughout our history, both sexes have been placed in very rigidly defined roles. Men were expected to be the major breadwinners in the family. They were expected to be aggressive, dominant, highly sexed, and competitive. Women, on the other hand, have been alternately seen as highly sexed and dangerous or as essentially uninterested in sex. Motherhood has been presented as the only viable role for women. The woman of the house, at least in the upper classes, was expected to be weak, submissive, nurturant, and willing to put up with sex as one of her conjugal duties.

In trying to ascertain the sexual climate and sexual activity during the Victorian age, the very repressiveness of the era makes specific activities difficult, if not impossible, to document. Sexual activity or any signs of such activity were hidden during this era. Even pregnant women were not seen among the "polite" public during this time, since pregnancy was a very definite outward sign that sexual activity had taken place (Gordon, 1976).

Women were taught that their genitals were dirty and should not be touched. This prohibition, which of course extended to masturbation, was also probably responsible in part for the failure of women of the day to utilize the birth control methods that were available, as these devices required handling of the genitals. Since women were taught that their proper place was in the home as wives and mothers, and that women did not enjoy sex, women may have demonstrated lower sexual drives than men, who were expected to be highly sexed.

Men also had a difficult time during this era. The wife was not seen as an individual in whom the husband could confide about the worries of his world. He was always expected to be the strong one in the family. Displays of affection and sensitivity were considered unmasculine and inappropriate. Although men had more freedom to move about in the outside world, the rigidly defined behaviors expected of them were probably as difficult to adhere to as were those of the women.

By the start of World War II, it was more acceptable for single women to work outside the home. The expectation existed then, as now, that most women would work for a few years after they finished their education, and would then marry and devote the rest of their lives to caring for their families and homes. Following World War II, there seemed to be a trend toward earlier marriages, and it became more common and acceptable for both single and married women to work outside the home for economic reasons (Lewis, 1978).

In a study of marriage and divorce patterns in the United States, Lewis (1978) found that the trend toward earlier marriages has now reversed itself. Women tend to marry later now than they did in the World War II era. In addition, the divorce rate has dramatically increased. As a result, more and more women are working outside the home, being exposed to more people than would have been possible in earlier times. This greater exposure to the outside world has been thought to have been a contributing factor to the increasing acceptance of female sexuality.

RESEARCH IN HUMAN SEXUALITY

The scientific study of sexual behavior did not really begin in this country until the early research of Alfred Kinsey in the 1930's. Most of Kinsey's interview data was later confirmed by the laboratory findings of Masters and Johnson in the 1950's and 1960's.

Since the early researchers in human sexuality began their preliminary data gathering and reporting, the subject of human sexuality has become more acceptable as a topic for research. Many recent researchers have attempted to replicate the findings of Kinsey and Masters and Johnson. The use of survey data is still commonly employed as a research technique.

Not all research in the field of sexuality has been of high quality. Some has tended to reinforce inaccurate notions about the activities and desires of many people, and has contributed to the formation of new myths about sexual function. For example, the old myth surrounding orgasm was that women rarely had them. If they did, it was the vaginal orgasm that was valued. The newer mythology surrounding female orgasm now requires that the woman experience multiple orgasms at each sexual encounter. This mistaken notion has placed much greater emphasis on performance during the sexual act. Its negative effects can be profound.

Kinsey

Alfred Kinsey and his associates participated in what was probably the first systematic research into the field of human sexuality. Kinsey based his findings on a series of interviews and extensive case histories obtained during the interviews. The sample size for the Kinsey research was over 10,000 and spanned a period from 1938 to 1953. Men and women were relatively evenly represented in the survey. The population was approximately 60 per cent Protestant, 12 per cent Catholic, and 28 per cent Jewish. The religious distribution is not representative of the religious distributions in the United States at the time. The Jewish population is over-represented and the Catholic population is under-represented (Kinsey, 1953).

In general, the Kinsey researchers found that men reported more sexual activity than women at all ages, but the form of the activity and frequency varied for different ages. Male frequency was found to peak in the early twenties, while the female peaked in sexual activity between the ages of 30 and 45. Although there was a marked difference in the age at which the individuals reported the greatest sexual activity, the males aged 30 to 45 still reported more sexual activity than the women at their peak of sexual activity. There was the least difference in frequency reported at this age group than at any other (Kinsey, 1953).

In addition to sexual frequency, subjects in the Kinsey studies were asked about the forms of sexual activity in which they participated that led to orgasm. Masturbation was reported most frequently among unmarried women. Of these women, 95 per cent reported that they achieved orgasm from masturbation. The most commonly cited source of sexual activity for married women was intercourse. More than 80 per cent of the sample reported genital petting by age 18, and 68 per cent of college men and 60 per cent of college women reported having premarital intercourse.

In researching premarital sexual relationships, oral and anal sex were rarely reported, although married couples did report manual stimulation during foreplay. Interestingly, married couples reported multiple orgasms in women. This finding was ridiculed by many in the field. It was not until Masters and Johnson demonstrated this potential under laboratory conditions that the idea of multiple orgasms for women became accepted (Frieze, 1978; Kinsey, 1953; Masters, 1966).

Homosexuality was found to be more prevalent than had been expected by the Kinsey researchers, with 10 per cent of the males over 15 years old and 1 per cent of the females of this age reporting that they were exclusively homosexual (these percentages were corrected for bias by the researchers) (Frieze, 1978). In addition to those reporting that they were exclusively homosexual, 25 per cent of the men and 3 per cent of the women reported that they had participated in overt homosexual experiences at least one time.

The effect of the Kinsey research was profound. For the first time people were researching sexual activity and finding that the previously held notions regarding masturbation, female sexuality, premarital intercourse, and sex play among the young unmarried population were incorrect. The research was survey type data, however, and still lacked the "scientific" label of controlled laboratory research.

Masters and Johnson

Masters and Johnson published their findings in their first book, *Human Sexual Response,* in 1966. Their work represented the first comprehensive scientific study of what actually occurs in men and women during the sexual arousal cycle and during orgasm. It was demonstrated in the laboratory that sexual response in both men and women involved the entire body. Breasts, skin muscles, rectum, heart rate, blood pressure, and respiratory rate were found to change during sexual arousal and response in both sexes. In terms of genital changes, women evidenced changes in the clitoris, vagina, uterus, and labia, while men showed changes in the penis, scrotum, and testes (Frieze, 1978; Masters, 1966).

The impact of the findings of Masters and Johnson were tremendous. For example, Kinsey's findings about multiple orgasm in women were confirmed. In addition, it was demonstrated conclusively that failure to reach orgasm has biological consequences for the woman. Previous to this, it was thought that only men suffered from the discomfort of vasoconstriction if not relieved by orgasm. Women too were found to experience physical discomfort, usually pelvic in origin, due to vasoconstriction. It was also proven that all orgasms involved the vagina and the clitoris, as well as other parts of the body. This finding effectively disproved the Freudian notion of vaginal versus clitoral orgasm.

A significant finding regarding the male partners in sexual activity was that a large penis did not necessarily mean better sex for the female partner. In fact, a very large penis was found to be potentially painful to the woman and could actually reduce her enjoyment.

By use of their laboratory and camera techniques, the Masters and Johnson team were able to show that the woman's vagina expanded to fix the size of the penis within normal size ranges. They also found that there was no correlation between nonerect and erect penis size. Withdrawal was shown to be an ineffective birth control technique, as it was found that most men have what is called a "pre-ejaculate" fluid that contains sperm and could not be subject to voluntary control by the man.

In their research, pregnant and elderly couples were investigated to document changes in the sexual response cycle that occured during these times. It was demonstrated that intercourse during pregnancy was not harmful to the unborn child, and that the elderly did indeed continue to have sexual drives and the ability to express these drives (Frieze, 1978; Masters, 1966).

The Sexual Response Cycle. In describing their findings, Masters and Johnson chose to divide the sexual response cycle into four phases: excitement, plateau, orgasmic, and resolution (Masters, 1966).

The *excitement phase* of the sexual response cycle can begin as a result of any source of reflexogenic or psychogenic stimulation. This is potentially one of the longest phases of the cycle, which continues and progresses unless the stimulation is removed or interrupted.

If the stimulation from the excitement phase continues, the individual will pass into the second stage, the *plateau phase*. The length of this stage is dependent upon the effectiveness of the stimulations and the individual's drive for culminating the increment of sexual tension. If, during this stage, the stimulus or drive of the individual is inadequate or removed, the individual will decrease in sex tension from the plateau phase tension levels into a prolonged resolution phase without orgasmic relief. If the stimulation continues, the sexual tensions increase and are intensified until they reach an extreme level from which the individual ultimately may move to orgasm.

Orgasm has been defined by Masters and Johnson (1966) as those few seconds during which the vasoconstriction and myotonia developed from sexual stimuli are released. The orgasm is an involuntary climax at any level that represents the maximum sexual tension increment for the particular occasion. The subjective awareness of orgasm is pelvic in focus. In women, the orgasm is felt in the clitoris, vagina, and uterus. Men experience orgasm in the penis, prostate, and seminal vesicles.

Laboratory research on orgasms demonstrated that women tend to have greater variation in the duration and intensity of the orgasmic experience. Less individual variation in the ejaculatory reaction in men was found (Masters, 1966).

Following orgasm, the individual begins the *resolution phase,* which is an involuntary period of tension loss. Basically, the individual goes through the levels of arousal in reverse, from plateau to excitement to an unstimulated state.

Women have been found to have the potential for multiple orgasm. This potential to return to an orgasmic state can occur from any point in the arousal cycle, including the resolution phase. It is most likely to occur (with effective stimulation) during the plateau phase.

Men, on the other hand, have been found to experience a *refractory period* during the resolution phase. Effective restimulation of the man is not possible until this refractory period is over. In some cases, the refractory phase may last as long in the reverse arousal stages as the excitement level. Even following the refractory period, Masters and Johnson (1966) found that, with few exceptions, the physiologic ability of the male to respond to restimulation is much slower than that of the female.

As previously mentioned, the sexual arousal stages involve body changes in both the male and the female. Table 3–1 (Female Sexual Response) and Table 3–2 (Male Sexual Response) more specifically outline the changes that occur in the four stages listed above.

The basic physiological responses to sexual stimulation, according to Masters and Johnson (1966), are vasoconstriction and myotonia. The vasoconstriction, congestion of the blood vessels, may be superficial or deep. For example, the sex flush which occurs on the skin is an example of superificial vasoconstriction. Deeper vasoconstriction is more evident in the plateau and orgasmic phases. Myotonia, the generalized increase in muscle tension, can be either voluntary or involuntary. Most of the time, the involuntary myotonia occurs in the plateau and orgasmic phases.

Kaplan

Kaplan (1974) has proposed an alternative way of viewing the sexual response cycle which utilizes the concepts of vasoconstriction and myotonia. She suggests a two-phase, or biphasic, sexual response cycle. The first stage is the vasoconstriction phase, which produces male penile erection and female vaginal lubrication. The second phase refers to the clonic muscle contractions that constitute orgasm. The biphasic model allows for a more clearly defined response in terms of nervous system responses but is generally not as well known or accepted as the four-level response cycle outlined by Masters and Johnson (1966).

HUMAN SEXUAL DYSFUNCTION

Following their research on the normal sexual response cycle, Masters and Johnson began to move into the area of disturbed sexual response–dysfunction. Prior to the Masters and Johnson approach, sexual dysfunction had been viewed by traditional psychotherapists as a symptom of some underlying psychological problem of "neurosis." Individuals with sexual dysfunctions were usually referred to a psychotherapist to deal with their "real problem," which had manifested itself in sexual dysfunction. It was thought that once the basic problem was remedied, the sexual one would disappear (Barbach, 1975).

Masters and Johnson rejected the notion that all sexual dysfunction was a result of neurosis. They advocated psychotherapy only when organic factors had been identified or ruled out (Masters, 1976). The sex therapy proposed by Masters and Johnson involved treating couples together, as a unit, by a dual-sex therapy team. The treatment was usually intensive for a short period of time and included education about sexual functioning and verbal and non-verbal communication. The basic premise in the treatment was that the sexual response is a natural function. Sexual functioning is influenced by psychosocial input and can be disrupted by anxiety, depression, or physical stress (Masters, 1976). For example, penile erection and vaginal lubrication, given appropriate stimulation, were viewed as inborn reflexes. Dysfunctions, such as vaginismus (involuntary spasms of the vagina resulting from any attempted penetration) and premature ejaculation were seen as conditioned reflex responses that could be reconditioned.

From the start of their treatment and study of sexual dysfunction, Masters and Johnson insisted on treating couples rather than the dysfunctional partner. They felt that "there is no such thing as an uninvolved partner in any committed relationship where there is sexual dysfunction" (Masters, 1976). Sexual dysfunctions were seen as arising from hostility, poor commu-

Table 3–1. Female Sexual Response

Area of Response	Stage of Arousal			
	Excitement	Plateau	Orgasm	Resolution
Breasts	Nipple erection Increased breast size	Reach maximum size	No change	Slow decrease in size and nipple erection
Skin flush	Begins at abdomen, neck, and throat	Spreads over body	Intensity correlates with orgasm (75% incidence)	Disappears in reverse order — rapid
Muscle tension (Myotonia)	Begins throughout body, mostly voluntary muscles (some involuntary)	Increases, contractions in face, abdomen, and intercostal muscles	Many involuntary contractions	Rapid decline
Rectum	Irregular contractions	Contractions — usually voluntary, of sphincter to increase stimulation	Strong involuntary contractions — correspond to orgasmic platform	No changes
Heart rate, blood pressure, breathing	Increased — in direct parallel to tension regardless of technique of stimulation	Continues to increase; hyperventilation	Increases more	Return to normal; sweating over body
Clitoris	Some enlargement	Glans pulled back	No additional changes	Rapid return to normal
Vagina	Lubrication; inner 2/3 enlarges	Orgasmic platform; outer 1/3 of vagina	Strong rhythmic contractions 0.8 second intervals	Slow return to normal
Uterus	Partial elevation	Elevates into false pelvis	Rapid irregular contraction	Very slow return to normal
Labia majora	Lips separate (effects differ for women with and without children)	Increased engorgement in both nullipara and multipara	No change	Rapid return to normal
Labia minora	Enlarge	Color change	No change	Rapid return to normal

Modified from Masters and Johnson, 1965.

Table 3–2. Male Sexual Response

Area of Response	Stage of Arousal			
	Excitement	Plateau	Orgasm	Resolution
Breasts	Nipple erection inconsistent	More erection of nipples	No change	Slow return to normal
Skin flush	Begins on abdomen	Spreads	Well developed — intensity correlates with orgasm (25% incidence)	Rapid fading in reverse order
Muscle tension (Myotonia)	Begins — mostly voluntary, some involuntary (partial testicular elevation); tensing of abdomen and intercostal muscles	Increased contractions all over body	Very strong Loss of voluntary control	Total relaxation — usually within five minutes
Rectum	Some irregular contractions	Voluntary contractions	Rhythmic contractions — 0.8 sec intervals	No changes
Heart rate, blood pressure, breathing	Increased in direct parallel to tension regardless of technique of stimulation	Markedly increased	Increases more	Return to normal, sweating in palms and feet
Scrotum	Contractions	No change	No change	Reduction in size
Testes	Elevate	Strong elevation	No change	Reduction in size and return to normal position
Penis	Erection	Stronger erection with increased penile circumference	Rhythmic contractions of entire urethra at 0.8 sec intervals	Rapid loss of erection initially; slower decrease to flaccid state follows

Modified from Masters and Johnson, 1965.

nication, the maintenance of a double standard, unrealistic expectations, deception, and differences in reproductive goals, to name only a few. As a result of the partner orientation of these etiologies, Masters and Johnson became committed to the idea that through the education of both partners in communication techniques, the couple could recondition themselves, given appropriate guidance. Communication is seen as a direct catalyst to the pleasurable experience of satisfying, responsive sexual interaction (Masters, 1976).

Male Sexual Dysfunction

Impotence. Impotence is the most commonly encountered male sexual dysfunction. Masters and Johnson (1978) have divided impotence into two categories, primary and secondary impotence. Primary impotence occurs when the male has never been able to achieve or maintain an erection sufficient to accomplish coitus. (Note: Impotence is not restricted to heterosexual intercourse. Sexual dysfunction in homosexual relationships will be discussed in a later chapter.) In the experience of Masters and Johnson (1978), 12 to 15 per cent of the men seen for primary impotence suffered from some physiologic or metabolic problem that resulted in primary impotence. Some of the nonphysiologic reasons for primary impotence include traumatic first coital attempts, the individual's interpretation of religious orthodoxy, and performance fears. Clinically, the man with primary impotence presents as an individual who is fearful that he will not be able to perform, an attitude often resulting in low self-esteem.

Secondary impotence is diagnosed in cases where a male has had successful coitus on one or more occasions, but later develops difficulty in achieving or maintaining an erection. According to Masters (1978), if a man has the occasion, even once, to seriously question his sexual performance, he is well on the way to impotence. Premature ejaculation is often the cause of secondary impotence. The man fears that he will once again ejaculate too quickly. Because of his fears, he is unable to achieve and maintain an erection. Alcoholism is the second major cause of secondary impotence. Even one case of impotence after consuming a large amount of alcohol can be sufficient to lead to impotence on a more permanent basis (Masters, 1978).

The explanation and removal of what is called the "spectator role" during sexual activity is a major goal in the treatment of impotence and all of the sexual dysfunctions (Frieze, 1978; Masters, 1976; Masters, 1978). This behavior develops whenever one or both partners sacrifice their spontaneity and become detached spectators of their sexual action. This commonly occurs in cases where one or both partners fear sexual performance will be inadequate. The fearful individual tends to check to see his or her own response or the response to the partner. This checking leads to less involvement and therefore to decreased sexual function, which serves as something of a self-fulfilling prophecy. The treatment of impotence involves teaching the partners to communicate. Sensate focus, including exercises performed by the couple with no pressure for coitus, is practiced in order that the couple can be more aware of themselves. Individuals are taught that they will never lose the fear of performance, but that any fears they have should be discussed. In terms of the spectator problem, the man is advised to watch the reactions of his partner rather than his own responses. By seeing that the partner is aroused, the man will receive the added stimulation of her arousal, and will stop worrying about himself. This explanation is by necessity somewhat superficial. A full explanation of the Masters and Johnson treatment for impotence is beyond the scope of this book. Interested readers are encouraged to read the texts available on the treatment of sexual dysfunctions for further, more detailed information.

Disorders of Ejaculation. A second commonly encountered sexual dysfunction in men actually represents several dysfunctions, the disorders of ejaculation. Included in this catetory are premature ejaculation, ejaculatory incompetence, and retrograde ejaculation. *Premature ejaculation* is difficult to define precisely because of its subjective nature. For the purposes of explanation, it is defined here as occurring when the man ejaculates more than half of the time before his partner is satisfied (Frieze, 1978). Masters (1978) states that any situation that places value on the speed of ejaculation can lead to later premature ejaculation. For example, if the man is with a prostitute or having intercourse in the back seat of a car, the value of rapid ejaculation is apparent. Some men, having performed in this fashion the first few times they have had intercourse, find that they are unable to delay ejaculation in subsequent intercourse. The traditional idea of trying to distract the mind with other things in order to prevent ejaculation has some negative effects, including secondary impotence. The man may become so distracted that the sexual stimulation will not be adequate to enable him to maintain his erection. Distracting himself from the sexual experience may also contribute to his becoming a spectator to his own sexual activity.

The usual treatment employed by Masters and Johnson for premature ejaculation involves the "squeeze technique". The penis is stimulated with the partner's hand. When the man begins to be excited and in the plateau phase, the partner's thumb is placed on the frenulum of the penis (on the ventral side) and the first two fingers of the hand are placed above and under the glans. The partner then squeezes, with enough pressure that the man can feel it, but not enough to cause discomfort. This squeezing will prevent ejaculation. During the second week of the therapy, this technique is practiced and learned. It is thought that by this type of "reconditioning" the man will learn to ejaculate more appropriately (Masters, 1978). There is a second type of squeeze called the basilar squeeze that may be utilized during intercourse to help decrease the feeling of impending ejaculation (ejaculatory inevitability). In this technique, the base of the penis is anteriorly and posteriorly squeezed. Not all cases of premature ejaculation are improved by the use of the squeeze technique, although it has been proven to be highly effective. Counseling is an integral part of the treatment of this and all dysfunctions. The activities alone are often insufficient to result in a cure.

Ejaculatory incompetence is defined as the inability of the man to ejaculate with the penis contained in the vagina. This can include inability to ejaculate under any circumstances or may just refer to the inability to ejaculate with a given partner. If the individual has never ejaculated, he is usually sent to a urologist to check for congenital absence of ejaculatory ducts. For those individuals who can ejaculate with manipulation, the treatment usually involves having the woman insert the penis into her vagina just prior to ejaculation. It has been found that if this is accomplished one or two times, the man can usually ejaculate within the vagina on subsequent occasions (Masters, 1978).

Retrograde ejaculation, ejaculation into the bladder rather than out of the urethra, may be a result of surgery or some physiological condition and will be discussed in the chapter on medical conditions.

Female Sexual Dysfunction

Anorgasm. The most commonly encountered female sexual dysfunction is lack of orgasm, or *anorgasm*. Nonorgasmic women are classified as exhibiting primary, situational, random, or secondary anorgasmia. Orgasm, as defined earlier, refers to the endpoint release of maximum increment of sexual response. A women suffering from primary anorgasmia does not experience orgasm by any means under any circumstances. In determining this diagnosis, much time may be spent educating the client in terms of what actually is an orgasm. Some women learn that unless they have the experience of "fire works" they are not having an orgasm. It is important to determine what the woman actually does experience. Situational lack of orgasm occurs when women experience orgasm only in response to a limited pattern or patterns of stimulation. For example, a woman may experience orgasm only with masturbation. Random orgasmic experiences occur unpredictably and unreliably. Often the woman will be orgasmic on vacations or special events but not consistently. Masters and Johnson (1978) have found that secondary loss of orgasmic activity is a rare occurrence. It may be brought about by the sudden loss of a partner, a change in the general physical well-being, or a loss of self-esteem that in turn leads to a loss of the previously established pattern of response to stimulation (Johnson, 1978).

Anorgasmia can be due to organic as well as psychological problems. Some potential organic explanations include insufficient vaginal lubrication, dyspareunia, and chronic pelvic congestion. Psychological factors that may contribute include the person's sexual value system, present sources of sexual arousal, personal values, and cultural influences. The treatment for this dysfunction begins, as do most of the Masters and Johnson types of treatments, with complete removal of performance pressure from the woman. Together the couple explore, define, and communicate erotic resources, needs, preferences, and inhibitions. During the treatment much education takes place. Specific physical activities are suggested. These are balanced with discussions, insights, and sex information. The progression of the activities is determined by the previous day's experience (Johnson, 1978).

Recently, with the so-called sexual revolution, and in part due to the increased knowledge about the sexual potential of women, orgasm has become more of a problem for some. The trend seems to place both women and men in a position where they are obligated to see that the woman not only enjoys sexual activity but also has multiple orgasms on every occasion. This goal orientation can lead to a mechanization of the sexual responsiveness of the woman (Johnson, 1978). Subjective pleasure for both partners without keeping score of the numbers and types of orgasms is probably a more realistic goal.

Vaginismus. A second dysfunction found in women is *vaginismus*. This condition is defined as involuntary constriction of the pelvic musculature that involves the outer one-third of the vagina and the perineum. The constriction is spastic, and, at least until the woman learns how to control it, is not under her control. The reflex is stimulated by an imagined, anticipated, or real attempt at vaginal penetration. The severity varies from a situation in which penetration is impossible to one in which there is mild dyspareunia and stinging upon penetration. The condition is not always associated with nonorgasmic dysfunctions and is not the same thing as dyspareunia. Painful intercourse (dyspareunia) can, however, lead to vaginismus, and will be discussed next.

The most frequent causes of vaginismus are psychogenic in origin and include severe psychosocial conditioning against intercourse, religious ortho- doxy, rape or gang rape, trauma associated with first pelvic examination, and male sexual dysfunctions that repeatedly leave the woman suffering from pelvic congestion (Biggs, 1978).

In diagnosing vaginismus, history data are very important. Therapists can get a "feel" for the woman's attitudes about herself, her partner, and other people with whom she has been associated sexually in the past. In addition, they can learn what intercourse means to the client. The diagnostic assessment of vaginismus is made during the pelvic examination with the attempt to insert one finger into the introitus. If evidence of the muscular contractions diagnostic of vaginismus is found, the nurse or therapist can demonstrate the spasm to both partners, utilizing a mirror for the woman. Demonstrating this spasm to the partner can help to reassure him that the response is indeed involuntary and not a result of the woman's feelings for him. Treatment of vaginismus includes the use of progressively larger dilators by the client, the examiner, and finally the partner when the woman is ready. Slowly the couple progresses to intercourse (Biggs, 1978).

A commonly encountered reason for the cessation or decrease in sexual activity in women is painful intercourse, *dyspareunia*. Unfortunately, many women are too embarrassed to discuss this with a nurse or physician and may instead decrease their activity. Dyspareunia can be attributed to many causes, most of which are easily remedied. For example, undiagnosed vaginal infections can often lead to pain during intercourse. In most cases, these infections are easily cured and the cause for the dyspareunia eliminated. Frequent douching, which is not necessary in any event, can also lead to painful intercourse. Some women suffer from allergic reactions to vaginal products, including some vaginal spermicides. Eliminating these products will often eliminate the pain. Tearing of vaginal tissues or improper healing following delivery of a child may also lead to dyspareunia. Finally, many older women approaching or experiencing menopause complain of dyspareu- nia, which is often very responsive to the use of an artificial sterile lubricant. The increased sensitivity in the vagina at this time is due to a decrease in the estrogen level in the vagina, which leads to a thinning and greater sensitivity of the vaginal mucosa. In cases where the sterile lubricant does not help the dyspareunia, an estrogen vaginal cream is almost always effective.

The preceding discussion of sexual dysfunctions is by no means exhaus- tive. It does, however, illustrate the very popular Masters and Johnson techniques. The reader should not think that these are the only treatment modalities available, however. Some very significant problems regarding the Masters and Johnson treatments exist. First, the treatment is often very expensive, involving thousands of dollars and requiring several weeks away from the home environment. For many, the treatment is impossible. For example, the great majority of the couples treated by the Masters and Johnson Institute are married. This necessarily eliminates a great number of people. Even if unmarried couples are accepted for treatment, individuals who do not have steady sexual partners are eliminated, as are those whose partners are unwilling or unable to attend. Until very recently, homosexuals were not treated. The number of homosexual couples seen is still very small. Finally, those who do not wish to involve their partners are not accepted for treatment (Masters, 1978).

One alternative treatment technique for treating nonorgasmic women has increased in popularity. This method involves the use of what are called "pre-orgasmic women's groups." In her book on female sexuality, Barbach (1975) describes the treatment that she originated. The treatment involves group meetings of approximately five to seven women, who meet twice weekly for 1-1/2 hours over a five week period. Two female coleaders run these group sessions. Most of the women in the initial studies of these groups were Caucasian, American born, and heterosexual. The groups were called "pre" rather than "non-orgasmic" because the leaders felt that this terminology implied to the clients that there indeed was hope, and that they would become orgasmic following their treatment (Barbach, 1975).

Utilizing the group experience for sharing sexual difficulties and feelings as well as for disseminating information, the women benefitted from the support of the group. In addition to the group meetings, the women were given "homework" assignments, beginning with a nine step masturbation program to help them get in touch with their bodies and sexual feelings. After the women were orgasmic through self-stimulation (93%), their partners participated in the homework assignments as much as possible. In a three-month followup, Barbach reported that more than 50 per cent of the women who had attended the groups reported that they were orgasmic with their partners.

Obviously, pre-orgasmic women's groups do not answer all of the needs of sexually dysfunctional people, but they do offer at least some alternative for those who had previously been excluded from treatment. It is hoped that, as more people and more professionals become knowledgeable in the field of human sexuality, new programs for dealing with people with sexual dysfunctions will become available.

NURSING PERSPECTIVES

Myths

In preparing to educate clients about some of the commonly encountered misconceptions that prevent people from realizing their full sexual potential, nurses can examine some of the myths they have heard recently and in the past. One of the most harmful myths that has become popular, perhaps as a result of increased coverage of sexuality by mass media, is that sexual behavior comes naturally. As Masters and Johnson have stated, sexual response is an innate behavior. The sexual behavior, including attraction, stimulation, and the actual sexual interaction requires information, practice, communication, and cooperation to be fully realized (Barbach, 1975).

A second myth concerns vaginal orgasm. Despite the evidence that orgasm is experienced by both the vagina and the clitoris, some people still feel that only vaginal orgasms "should" be experienced. More pressure has been placed on both partners regarding orgasm. The idea that mutual orgasms, in which both partners experience orgasm at the same time, epitomized good sexual functioning became popular in the late 60's and early 70's. Orgasm is also thought by some to be "natural" only if it occurs during intercourse. Individuals who hold these beliefs about the proper time and place for orgasm necessarily limit the potential for orgasmic experiences. Nurses are not the appropriate individuals to try to change the client's perceptions, but they are in a good position to indicate to the client that other methods of sexual stimulation can lead to very pleasurable orgasmic experiences for both partners, and that these practices, such as oral-genital sex and mutual masturbation, are very common.

The final misconception regarding orgasm to be discussed here is that the man is responsible for the woman's orgasm. All people are responsible for themselves and their pleasure during sexual activity as in any other action. When the responsibility for one partner's enjoyment is placed on the other partner, the tendency is to reduce the act to one in which one person "makes" the other have an orgasm and is potentially highly unsatisfactory to both. Instead, couples should be encouraged to communicate what things are pleasurable. In this way, both can enjoy the experience, being responsible for themselves only. For example, the man may assume that direct clitoral stimulation is the route to orgasm for all women. In the effort to meet the expectation that the woman must experience multiple orgasms, her partner may stimulate the clitoris directly, causing pain and a decrease in sexual excitement. This can lead to frustration in both partners, with the male trying even harder to force an orgasm that cannot occur. By communication and by suggesting that the direct clitoral stimulation is not effective, or by suggesting some other activity that is pleasurable, the woman relieves the man of the sole responsibility for her orgasm. He is also no longer placed in the position of having to be all-knowing about sexual activity.

The search for substances that increase the sexual desire and potency of men and women has continued throughout time. In our culture a popularly held misconception is that alcohol is a sexual stimulant, particularly in the male. While it is true that alcohol may act on an individual to decrease inhibitions, it has a markedly negative effect on sexual performance. Alcohol is, after all, a depressant. The effect on the man's potential to achieve and maintain an erection is not at all in the intended direction. Inability to achieve erection following an excessive alcohol intake is often cited as a major contributing factor in cases of secondary impotence (Masters, 1978). At other times various foods have been thought to have an aphrodisiac effect. Some of these are oysters, organ meats, and a substance called "Spanish fly." None of these have been found to have the desired effect, except in the sense that they may function as placebos. Individuals believe that their sexual function will be improved, and as a result of increased confidence, actually do perform better.

Role of the Nurse

The list of myths held out about sexuality and human sexual functions could fill volumes. Nurses must educate themselves, both formally and from clients, regarding sexuality in this culture. They must be available to teach, counsel, and refer, if necessary, any clients who need sexual health care. If, in the course of the physical examination, it is determined that a client is suffering from a sexual dysfunction that is not within the competency of the nurse to treat, referral should be made by the nurse after discussing this with the client. Nurses must be knowledgeable about the referring agency and the individual, so that they can adequately prepare the client for what to expect.

Perhaps the most important precaution that nurses must take in dealing with the sexual health care of clients is to avoid assuming anything. Because clients report that they are sexually active, nurses cannot assume that intercourse is taking place. The individual may be involved in mutual masturbation, heavy petting, or may consider kissing to be a sexual act. To assume that all clients are heterosexual is also unfair and can be a significant block to the establishment of a working relationship between nurses and clients. Nurses must clarify sexual preference so that both the nurse and the client are clear on the sexual orientation of the client. Having done this, nurses must avoid judging whether this is the "proper" orientation. If clients report that they are unhappy with their sexual orientation, the nurse and the client can investigate this issue further. It is inappropriate for nurses to judge sexual activity as "wrong." In order to give good care, what is necessary is not that nurses agree with the behaviors or moral attitudes of clients, but that they are able to put aside biases and give clients the best nonjudgmental care possible.

It is only recently that people have felt free enough to discuss sexual behavior openly. The nurse is in an excellent position to educate, reassure, and counsel clients of both sexes regarding their sexuality.

References

Barbach, Lonnie Garfield: *For Yourself: The Fulfillment of Female Sexuality.* New York, New American Library, 1975.

Barker-Benfield, G. L.: "Sexual Surgery in Late Nineteenth Century America: *In* Dreifus, Claudia (Ed.): *Seizing Our Bodies: The Politics of Women's Health.* New York, Vintage Books, 1977.

Biggs, Mae A.: "Vaginismus." *Human Reproductive Biology Institute Seminar on Human Sexuality for Nurses,* Boston, 1978.

Ehrenreich, Barbara, and English, Deirdre: "Complaints and Disorders: The Sexual Politics of Sickness." *In* Dreifus, Claudia (Ed.): *Seizing Our Bodies: The Politics of Women's Health.* New York, Vintage Books, 1977.

Frieze, Irene H.: "Sexual Roles of Women." *In* Frieze, Irene H., Parsons, Jacquelynne E., Johnson, Paula B., Ruble, Diane N., and Zillman, Gail L. (Eds.): *Women and Sex Roles: A Sociological Perspective.* New York, W. W. Norton and Co., 1978.

Fortier, Lisa; "Women, Sex and Patriarchy." *Family Planning Perspective,* Vol. 7, No. 6, Nov/Dec 1975.

Gordon, Linda: *Woman's Body, Woman's Right.* New York, Penguin Books, 1976.

Johnson, Virginia: "The Nonorgasmic Female." *Human Reproductive Biology Institute Seminar on Human Sexuality for Nurses,* Boston, 1978.

Kaplan, H. S.: *The New Sex Therapy.* New York, Brunner/Mazel, Inc., 1974.

Kinsey, Alfred C., Pomeroy, Wardell B., Martin, Clyde E., and Gebhard, Paul H.: *Sexual Behavior in the Human Female.* Philadelphia, W. B. Saunders Company, 1953.

Lewis, Gwendolyn L.: "Changes in Women's Role Participation." *In* Frieze, Irene H., Parson, Jacquelynne E., Johnson, Paula B., Ruble, Diane L., and Zillman, Gail L. (Eds.): *Women and Sex Roles: A Sociological Perspective.* New York, W. W. Norton and Company, 1978.

Marieskind, Helen I.: "The Women's Health Movement: Post Roots." *In* Dreifus, Claudia (Ed.): *Seizing Our Bodies: The Politics of Women's Health.* New York, Vintage Books, 1977.

Masters, William H., and Johnson, Virginia E.: *Human Sexual Response.* Boston, Little, Brown and Company, 1966.

Masters, William H., and Johnson, Virginia E.: "Principles of the New Sex Therapy." *American Journal of Psychiatry,* Vol. 133:5, May 1976.

Masters, William H.: "Disorders of Ejaculation." *Human Reproductive Biology Institute Seminar on Human Sexuality for Nurses,* Boston, 1978.

Walum, Laurel Richardson: *The Dynamics of Sex and Gender: A Sociological Perspective.* Chicago, Rand McNally Publishing Company, 1977.

Weidger, Paula: *Menstruation and Menopause.* New York, Alfred A. Knopf, 1976.

Development and Expression of Sexuality

SEXUAL DEVELOPMENT—BIRTH TO ADOLESCENCE

All people have ideas regarding similarities and differences between men and women. Boys and girls are seen as having basic differences beyond the purely biological. Sex roles, the sum of socially designated behaviors that differentiate men and women, are both persistent and pervasive in our society (Broverman, 1972). In the past, the positive values for stereotypical sex roles have rarely been questioned. More recently, with the advent of the feminist movement, greater attention has been focused on the potentially damaging effects of sex role stereotyping.

Despite the increased awareness of the dangers of sex role stereotyping, studies show that sex role stereotypes continue to exist (Broverman, 1972; Guttentag, 1976; Moss, 1972; Rubin, 1974; Weinberg, 1980). A strong consensus concerning differing characteristics of men and women was found across groups that differed in age, sex, religion, marital status, and educational level (Broverman, 1972). In describing women, both men and women tended to place women in what Broverman has called a "warmth and expressiveness" cluster. Women were described as gentle, sensitive to the feelings of others, tactful, religious, quiet, interested in art and culture, and able to express tender feelings. These traits were considered to be highly valued in women. Men were most often described around a "competency cluster," which included such descriptors as independent, objective, active, competitive, logical, skilled in business, worldly, adventurous, able to make decisions easily, self-confident, always acting as leader, and ambitious. These competency cluster variables were highly valued in males. Males were considered to be lacking in warmth and expressiveness cluster items, while women were seen as generally lacking the masculine traits.

In attempting to evaluate the effects of sex role stereotypes, studies to determine general standards for mental health have been conducted. When therapists were asked to describe a healthy male adult and a healthy female adult, differences similiar to those outlined above were obtained. When the therapists were asked to describe a normal adult, without specifying the sex of that adult, therapists more often identified characteristics attributed to the healthy male adult. The implications of this are striking. The general standards of health for adults are actually applied to men only, while healthy adult women are perceived as significantly less healthy by adult standards (Chessler, 1972; Broverman, 1972).

Arbitrary decisions about appropriate sex role behaviors serve to limit the development of fullest potential in any person, and are therefore of negative value. In response to this rigid stereotyping, the concept of androgyny has become popular. All people are viewed as individual blends of capabilities considered both masculine and feminine according to the traditional stereotypes. An adult of either sex is seen as possessing both "masculine" and "feminine" traits. Viewing individuals as androgynous allows them an expanded range of acceptable behaviors (Bem, 1975; Guttentag, 1976).

As the earlier chapters of this text have discussed, individuals experience sexuality physiologically, culturally, socially, and psychologically. Sexuality is not limited to the reproductive organs or to sexual intercourse. An explanation of sexuality and its development is complex. Four sources for sex differences will be identified and discussed here. Biological differences will be discussed first, followed by a consideration of three theories of sex role learning. Although this division seems to imply a nature/nurture controversy, neither the environmental nor the biological explanations alone are sufficient to explain the differences in the sexes. The effects of both must be examined and evaluated together. Only for ease of discussion are they separated here.

Following a discussion of theories of sex differences, the socialization processes likely to be encountered by children from the time of birth until adolescence will be covered. Particular attention will be given to the developing awareness of sexuality. Finally, the role of the nurse will be discussed. Particularly, the relation of the teaching functions appropriate for clients, their parents, and educators in the aforementioned age groups will be considered.

SEX DIFFERENCES—THEORIES

Biological Sexuality

Biological sexuality has been defined by Leach (1978) as referring to the chromosomes, hormones, and primary and secondary sex characteristics that distinguish males from females. This definition forms the basis for discussing biological sexuality.

The sex of an individual is determined at the moment of fertilization. This is the first step in sex determination of the fetus. The chromosomes for a male offspring are of the XY combination, and those for a female offspring are of the XX combination. These chromosomal combinations determine whether the undifferentiated fetal gonads become ovaries or testes at around four to six weeks of gestation. At this point, the individual is either chromosomally male or female. The second step involves the secretion or lack of secretion by the fetal gonads. This determines whether the male or female genital pattern will develop. If the male testes secrete fetal androgen between the seventh and twelfth weeks of gestation, male structures will develop from the wolffian ducts. Even in a chromosomally male fetus, if androgens are not present, the fetus will develop female reproductive structures. In addition to the development of male structures from the wolffian ducts, a mullerian-inhibiting substance is secreted that prevents further development of the mullerian, or female, duct system. The female fetus, unexposed to fetal androgens, develops mullerian ducts rather than wolffian ducts. Finally, the pattern of release of pituitary gonadotropins is established in what Money (1972) has called the "sex typing" of the brain. This is the third step in biological sex determination. Sex typing is thought to occur at a critical period of development. The brain becomes especially sensitive to testosterone, a male hormone. If the brain is influenced by testosterone, a noncyclic pattern for the release of gonadotropins is established. If the brain is not influenced by testosterone, as in the female fetus or nonfunctioning male fetus, a cyclic pattern of gonadotropins is established, following the release of estrogen. Money postulates that after this critical period, the individual becomes resistant to testosterone or estrogen, depending on the sexual differentiation. The development of the internal and external genitalia that occurs as a result of exposure to or lack of testosterone, as in steps one and two above, are identified by Money as the first critical point in the establishment of gender identity.

Maccoby, in a thorough review of the literature on sex differences, has identified two other factors related to biological differences between men and women: aggression and visual-spatial ability (Maccoby, 1974). The idea of aggression being biologically based is defended on the basis that the sex differences identified in humans also exist in subhuman primates. In addition, the sex difference is cross culturally universal. Finally, levels of aggression have been shown to be responsive to sex hormone levels. Maccoby concludes, then, that the greater aggression of males is biologically based.

Visual-spatial ability has been identified as a recessive sex-linked gene, in which 50 per cent of males and 25 per cent of females show the phenotype. This is not to say that men are innately superior to women in mathematics. Indeed, this visual-spatial ability is only one aspect of some types of mathematical problems.

Sex Role Learning Theories

When people search to find the one true method by which children learn the "proper" sex role behaviors, they tend to become confused. Many rationales have been provided to better explain the processes necessary to ensure these learnings. Four broad theories frequently encountered in the literature will be discussed here. Although these theories are not the only explanations for the learning of sex role stereotypical behavior, they are generally accepted as contributing to the prevalence of sex role stereotypes (Guttentag, 1976; Seiden, 1976).

Freudian Theory of Sex Role Behavior. According to Freudian theorists, young children of both sexes initially identify with the mother. The female child continues in this relationship with what is seen as the "castrated" mother. The male, however, gives up his love for his mother because of his fear of arousing the wrath of the father. The male child is seen as fearing that the father will castrate him, as he believes the father has castrated his mother. The male child, to avoid this wrath, identifies with the father, rejecting the values of the mother. According to the Freudian theory of sex role behavior, the major process for learning appropriate sex role behavior is direct imitation of the appropriate parent (Erikson, 1963; Leach, 1978).

Social Learning Model of Sex Role Behavior. The social learning model proposes that the concepts of masculine and feminine characteristics are fixed in the minds of the parents. The behaviors exhibited by the child are compared with the "ideal" sex role models by the parents. The child's behaviors are then either rewarded or punished, depending on the activity and sex of the child. This reinforcement by the parents is not thought to be on the conscious level. In addition, the idealized male and female behaviors may not be consciously applied to the child's behavior (Bardwick, 1971; Moss, 1972; Seiden, 1976).

Cognitive Development Theory of Sex Role Behavior. Sex role identity is seen by the cognitive development theorists as an important part of internal cognitive development. In fact, it is considered to be as important as gender identity development. When children are able to label themselves as males or females (which is a cognitive step) they will choose to do those things that emphasize maleness or femaleness. The sex typed behavior and the sex role concepts are seen as paralleling the child's conceptual growth and can be predicted by it (Money, 1972).

Cultural Model for Sex Role Behavior. According to the cultural model, children are influenced by forces in their culture, such as peers, schools, and mass media. Family and socioeconomic status are seen as having little effect on this process. The stereotyping is not seen as a part of the development of gender identity as it is in the cognitive development model (Bardwick, 1971; Kohlberg, 1966; Komisar, 1971; Walum, 1977).

These are four models of sex role learning behavior. While none explains learning completely, each has something to contribute to the understanding of sex role learning. In addition, people's biology and experiences will determine the sex role stereotypes that they will carry.

SEXUAL DEVELOPMENT: INFANCY TO ADOLESCENCE

Infancy

Sex typing of behavior has been observed as early as in newborn nurseries. In many hospitals, it is still common practice to wrap newborn girl babies in pink blankets, while blue blankets are used for boys. Studies have shown that female babies are handled more delicately and cooed at more, while male babies are handled more roughly. This has been found even in the first days of life (Walum, 1977).

Parents' perceptions and sex typing have already begun at birth, according to a study by Rubin (1974). In this study, 30 newborns were rated by their parents 24 hours after delivery. Parents identified their female children as softer, finer featured, smaller, more inattentive, more awkward, and more delicate than did parents of male infants. The parents of the male children described their sons as firmer, larger featured, better coordinated, more alert, stronger, and harder. This early sex role stereotyping has been found to continue throughout the first year of life. When infants are dressed in "male" or "female" outfits, and the subjects are told that the child is the appropriate sex for the clothing, studies have consistently found that people act differently and evaluate the infant differently, according to their perceptions of the infant's sex (Condry, 1976; Weinberg, 1980; Will, 1976).

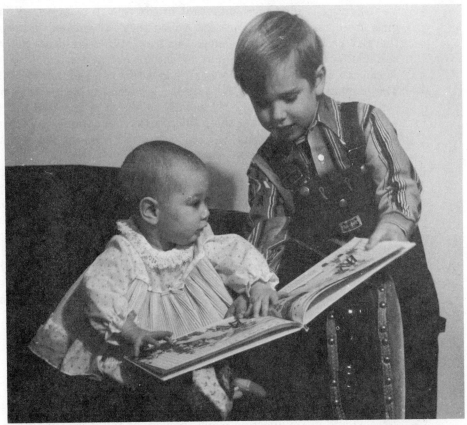

Photograph by Jim Tackett

"Sugar and spice and everything nice; that's what little girls are made of."　　*"Snips and snails and puppy-dog's tails; that's what little boys are made of."*

The traditional rhyme still reflects society's differences in attitudes toward boys and girls. Although some parents consciously try to raise their children in ways they consider to be nonsexist, other parents sincerely believe the appropriateness of sex role differences and choose their children's clothing in accordance with their beliefs.

Toddlers

By the time children reach two or three years old, they know which sex-linked behaviors are expected of them. Gender identity, the individual's sense of himself or herself as male or female (or ambivalent), is usually established by this time (Guttentag, 1976; Leach, 1978; Money, 1972; Seiden, 1976). Gender role is defined as the expression of gender identity. Everything that individuals say and do to indicate to others or to themselves the degree to which they are male, female, or ambivalent is the gender role. Various theories attempt to explain the source of gender identity, but most studies deal with gender role, the public expression of gender identity.

Different behaviors are expected from males and females from infancy. Boys are encouraged to participate in physical activity. Aggressive behavior is tolerated in boys, while crying is treated very negatively. Strangers have a great effect on this stereotyping, while parents tend to view their children at this stage (1-3 years old) more as individuals with specific temperaments and talents. Teachers, babysitters, and relatives may have the greatest role in perpetuating stereotypes, at least during this stage of development (Maccoby, 1974).

Clothing is also very important in sex role stereotyping. From infancy, girls are dressed in frilly dresses, which they are warned to keep clean. As the girl passes through infancy, she may still wear dresses that are not suitable for rough play. She may be encouraged to participate in quiet play, so she can behave more like a "girl" and so she can look her best at all times. The emphasis on physical appearance for females begins this early! Boys' clothing, on the other hand, is usually tough. It is expected that little boys will get dirty as a result of their "naturally" rough games (Walum, 1977).

In reading this section, the reader may be thinking, "But that's not the way it is anymore! Girls wear jeans and t-shirts now, too." Although this is becoming more and more common, a trip to a children's clothing store will reveal that, especially for three-year-olds and up, clothing is separated by sex. Girl's outfits, even jeans, often have ruffles, and are generally fancier and less sturdy than clothing for boys of the same age. Clothes for fancy occasions are frilly, "feminine" dresses for girls and "suits" for boys. Another interesting factor is that although girls, and indeed women, can be seen wearing traditionally male clothing, we never see men or boys wearing traditionally female clothing. This may be because male clothing is generally more utilitarian than female clothing, or it may be due to a more subtle status difference associated with particular types of dress.

Preschool

From about the age of two until school age, crying behavior is reacted to quite differently by adults depending on the sex of the child. Girls are often consoled and given affection when they cry at this age. They are usually not encouraged to be "strong," but, in fact, learn that they will be taken care of by some adult or other more powerful person if they engage in some kind of emotional display. Boys, on the other hand, are not "coddled" when they cry. In fact, they may be embarrassed by others if they cry. The boy may be called a "sissy" or told that "big boys don't cry." Not only does the boy get the message that he must conceal his emotions but he is also taught that he must learn to stand up for himself. This is especially apparent in regard to fighting behavior. Although fighting and aggression of all types are usually verbally discouraged (Guttentag, 1976; Maccoby, 1974), they are, in fact, subtly reinforced in boys. If a boy tells his parents that he was involved in an argument that was leading to a fight, but ran away, the parents may express disappointment that the boy didn't "stick up for himself." If the boy did fight and win, the parents may show pride in his achievement. Even if he fights and loses, he is rewarded for his effort.

Conversely, fighting of any kind is discouraged in girls. Confrontation is also discouraged. Parents may tell a child to tell the teacher (who will then take care of her) or to tell the parents if someone starts a fight with her. The parents may then speak to the parents of the child who ostensibly started the fight. The message to the girl is clear. She learns that she needs protection, and that fighting is not "ladylike."

Obviously, some extreme cases of stereotypical behavior have been presented here. Behavior of this type continues to exist and must be recognized for the potentially harmful effects that it may have on both sexes.

Competition and its expressions differ between boys and girls. Girls learn that they are valued for the way they look, not for what they do. They are usually compared to other girls. Their goal is to be the prettiest or the most popular (Guttentag, 1976). Boys learn that they must be "winners." They are told by their parents that they are the best or can be the best if they try. Expectations that the boy will be successful are established. When a boy wins at something, pride is shown by the parents, and when he loses, disappointment is shown. The little league baseball experience is a good example of this. Some parents become very involved in the competition of the sport, and may even embarrass a son if his team doesn't win, or if he plays badly. (Despite the fact that girls are now allowed on little league teams, their participation in such sports is rare.) The drive to win may become overly important to the boy, who wishes to achieve his parents' approval. He may fear rejection if his performance is less than excellent.

Sexual behavior of their children is often first noticed by parents during this time (age group 2–6). Actually, many children find that stimulating their genitals is pleasurable long before the age of two. If the parents notice that their children are doing this, they may become concerned that the children have premature adult sexual feelings. In order to prevent what the parents may perceive as an abnormal interest in sex, the children may be punished, either by being scolded or by being slapped on the hand every time the genitals are handled. In fact, masturbation has been demonstrated to be a part of the normal process of sexual development in both sexes. It has not been found to cause any harm to the individual, other than perhaps the harm that can come from guilt feelings (Taylor, 1978; Goldstein, 1976; Leach, 1978; Wilbur, 1973; Woods, 1979). Masturbation as it is defined here refers to the sexual arousal of oneself through stimulation of the sex organs. Orgasm is not a requisite. However, orgasm is, in fact, reached during masturbation in some children even before the age of puberty. No ejaculation accompanies the orgasm in the prepubescent male.

Historically, many conditions have been attributed to "excessive" masturbation, or even to any masturbation. For example, it was thought that masturbation could lead to insanity, nervous disorders, blindness, and criminality, to name only a few. As attitudes towards masturbation relaxed, it became acceptable for adolescents to masturbate until they were married. At that time it was no longer considered necessary. Even for adolescents, though, the warning that it must not be indulged in "excessively" was always there. Sadly, for concerned adolescents no one ever defines "excessive."

Following the findings of Kinsey, masturbation came to be more acceptable behavior. With the advent of the studies of Masters and Johnson, masturbation has been accepted as part of the treatment for many sexual dysfunctions. Although the scientific world seems to be more accepting of masturbatory behavior, many people still feel uncomfortable about this and actively discourage their children from such activities. The nurse is in a good position as teacher and counselor to educate parents about the normality of masturbation, even in very young children. Masturbation is a normal function that begins in infancy and continues throughout life for the majority of people.

During the toddler period, children begin to learn about modesty. They are taught that the genitals are to be covered at all times, and that it is not polite to be exposed when others are around. For girls, this modesty is reinforced even more extensively than for boys, partially because of the differences in clothing. Girls learn not only that no one should see their genitals but also that even letting someone see their underwear (under their dresses, of course) is unacceptable. This modesty about underwear also exists for boys, who may be terribly embarrassed if their zippers are open and this is noticed by someone else. However, the likelihood of this occurring is far less than that of little girls having their underwear seen. Children of both sexes learn that their genitals are considered unacceptable, and some learn that they are "dirty." Viewing the genitalia as dirty can certainly impede normal sexual pleasure later in life, particularly if such beliefs continue.

In addition to what children learn in their homes from their families, children learn a great deal about sex roles and behavior from the media. Guttentag (1976) found that mass media, peers, and schools were actually more powerful in their influence on sex role stereotypes than were parents. For preschool children, the major source of media exposure comes through watching television. Television programs, such as the Saturday morning cartoons and Sesame Street often reinforce gender stereotypes. Even the Muppets, who are generally asexual, often tend to have male voices. The major characters on Sesame Street, Ernie and Bert, are both male. Although some progress has been made, scenes in which boys play actively and girls watch continue to exist. In cartoons, female characters are usually in traditional "mothering" or "feminine" roles (Walum, 1977).

It is in the commercials, however, that the most blatant stereotyping can be observed. Advertising does not create the stereotypes but it does serve as a powerful reinforcer (Komisar, 1971). In toy advertisements, most girls are seen as wanting a ballerina doll or some other doll they can love and dress in fashionable clothes. The message is obvious. Little girls learn that the way they look and what they wear is of great importance. In addition, the girls shown playing with these dolls are always wearing dresses and are seen playing quietly, either alone or with one other girl.

As the advertisements allow the girl to age somewhat, she is presented as a combination sex object, wife, and mother. Fulfillment is promised to girls and women who can look alluring and beautiful for boyfriends and who can cook, clean, wash, or polish for husbands and children. Indeed, even cleaning is most often taught by a man. It is a man in the commercial who shows a woman how to get her husband's shirts whiter. It is a man who creates the scientific wonders that allow her house to sparkle. In fact, there is even a commercial in which a man tells women what to look for in their brassieres (Komisar, 1971; Walum, 1977)! The rationale for this preponderance of males teaching females to fulfill the roles that females were stereotypically "made" for lies in the fact that the male voice is considered by advertisers to carry more authority than the female voice, and is therefore utilized for its greater persuasiveness.

Although over half of the women in the United States work, advertisements do not reflect this (Komisar, 1971). Most mothers are portrayed as always being home, ready to put aside all of their interests and talents in order to place their husband and family ahead of themselves. Those who do work are usually seen in low status jobs.

In addition to reinforcing mens' concepts about the womans' place being in the home and woman's role as being submissive, advertisements say a great deal about the man's role. In addition to legitimizing male dominance, advertising of this type actually questions the manhood of men who don't wish to go along with the stereotypes of women. Men are made to feel henpecked or inadequate in any relationship in which the man shares the traditional female roles such as child care and dishwashing.

Recently, advertising has begun to reflect the realities of women in the working world more than they have in the past. Even now, however, the stereotypes abound. For example, most of the working women with families are still shown as having the primary responsibility of preparing dinner and shopping for food. In the advertisements where this is not true, the husband is pictured as "helping out" for the night. The idea of sharing the responsibility for the family has not yet reached the television advertising policies.

As children enter school, they are exposed to a new type of stereotyping—that of textbooks and storybooks. Generally, female characters are far underrepresented in children's books. The characters that are female are most often portrayed in aprons. Even animals wear aprons to distinguish males from females. In the pictures, males are shown as active, while females are shown as passive. The adult woman is stereotyped as passive and dependent, performing activities of service to men and children in the home. Motherhood is represented as a full time, lifelong job. Fathers never share the cooking. If the mother is for some reason not available to do the cooking, the father is most often seen taking the children out to dinner. The ultimate goal presented for women is motherhood and marriage, while the goal for men is to become President (Guttentag, 1976; Sprung, 1975; Walum, 1977).

School Age

Play during the school age years is also differentiated by sex. Boys are encouraged to participate in competitive and cooperative sports. Team sports such as football and baseball are encouraged. Although at some elementary schools girls also participate in these sports, they are not encouraged to compete. In fact, girls are taught that they should not win in competition with boys. For a boy, the worst insult is to be beaten by a girl. Girls learn that they are not "feminine" if they are better than a boy in some competitive sport. The group cooperation and competition that is stressed so much in boys is not valued in girls. Girls learn that boys are in general more valuable than themselves. In fact, when dating begins, many girls will make arrangements to spend time with a girlfriend only if they have not been invited to spend time with a boy. This is a clear example of the value that girls learn to place upon themselves.

Sexual curiosity may also begin quite young in children. During the preschool ages of 3 to 6, the parents may discover that children explore and generally compare their genitals with those of other children of the same age and opposite sex. This type of interest and curiosity is a normal, natural part of development of children, and should be accepted by the parents on that basis.

In discussing sex role stereotyping from infancy to adolescence, some major socialization differences have been presented and will be summarized here (Maccoby, 1974):

1. Boys are handled and played with more roughly than are girls.
2. Clothing has an effect on the behavior of adults toward children, according to the sex appropriateness of the behavior displayed by the child.
3. Boys receive more praise and criticism from caretakers. Girls receive more protection and consolation.
4. Parents show more concern over a boy's being a "sissy" than over a girl's being a "tomboy." (Note: This is especially true of fathers.)
5. Relative strangers may exert more stereotyping pressure on children than their own parents. Teachers, television, and peers have been described as highly influential.

FEELINGS OF THE NURSE

In taking the sexual history, or in beginning to provide anticipatory guidance regarding the sexuality of children, nurses will be asking the parents what they first learned about the sex act and the issues of sexuality. Before they are prepared to listen fully and attend to the information provided by the clients, nurses must have already answered those questions about themselves. The information, both verbal and nonverbal, about masturbation that nurses received as children is an important issue that must be considered in terms of the nurses' biases and attitudes. If, for example, they were punished for masturbating and informed that the genitals were dirty places that should not be touched unless absolutely necessary, they will have to deal with these feelings before they will be able to discuss them with clients.

Cultural biases must also be examined. For example, in asking clients about how affection was demonstrated in their homes when they were children, nurses must be able to put aside their own cultural expectations and to understand the client through his or her culture.

Nudity is another issue that often comes up for parents. Some parents feel that this is natural, and that there is nothing wrong with allowing children to see their parents naked. Others feel that this is not appropriate, and would feel embarrassed walking around unclothed in front of their children. Nurses must allow clients to decide issues of morality and what is right for them. The nurse must respect the right of clients to have values that may differ from those of the nurse.

At times, because of early socialization or experiences, nurses may find that they are unable to deal comfortably with the questions of sexuality in young children. At times, nurses may have to deal with the issue of sexual molestation of children. This is an unpleasant task, but one that must be dealt with. If the nurses involved feel unable to continue to be therapeutic in this or any other situation involving the sexuality of children and their parents, it is essential that the topic be dropped, but that the clients be referred to someone who is able to deal effectively with these issues. Nurses must be honest with themselves regarding their abilities and must be honest enough with clients to be able to admit that perhaps someone else would be better equipped to handle this aspect of their care. As always, the nurse must be sure that the client will receive quality care even if they are referred.

Nurses who deal with the issues of sexuality throughout the life span accept sexuality as a normal part of life. They must be in touch with their own feelings to be effective.

NURSE AS TEACHER

Nurses, because of their knowledge of health, anatomy, growth and development, sociology, and psychology, are among the primary providers of instruction and guidance to parents to help them to teach their children about human sexuality. Because the nurse is often involved in prenatal care, prepared childbirth classes, and well-child visits, opportunities for discussion of sexuality in both adults and children can arise. Before discussing some specific situations in which the nurse can serve as teacher, some general principles in dealing with parents about the sexuality of their children will be reviewed (Rybicki, 1976; Wilbur, 1973).

In discussing the sex education of young children, nurses must be aware that the parents of these children probably received inadequate sex education from their own parents and will most likely need a thorough review before they are prepared to discuss this information in a relaxed manner with their children. Parents should be reassured that children have a natural curiosity about their bodies and the bodies of others, and will probably ask questions about sexuality on their own. Giving sex information to children does not, as some believe, "put ideas into their heads" or encourage early promiscuity. The sex experimentation that does occur is a normal part of growth.

When parents give sex information to their children, the information need not be separated from other information, as if it were improper to discuss it in any other setting than a quiet, serious one. Questions about sex and sexuality should be answered by the parent like any other question in order to assure the child that sex is not more mysterious than other subjects. Some parents become concerned when their children ask the same questions over and over again. They should be reassured that children, like adults, need time to assimilate information, and that this questioning does not indicate a preoccupation on the part of the child.

Children tend to discuss with their friends what they have learned. A tremendous amount of misinformation can be accumulated in this way. If children are educated well by their parents they will be equipped with the facts about sex and reproduction, and will be less likely to believe erroneous information. Children who have had open discussions with parents about sexuality in the past are more likely to bring information that they are not certain of back to the parents for validation.

Children learn from the emotional atmosphere in situations as well as from the actual information obtained. For example, a child's attitudes and conclusions will be affected by how the child hears sex referred to in the home. The manner in which the parents demonstrate affection toward each other and their children is also a means through which children learn about sexuality. Breast feeding, which will be discussed more specifically shortly, is another vehicle through which children can learn attitudes about sexuality.

"Where Did I Come From?"

When a child asks a question, the parent must determine exactly what it is that the child wishes to know. For example, if a child asks where he came from, as the joke goes, he may wish to know only what hospital or city he was born in. There is a tendency to overload the child with information based on what may have been a very different question than the one asked. This overloading may be due to the parents' anxiety about the topic. Feeling that their child has finally asked the question that they had feared, some parents feel that they are "ready" to discuss the whole thing, then and there. In their nervousness, they may miss the message that the child is not ready for or interested in their speech. A good rule of thumb for parents and nurses is to answer exactly the question asked, without providing additional, unrequested information. If children wish additional information, they will usually ask for it, provided a comfortable atmosphere for discussing sex has been established.

In discussing sex and sexuality, the use of correct terms is preferable. Euphemisms tend to confuse children later, when they hear correct terminology utilized. In addition, using vague terms may be interpreted as discomfort with the topic. The message given, although unintentional, may be that it is not "OK" to talk about sex. Since children will have to learn some new terminology in dealing with sexuality, why not teach the child the right terms from the beginning?

When a child asks questions about reproduction in humans, answering in terms of birds or bees or some other animals will at best be confusing to the child. Such an answer does not answer the question the child has asked. It may also tend to make the child suspicious that there is something very mysterious and perhaps bad about reproduction in humans.

For most adults and parents as well as professionals, the most difficult questions to answer are those that deal with sexual intercourse. Although generally children understand far more than adults expect them to, at some ages children are not yet capable of understanding the feelings that accompany sexual intercourse. By the time children are asking questions, they are usually able to understand simple explanations of the physiology of sexual intercourse but it may be beyond their understanding why two adults would want to do such a thing. Because the feelings that accompany intercourse are often avoided in discussions of reproduction, most children leave their early lessons on intercourse and reproduction with the mistaken notion that conception takes place after every intercourse and that intercourse is something adults do only when they wish to enlarge their families. One way to avoid such misunderstanding is to explain that fertilization does not occur after each intercourse. It is appropriate to tell children that as they grow older they will change in ways they cannot understand now, and will start to have new, grown-up feelings. They can be told that one of the new feelings that they will have is the desire to express their love for another person physically, in a way that seems strange to them now, but in a way that is very pleasurable for both of the adults involved. In discussing sexual intercourse and the feelings that accompany it, parents should be reminded that discussion of sexual morality is beyond the comprehension of a child under six years old, and is therefore inappropriate. The parent can discuss morality with the child at a later time, when the child is better able to understand. Morality regarding sexual activity should be discussed before the child reaches puberty.

If possible, both parents should be available to give information about sexuality and sexual activity. Prior to the time in which children begin to ask questions, parents should be encouraged to work together to develop a basic philosophy and their own methods of teaching their children that they can implement as the situation arises. Single parents should also be encouraged to examine their philosophies and devise teaching methods.

Many parents first encounter questions about sexuality and reproduction from their children when another child is on the way. Older children may notice that their mother is beginning to look different, and may question her about this change. (Although this sounds like a gross understatement, many children do not notice such changes, since they are generally so gradual that they may not seem odd.) The nurse can be of great support to parents during this prenatal period in determining how to answer the questions that children may ask. A question commonly asked by three- to six-year-old children is, "Where do babies come from?" (Wilbur, 1973). When it has been established that the child does not want to know that children are born in hospitals or at home, a good answer for the parent to give is, "In a special place in the mother called the uterus." Telling a child that the baby grows in the mother's stomach is incorrect and may lead to several confusing thoughts in the child. The child may think that pregnancy is achieved through eating or may have a mental picture of the food the mother eats falling on the head of the baby that is occupying her stomach. Nurses and parents must keep in mind the concreteness of thought in children of this age.

Another commonly asked question, often following the first question, is, "How does the baby get out?" Once again, the person talking to the child should avoid answering more than has been asked. Often, telling the child that there is a special place or opening through which the baby can get out is sufficient. Children should not be told that the baby gets out from the same openings used for urination and bowel movements. Mistaken thoughts about bowel movements and childbirth may cause a child to retain bowel movements (Erikson, 1963). If the child asks for the location of this special opening, the teacher can tell the child that the opening is located between the mother's legs.

The above questions are generally encountered in preschool age children. Simple answers are usually sufficient at this stage and are appropriate for the child's level of understanding. Of course, individual children may differ in their curiosity and ability to understand, so these general examples should not be used inflexibly.

By the time a child reaches school age, simple answers to simple questions may no longer be sufficient. Children may now wish to know how the baby got into the mother's uterus in the first place. It is at this point that parents often become unsure of how much information to give their children. In counseling, parents are shown ways to avoid overloading their children with information. The nurse can advise that the parents follow a simple three-level answer to this question (Wilbur, 1973).

When children ask how the baby got into the mother's uterus, the first level answer is that the cell from which the baby grows is in the mother. If children wish to know more precisely how the cell got there, they will usually repeat the question. At this point, the parent can begin the second phase answer for this question, which involves a simple explanation of the reproductive system of women. The parent can tell the child that within girls and women there are two bodies that bear tiny eggs, and a special sac, the uterus, in which the baby grows until it is old enough to live in the outside world. This explanation of the presence of ovaries in both little girls and women reassures girls that they do not lack anything in terms of sexual equipment, and that theirs is located inside their bodies where it cannot be seen. The information is also reassuring to boys, in that they learn that girls have something different from them, and do not merely lack a penis.

The third level answer is appropriate if children ask what it is that makes the egg in the mother start to grow. Telling children that a special cell from the father called the sperm causes the growth of the egg may not be sufficient. Children may be satisfied with this answer, which does serve to help them understand the father's part in reproduction. If they continue the questioning with, "How does the father's cell get into the mother?", they are generally ready to hear an explanation of intercourse. Children can be told that parents like to do things together, and when they sleep together, it is often natural and pleasurable for the father's penis to fit into the mother's vagina. When this happens, the father leaves cells in the mother that can stimulate the growth of the egg. Intercourse and reproduction should not be connected in such a way that children believe that pregnancy results from all acts of sexual intercourse. When children are told that intercourse occurs between their parents, they learn about sexual activity as being within the context of a committed relationship. Some parents, in an attempt to instill values, may say that when two people are in love and are married they have intercourse. This places intercourse within the institution of marriage.

The Nurse and Sex Education

In educating parents to deal with their children's inevitable questions about sexuality, the issue of who should actually teach children about sex and reproduction may arise. Parents may feel that they are the only ones who should have this responsibility, and that neither schools nor churches have the right to participate in the sexual education of their children. This can be a dilemma for both the nurse and the parents. For those who feel that sexuality is an integral part of all that people do, separating information about this vital aspect of all individuals seems inappropriate and nearly impossible. In addition, the fact that so many parents are poorly prepared to participate in adequate sex education for their children has caused alarm in those who are committed to educating youth about their own sexuality and the sexuality of their peers (Schiller, 1968). On the other hand, some parents feel too embarrassed to deal with the questions that may be raised by their children and wish to have someone else take the responsibility of teaching their children about human sexuality. Still others may feel that children do not need to learn such things, and that they will learn them on their own when they are older. Nurses in their positions of authority and given their knowledge may be pivotal people in helping parents deal with their feelings about sex education and their children. Nurses may serve as liaisons between schools and parents in establishing sex education in the schools. They must remember that each individual has the right to his or her own views, and that the ability to be nonjudgmental is a necessary prerequisite to helping others. By providing an atmosphere in which parents feel relaxed enough to discuss their sexual concerns, nurses have taken a large step toward helping parents deal with the developing sexuality of their children.

If nurses are to participate in the development of a sex education program in the school, the following guidelines can be very useful in making this development as smooth as possible (Schiller, 1968). First, and perhaps most importantly, the school should enlist parental support and involvement throughout the planning and operation stages of the program. By providing for such participation, the educators can be sensitized to the concerns and attitudes of the parents. Some parents fear that sex education programs will teach new values, standards, or behavior patterns that they feel will be different from those they feel are important for their children. By encouraging their participation in all stages of the program, parents are reassured that their input is valued and respected. If at all possible, parents should be involved in separate group discussions, study groups, lectures, or seminars at the same time that their children are receiving sex education. This serves the purpose of educating the parents and, hopefully, will lead to more open explorations of feelings, based on sound knowledge, between the parents and the children.

Secondly, sex education programs should be appropriate for each age level, and should be included as an integral part of the curriculum from preschool education to the college level. In the school-age years, prior to adolescence, children should receive information regarding reproduction and puberty. This information is not sufficient, however. In addition, family roles and relationships should be discussed, being careful to avoid restricting stereotypes. Children of this age are able to understand and participate in discussions regarding emotions, especially love, anger, and aggression. Anxiety and guilt can also be discussed with children of this age group. These topics are not related directly to anatomy and physiology or reproduction but are an integral part of sex education and the development of the sexual self.

Even if nurses are not involved in the school system, they still have a great deal of input into the sex education of children. The prenatal period may serve the valuable function of early sex education for the older siblings. Parents should receive anticipatory guidance from nurses on how to deal with the questions they may be asked, and how to deal with their own changing sexuality at this time. (More on the sexuality changes during pregnancy will be discussed in a subsequent chapter.) If the parents decide that the new child will be breast-fed, other issues arise that should be discussed. For example, the parents themselves must decide how they feel about women breast-feeding in public. In our society the breast is still considered a sexual organ, and many people feel uncomfortable either exposing their own breasts to nurse an infant or seeing someone else do so. The feelings and questions of older children when they see the mother breast-feeding the new baby are the focus for discussion here. The comfort of the mother at this point is very important. Most children will ask the mother what she is doing. After being told that this is the way that the baby eats, and perhaps that this is the way they ate when they were babies, older children may decide that they would like to do this again. For many parents, this decision can be upsetting. The desire is usually recognized by parents as a part of the jealousy felt by the older sibling toward the new baby because of the loss of the older child's role as the baby. Beyond this, however, the parents often feel decidedly uncomfortable in what they may perceive as the sexual feelings inherent in such a request. If children are not allowed to try nursing once at this point, they may become quite insistent and babyish until allowed to do so. This regressive behavior may be even more upsetting to both the parents and the older child. Most children, if allowed to try the breast, will decide that breast milk is not so great, and that they, in fact, prefer their own peanut butter and jelly. By allowing children to try the breast, and by accepting the fact that the desire is sexual in that the child wishes to once again be the main focus for the mother, an atmosphere in which these feelings can be discussed is provided. Discussion and reassurance by the parents that the new baby has not replaced the older sibling and that he or she is still of great value and importance to the parents will usually lead to the disappearance of this type of behavior.

In earlier discussion, it was noted that in the hospital, nurses have been shown to contribute to the sex role stereotyping of newborn infants. Since stereotypes of any kind are limiting, the blatant stereotyping that exists should be eliminated. Nurses should be careful when expressing positive aspects of a child to the parents to avoid stereotypical remarks such as, "What a strong boy he is," or, "She's so delicate." It is important for nurses to be aware of their own prejudices and biases and to prevent them from interfering with provision of the best care possible. This includes avoiding the perpetuation of stereotypes.

Whenever possible, fathers should be included in the teaching of infant care provided for the new mother in the hospital, or in home visits made by the nurse. Many men wish to know how to care for their new babies but may be embarrassed to ask, or feel that it is not proper for a man to participate in this care. If the man does share in the care of the infant, he may be the subject of ridicule from peers for not fulfilling his "masculine" role. The nurse is a good source of a supportive atmosphere and for reinforcement of the attitude that the role of caring for children is one that can and should be carried out by both parents. At times, both professionals and lay people lose sight of the fact that it is only in the first nine months of life that the mother has a unique role in caring for the baby. Once the baby is born, the necessary uniqueness of this function no longer exists, except perhaps in breast-feeding. By including the father in the teaching of infant care, the nurse removes the expectation that, after the baby is taken home, the mother will know what to do in all situations, since she was the one who received the training. Both parents often fall into this trap. If both receive teaching together, they will realize that there will be times when they just will not know what to do and may feel overwhelmed with the responsibility of a new child. Having both received the teaching, they may be better able to support each other when the awesome responsibility of infant care becomes a reality. As the child grows and is brought to well-child visits, the nurse is once again in a good position to reinforce past teachings about sexuality in children and to provide some anticipatory guidance for the parents regarding what to expect next.

SUMMARY

Much of the information in this chapter has dealt with sex role stereotypes. One explanation for their tenacity in our society was explained by Maccoby (1974), who stated that if a generalization about a group of people is believed, whenever a member of that group behaves in an expected way, "the observer notes it and his/her belief is confirmed and strengthened; when a member of the group behaves in a way that is not consistent with the observer's expectations, the instance is likely to pass unnoticed, and the observer's generalized belief is protected from disconfirmation." This may be the explanation for the persistence of sex role stereotypes, despite the fact that some of these beliefs have been disproved.

Some sex differences that are fairly well established, and have been experimentally confirmed, follow (Maccoby, 1974):

1. Girls have greater verbal ability than boys. In the preschool years, verbal abilities of boys and girls are approximately the same. At about the age of 11, however, female superiority in this skill increases, at least through high school. College studies are very rare.
2. Boys excel in visual-spatial ability. This has been found to have a genetic base. This superior ability has been found to be fairly consistent in adolescents and in adults.
3. Males are more aggressive than females. This finding has been validated in studies of children as young as two or two and one half, and older. The greater aggressiveness has been found in both verbal and physical behavior.

Myths about sex differences abound, and are generally accepted, as we have seen. The following is a list of unfounded beliefs about sex differences (Maccoby, 1974):

Myth 1. Girls are more social than boys. Studies have shown that both sexes display equal interest in social stimuli and in their ability to learn through imitation of models. There is an equal response to social stimuli as well. The differences that have been uncovered regarding "sociability" between boys and girls are more in the kind of social activity than the amount. Boys have been found to be more highly oriented to the peer group, and have been found to congregate in larger groups, while girls tend to associate in small groups or in pairs.

Myth 2. Girls are more suggestible than boys. Both sexes have been found to be equally likely to imitate others spontaneously and equally likely to be susceptible to persuasive communication.

Myth 3. Girls have lower self-esteem than boys. Overall satisfaction and self-confidence evaluations between boys and girls have been found to be highly similar throughout childhood and adolescence. Girls tend to rate themselves higher in the social competence measures discussed earlier, while boys more often tend to evaluate themselves according to the competency cluster. Within the areas that each sex feels are important for themselves, however, the self-esteem ratings are the same.

Myth 4. Girls are better at role learning and simple repetitive tasks that require higher level cognitive processing and inhibition of previously learned responses. Studies have not confirmed this hypothesis.

Myth 5. Boys are more analytic. Boys have better visual-spatial abilities as a rule, but analytic abilities were not found to differ between the sexes.

Myth 6. Girls are affected more by heredity, boys by environment. Boys and girls are equally affected by their heredity and their environment.

The list of myths could fill pages and pages. Readers are encouraged to examine their own stereotypical ideas about the differences between men and women. All of us have these images, and recognizing them is a necessary first step to dealing with them. What can be done to change the sex role stereotyping that is so prevalent? First, people need to be educated and informed as to the stereotypes that are common. Many of us are unaware of these and may be perpetuating ideas about the roles of men and women that we would not wish to perpetuate. Advertising and textbooks could be reviewed (and indeed have been reviewed) with the idea of eliminating texts that are sexist. School programs for young children have been established, but education of parents as well as young children is essential (Guttentag, 1976). In many instances, the nurse is the appropriate and available person to fulfill this need for education of parents. The advantages of androgynous role possibilities can be stressed in this teaching. By viewing people as unique and valued blends of capacities and talents, all individuals can strive toward a fuller expression of themselves, unhindered by rigid, stereotypical expectations. If sex role stereotypes could be eliminated, people would be much further along the way to understanding and enjoying themselves and their sexuality.

References

Bardwick, Judith M.: *Psychology of Women: A Study of Bio-cultural Conflicts.* New York, Harper and Row, 1971.

Bem, Sandra Lipsitz: "Androgyny vs. the Tight Little Lives of Fluffy Women and Chesty Men." *Psychology Today,* Sept. 1975.

Broverman, Inge K., Vogel, Susan R., Broverman, Donald M., Clarkson, Frank, and Rosenkrantz, Paul S.: "Sex Role Stereotypes: A Current Appraisal." *Journal of Social Issues, 28*:2, 1972.

Chesler, Phyllis: *Women and Madness.* New York, Doubleday & Co., Inc., 1972.

Condry, John, and Condry, Sandra: "Sex Differences: A Study of the Eye of the Beholder." *Child Development, 47*:3, Sept. 1976.

Erikson, Erik: *Childhood and Society.* 2nd ed., New York, W. W. Norton & Co., Inc., 1963.

Goldberg, Susan, and Lewis, Michael: "Plat Behavior in the Year Old Infant: Early Sex Differences." *In* Bardwick, J. (Ed.): *Readings on the Psychology of Women.* New York, Harper and Row, 1972.

Goldstein, Bernard: *Human Sexuality.* New York, McGraw-Hill Book Co., 1976.

Guttentag, Marcia, and Bray, Helen: *Undoing Sex Stereotypes.* New York, McGraw-Hill Book Co., 1976.

Kohlberg, Lawrence: "A Cognitive-Developmental Analysis of Children's Sex Role Concepts and Attitudes." *In* Maccoby, Eleanor (Ed.): *The Development of Sex Differences.* Stanford, California, Stanford University Press, 1966.

Komisar, Lucy: "The Image of Women in Advertising." *In* Gornick, Vivian, and Moran, Barbara K. (Eds.): *Women in Sexist Society: Studies in Power and Powerlessness.* New York, Basic Books, 1971.

Leach, Anita M.: "Sex Theory and Application." *In* Harber, Judith, Leach, Anita, Schultz, Sylvia, and Sideleau, Barbara Flynn (Eds.): *Comprehensive Psychiatric Nursing.* New York, McGraw-Hill Book Co., 1978.

Maccoby, Eleanor, Emmons, Jacklin, and Nagy, Carol: *The Psychology of Sex Differences.* Stanford, California, Stanford University Press, 1974.

Money, John, and Anke Ehrhardt: *Man and Woman, Boy and Girl.* Baltimore, Johns Hopkins University Press, 1972.

Moss, Howard A.: "Sex, Age and State as Determinants of Mother-Infant Interaction." *In* Bardwick, J. (Ed.): *Readings on the Psychology of Women.* New York, Harper & Row, 1972.

Rubin, Jeffrey Z., Provenzano, Frank J., and Luria, Zella: "The Eye of the Beholder: Parents Views on Sex of Newborns." *American Journal of Orthopsychiatry, 44:4,* 1974.

Rybicki, Laura L.: "Preparing Parents to Teach Their Children About Human Sexuality." *Maternal-Child Nursing,* Vol. 1, May/June 1976.

Schiller, Patricia: "Sex Education that Makes Sense." *National Education Association Journal,* Feb. 1968.

Seiden, Anne M.: "Gender Differences and Sexual Reproductive Life." *American Journal of Psychiatry,* Vol. 133, 1976.

Sprung, Barbara: *Non-Sexist Education for Young Children.* New York, Citation Press, 1975.

Taylor, Carol: "Cultural Aspects of Human Sexuality." *In* Barnard, Martha Underwood, Clancy, Barbara J., and Krantz, Kermit (Eds.): *Human Sexuality for Health Professionals.* Philadelphia, W. B. Saunders Company, 1978.

Walum, Laurel Richardson: *The Dynamics of Sex and Gender: A Sociological Perspective.* Chicago, Rand-McNally College Publishing Co., 1977.

Weinberg, Janie S., and Weinberg, Sanford B.: "Influence of Clothing on Perceptions of Infant Sex Roles." *Journal of Applied Communication Research,* April, 1980.

Wilbur, Cornelia, and Aug, Robert: "Sex Education." *American Journal of Nursing,* 73:1, Jan. 1973.

Will, JerrieAnne, Self, Patricia A., and Datan, Nancy: "Maternal Behavior and Perceived Sex of Infant." *American Journal of Orthopsychiatry, 46:1,* Jan. 1976.

Woods, Nancy Fugate: *Human Sexuality in Health and Illness.* St. Louis, C. V. Mosby Co., 1979.

THE ADOLESCENT'S SEXUAL WORLD

PUBERTY

Puberty has been recognized throughout history as a difficult time for individuals experiencing it and for those around them. In many cultures, specific skills or duties must be performed as rites of puberty. Following these activities, the successful individual is thereafter considered an adult member of the community. Puberty rites are not confined to primitive cultures. In Jewish culture today, 13 is the age at which individuals are considered to be adult members of the community. In the Conservative and Orthodox denominations, when the male has reached this age he is Bar Mitzvah, and a ceremony is performed in which he is accepted into the adult Jewish community. The more liberal Reformed Jews also have a similar ceremony for the female members of the community, the Bat Mitzvah.

In American culture, however, there are no real rites to help individuals experience adolescence. The term "adolescent" encompasses all individuals from about 12 years old to about 20. The young adolescent experiences dramatic psychological and physiological changes, which can be sources of both great pleasure and embarrassment.

Male

At puberty, secretions of testosterone and small amounts of other male hormones lead to an increase in the size of the penis, scrotum, testes, prostate, and seminal vesicles in the male. Although this growth begins in early adolescence, it may continue until the male is 20 years old. Ejaculation, the emission of seminal fluid, usually begins one or two years after the start of the adolescent growth of the reproductive organs.

Testosterone causes other changes in the adolescent male, including the characteristic male hair distribution, the deep voice, the decreased subcutaneous fat, the increased muscle size, and acne. The increase in hair growth usually begins in the pubic area, followed by growth of the axillary, facial, body, leg, and arm hair. The deep voice of the adult male is caused by hypertrophy of the laryngeal mucosa and the vocal cords. The increased size, mass, and strength of skeletal muscles in the adult male is related to the stimulation of protein synthesis as well as to testosterone secretion. Finally, testosterone stimulates the production of sebum by the subcutaneous glands, making the adolescent male particularly vulnerable to acne (Tichy, 1976).

Penis size is a common source of concern for adolescent males. (This worry often continues well into adulthood.) The adolescent male may fear that his penis is not growing, or that it is not growing enough. Much covert comparison is made with other adolescent males. At times, viewing an adult penis can cause further worry in the adolescent, who may feel that he will never attain this adult size. He may not realize that there is no relationship between the size of an erect and a nonerect penis. The normal length of the erect adult penis is usually four to six inches (Gordon, 1971). This information can be distressing to the adolescent who is far from this adult size. When the male does have an erection, he may feel that it is not sufficient to satisfy a women sexually. He may have read books, seen movies, or heard other, older adolescents telling stories of great sexual potency and enormous penis size. The adolescent male may believe that it is only through having a large penis that sexual pleasure is possible (Gordon, 1971; McCary, 1971). In fact, the size of the penis has been found to have little or no effect on the ability of a man to satisfy a woman sexually (McCary, 1971; Masters, 1966; Gordon, 1971). The wrinkling and darkening of the skin in the genital region may also be disturbing to the adolescent. He may be upset to find that one testis is smaller than the other, or that one hangs somewhat lower than the other. If he does not know that these are normal occurrences, he may become quite anxious about his future potential for sexual performance.

Female

The physiological changes that occur in the adolescent female are no less striking. When the inhibition of gonadatropin release factor ceases, increases in follicle-stimulating hormone (FSH) and luteinizing hormone (LH) production lead to increases in production of ovarian hormones. With the release of these ovarian hormones, the often asymmetrical breast development in the young adolescent female begins. In addition, a layer of subcutaneous adipose tissue is deposited over the whole body, especially the breasts, buttocks, hips, and thighs. As the pelvis begins to take on the adult, gynecoid shape, the transverse diameter increases. The cyclic release of hormones leads to the start of menstruation (menarche).

A further effect of the estrogens is the closure of the epiphyseal plates, preventing further bone growth. The typical triangular distribution of female pubic hair is also due to the estrogenic effects. Finally, the soft, smooth skin characteristic of females is due to an increase in sodium and chloride retention, leading to an increase in body weight and mild edema (Tichy, 1976) secondary to estrogen effects.

Adolescent girls are as concerned with breast size as are adolescent boys about penis size. The normal asymmetrical growth of the breasts is often of great concern to the adolescent female, who may fear that her breasts will be of greatly differing sizes. In adult women, one breast is usually somewhat larger than the other, although the size difference is not striking.

In our society, the breast is seen primarily as a sexual organ. Adolescent girls may feel embarrassed by this obviously sexual part of themselves that previously did not exist. Girls who mature the latest are often the most upset about the changes in their breasts. Girls who feel that their breasts are too small may fear that they will be sexually inadequate in adulthood. The girl with the large breasts that develop far before those of her friends faces the problems of dealing with the mature body of a woman while still in early adolescence (Rosenthal, 1977).

For the first time in her life, the adolescent girl is being affected by cyclic hormonal changes. These cycles may cause mood fluctuations as well as physical changes. The most striking occurrence that a female experiences at puberty is the appearance of menstrual periods. Many girls who have not been prepared for the onset of menstruation may be frightened by the appearance of blood from within their bodies, and may be convinced that they have been injured in some way (AASECT[a], 1977).

Even the adolescent who has been prepared for menarche may experience her first menstruation and subsequent ones with mixed emotions. One reason for this ambivalence lies in the teaching that young girls receive about menstruation in our culture. In textbooks, television, magazines, and other media sources, the menstruating woman is portrayed in a certain way, usually negatively. Widespread cultural expectations and taboos regarding menstruation continue to exist, including the separation of menstruating women from the rest of the family and the prohibition on sexual intercourse during menstruation (Hyde, 1979; McCary, 1971; Weideger, 1976).

Learning About Menstruation

Prior to a full discussion about the mood changes and premenstrual syndromes in women, a study that analyzed introductory material intended for premenarcheal girls will be discussed at length to illustrate the subtle negative messages received by young adolescent females regarding their sexuality (Whisnant, 1975). Seven booklets (two intended for mothers, one for the mothers of retarded girls, and four for adolescent girls) and two films were reviewed for content. Several types of information are usually covered in these product-oriented books and films: 1) The stated purpose of the material; 2) the anatomy and physiology of menstruation; 3) pubertal changes; 4) the significance of menarche; 5) the experience of menarche; and 6) the product.

Most of the material reviewed implied a private, exclusive dialogue with the adolescent female that would initiate her into "complete womanhood." The language of these introductory comments was found to be vague and mysterious.

The anatomy and physiology of menstruation is usually described in technical medical terminology. Most of the booklets do have some sort of glossary attached. In describing ovulation, the girl is presented with a story about "the journey of the egg." In this journey the girl is seen as a passive participant, while the egg has the active role. Hormones and their potential effects on the emotions and physiology are not discussed. In anatomical drawings, the outline of a young woman is shown, with the internal organs, uterus, tubes, and ovaries in their approximate positions. However, rarely if ever does the young woman see a diagram that includes any connection between the internal organs of reproduction and the outside of her body. The vagina and vulva are not shown!

Pubertal changes discussed were aimed primarily at the appearance. For example, Whisnant (1975) quotes from one of the booklets, ". . . around the time of your first period you'll begin to develop the pretty curves that make older girls so proud of themselves." The increase in the girl's interest in a capacity for sexual arousal is not mentioned. Also absent are references to the development of new ways for the adolescent woman to deal with parents, siblings, and peers in light of these changes. Allusions to the other physical changes that occur (breast enlargement, pubic and axillary hair, etc.) are vague and brief.

In discussing the significance of menarche to the young woman, the material investigated carried the strong implication that menarche is related only to reproduction. The other changes that accompany it were not considered. The terms "womanhood" and "motherhood" were used almost interchangeably throughout. Never was there a mention of the possibility that the young woman might want to choose a lifestyle that would not include motherhood.

Menstruation itself was presented as an occurrence that is not to be acknowledged by the young woman or any of those around her. The information on how to conceal all evidence of menstruation was usually quite precise. In fact, it is assumed that the young woman would be embarrassed to have anyone know that she is menstruating, since that would mean that they either noticed the odor or the lines of the sanitary belt, or that someone had seen the menstrual flow. Although, to their credit, the books tended to depict menstruation as a normal part of the life of a woman, they tended to go overboard in some cases, implying that if the young woman encounters any difficulties or unpleasantness as a result of menstruation, they are somehow her fault. Instructions about sanitary protection are usually presented as rules to be followed without question. They promise control if they are followed and embarrassment if they are not.

The young woman is also held responsible for the control of her emotions during her periods. Positive mental attitudes are advocated. Instead of encouraging the menstruating woman to stay in bed as has been done in the past (Ehrenreich, 1973), the girl is shamed if she does this. The booklets state that some women use their periods as an excuse to be "lazy." The experience of what menstruation will feel like is not covered in the booklets intended for the normal adolescent. The booklets intended for retarded girls contain a simple vivid description.

Obviously, the major impetus for the booklet is the product to be sold; it is presented in terms of its attributes, which will help the young woman to "cope" with menstruation.

The extensive discussion of the results of this study are not presented here as an indictment of pharmaceutical companies. They have fulfilled a need for a certain type of education about puberty. After all, it is their purpose to sell their product. The information that they include can be seen as a bonus for the potential user of the product. Unfortunately, this brief, vague introduction to menstruation and puberty may be all that the young adolescent receives. While it provides a point of departure for future discussion, it is not sufficient for parents or educators to rely solely on information of this type to educate adolescents about sexuality.

Boys seldom receive even this much information about menstruation and female sexuality. In many schools, the girls are separated from the boys (usually in gym class) to view these films, which are shown by the gym teacher. Most of the time, discussion about the film does not ensue (AASECT [b], 1977).

Menstruation and Mood Changes

Menstruation has been used as an explanation for mood and activity changes in women. Recently, the term "premenstrual syndrome" has gained in popularity (Hyde, 1979). According to the theory of premenstrual syndrome, women's moods are positive around the time of ovulation and negative premenstrually. (The premenstrual time indicated here usually includes the four days immediately preceding menstruation and the four days of menstruation, making a total of eight so called premenstrual days.) Most of the data on mood changes during the menstrual cycle utilize the subjective reports of women. The reliability of these reports can be seriously questioned. Statistics that show that women commit a larger number of criminal acts of violence and suicide in these eight premenstrual days are often cited. In fact, however, although women are somewhat more likely to commit crimes during these ght days, they are consistently less likely to commit crimes of violence than are men (Hyde, 1979).

Hyde (1979) has proposed that mood changes be seen in a different light. Rather than viewing the premenstrual days as days in which the woman is suffering from a psychological deficit, she proposes that women may be psychologically normal during the premenstrual period, and subject to unusually positive psychological states during ovulation. Obviously, this is partly a matter of semantics, but the difference in interpretation can be profound. More research into this area will be necessary before a definitive answer can be found.

In the controversy about mood swings and their origin, the nature-nurture controversy again arises (Hyde, 1979; McCary, 1971; Weideger, 1976). To those who feel that the mood swings are part of the nature of women, the changes are directly attributable to hormonal fluctuations experienced by all women as a part of their cyclic nature. Studies have indicated that depression in women is more common premenstrually, at menopause, during the post partum periods, and in those taking oral contraceptives. These data suggest that female sex hormones may be related to depression, since the aforementioned times correlate with specific hormonal situations. Caution should be exercised to avoid attributing a cause and effect explanation with correlational data. The hormone-mood relationship is not currently known.

According to the cultural theory of the origin of depression and premenstrual syndromes, women learn that menstruation is negatively valued in our culture, and therefore begin to experience negative feelings about themselves during these times (Hyde, 1979; McCary, 1971; Weideger, 1976). During childhood or adolescence they may have heard menstruation referred to as "the curse" and may have been told that they were "unwell" during their menstrual periods. This terminology further reinforces negative attitudes toward menstruation. Tracing the cultural origin of menstruation taboos further, both McCary (1971) and Weideger (1976) suggest that the universal fear of blood is a contributing factor to the generally negative feelings about menstruation and about intercourse during menstruation. Blood is usually associated with violence, injury, and death.

In our culture, women learn that it is expected that they act strangely just before and during their periods. In fact, it is not uncommon, if a woman is acting somewhat depressed, or "down," for a well meaning friend to ask her if she is about to get her period. This question can act as a reinforcement that depression is expected to occur with menstruation.

After considering the preceding, the reader can better understand the ambivalent feelings with which most adolescents approach menarche. For boys the situation may be even worse, since they most often know that young women menstruate but may be filled with misinformation about the feelings associated with menstruation. They may think that this is a very painful experience for the young woman. Most adolescent males are too embarrassed with their own bodily changes to risk asking about the changes that young. women are experiencing. They may prefer to act knowledgeable rather than risk asking potentially embarrassing questions to gain information.

The massive body changes described are often rapid and frightening to the adolescent, who may not be prepared for the physical or the often more upsetting psychological changes that accompany puberty. The rapid changes make it necessary for adolescents to almost constantly revise their mental pictures of themselves. Body image has been demonstrated to be related to self-esteem in much research (Kolb, 1959; Rosen, 1968; Secord, 1953). The adolescent who is experiencing these tremendous changes is subject to much fear and doubt about himself or herself.

DEVELOPMENTAL TASKS OF ADOLESCENCE

Adolescents face many changes in their lives (AASECT[a], 1977; AASECT[b], 1977; Hyde, 1979). The first and perhaps most significant task is to become independent of parents, both emotionally and physically. As part of this striving for independence, the peer group becomes an important source of reinforcement and provides a sense of belonging for adolescents when they declare some independence from the family. Sexual behavior is one way in which adolescents can express their autonomy and independence.

Related to the use of sexual behavior as an expression of independence is the need of adolescents to develop their own moral system. Prior to adolescence, the child has unquestioningly accepted the moral attitudes of the parents. With adolescence, however, those previously accepted notions are severely questioned and often rejected. Adolescents must develop personal ethical systems and must decide how sexuality will fit into their close relationships with others. Decision making about nonmarital intercourse, birth control, and the possibility of unwanted pregnancies emerges here. Adolescents rely heavily on the media and peers during this time.

The third task faced by adolescents is to establish a sense of identity. They begin to look for a sense of a self, independent from the family, and begin to question the traditional male and female roles. The establishment of a sexual identity, be it heterosexual, homosexual, or ambiguous, becomes very important at this time.

Finally, adolescents are striving to develop their capacities for commitment, intimacy, and nurturance of others. This final task takes the place of the adolescent's previous childhood dependency and selfishness. He or she strives to learn to establish and sustain intimate relationships with another person during this period.

As adolescents begin to work to fulfill developmental expectations, they

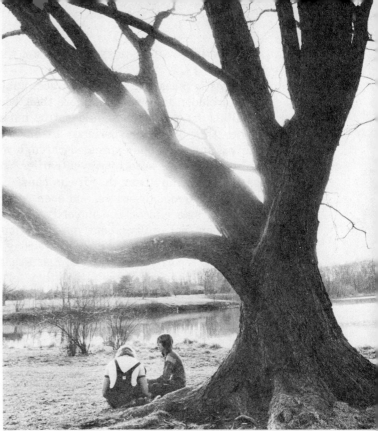

The adolescent must develop a capacity for establishing an intimate caring relationship—one that can be sustained—with another person. (Illustration courtesy of Courier-Post, Camden, New Jersey.)

Photograph by Evangelos Dousmanis

are continually subjected to the physiological changes occurring within their bodies. As they begin to have more intense sexual feelings, sex education begins to have a more special, personal significance. They are more likely to be interested in sex information and in sexual activities (AASECT[b], 1977). The period of early adolescence is usually a period of relatively self-centered sexual activity, including a great deal of fantasy, self-exploration, and masturbation. Later adolescence brings an increase in shared sexual experimentation, both homosexual and heterosexual. The following discussion will be divided roughly into these interests.

THE SELF AS A FOCUS FOR SEXUAL PLEASURE

In his landmark study on human sexual behavior, Kinsey (1948) found a sharp increase in masturbation in boys between the ages of 12 and 15. By the age of 12, 21 per cent of Kinsey's sample of boys reported that they had masturbated, and by the age of 15, 82 per cent had masturbated. Sorensen (1973), in his study of the personal values and sexual behaviors of adolescents from the age of 13 to 19, found that 58 per cent of the males had masturbated at least once before they were 14, while 39 per cent of the females had masturbated at least once by the age of 13. In the Sorensen study, a variety of sexual issues were addressed, including homosexuality, premarital sexual activity, and oral-genital sex. Of all the topics discussed, Sorensen reported that masturbation was the act about which adolescents were the most defensive and the most private.

The reasons for the reluctance to discuss masturbation are easy to predict. During childhood, children are taught that although stimulation of the genitals is pleasurable, it is not acceptable behavior. In fact, some children are forbidden to touch or explore their bodies, with the admonition that the genitals are dirty and should not be handled. As children approach adolescence, they begin to experience a tremendous surge of sexual energy, which almost invariably is expressed through masturbation, often combined with fantasy. At adolescence or even earlier, children learn myths about masturbation. They may hear that it can cause blindness, hair on the palms, acne, insanity, nervous disorders, and even venereal disease. Despite fears of these potential side effects, the majority of adolescents continue to masturbate. They may feel guilty about masturbation, but the guilt and fear are not usually sufficient to overcome the strong sexual urges felt at this age. Of those who reported that they did masturbate, 83 per cent of the males and 78 per cent of the females said that they felt at least rare guilt feelings about masturbation (Sorensen, 1973).

The more fortunate young adolescents may not have heard or believed the myths. Instead, they may have learned that masturbation is considered normal as long as it is not "excessive." Most adolescents feel that masturbation of any amount is excessive, so they may once again fear that they are in some way abnormal. Sorensen (1973) found that only 18 per cent of the males and 16 per cent of the females reported that they had been told about masturbation by their parents.

In a more recent study (Chess, 1976) involving 15- to 19-year-old adolescents in indirect questioning interviews about sexuality and sexual behavior, masturbation was never brought up by the parents or the adolescents themselves. The authors interpreted this to mean that masturbation was not a topic of concern to either the parent or the adolescent. Given other study results, this conclusion is unwarranted.

By the time individuals reach late adolescence, masturbation has become a part of their sexual life. Many still feel that it is dangerous, immoral, or immature (AASECT[a], 1977). They think that most adults do not masturbate. Adults who do are viewed as inadequate, weak, or abnormal.

In the light of this information it is easy to understand why the normally open subjects in the Sorensen study (1973) were less willing to talk about masturbation. Masturbation is a normal part of sexual development and expression in all people. It is not physically harmful regardless of how often it is practiced (Gordon, 1971; Masters, 1970). It becomes abnormal only when it becomes a compulsive act in which the individual feels a loss of control or becomes so guilt-ridden or fearful that the masturbation and attendant feelings cause interference in other aspects of the individual's life (Gordon, 1971; Masters, 1970; Rosenthal, 1977).

Prior to adolescence, most children are taught that sexual activity takes place only within the context of marriage. When individuals enter adolescence, then, they are usually oriented toward nonmarital chastity. At least a part of the questioning regarding moral aspects of nonmarital sexual activity originates in the bombardment of sexual stimuli directed toward adolescents (Crist and Gale, 1978; Weinberg, 1979). Television and magazine advertisements emphasize sexuality and sexual expression as an integral part of the young culture (Weinberg, 1979). Women are portrayed as perpetually desirable to and desirous of men. Products show women how to make sure that a man "can't get her out of his mind." The advertisements encourage seductiveness, teaching women (particularly adolescents) that if they want their man to be "more of a man," they must use some product that will make them "more of a woman." All adolescents in advertising, both male and female, are physically attractive. Even commercials for acne preparations somehow seem to avoid using adolescents who actually have pimples. Adolescent males are portrayed as active, "manly" men. Toughness and physical sports are encouraged by men in these advertisements. They are encouraged to be desirable to women, but in a more traditionally "masculine" manner.

Given these ambiguous messages regarding sexuality and sexual activity, adolescents are understandably confused. Their feelings about virginity have been investigated to determine how adolescents deal with the daily ambiguities of their world. Fifty-eight per cent of the female respondents in the 13- to 15-year-old age group agreed with the statement, "A girl should stay a virgin until she finds the boy she wants to marry." Forty-three per cent of the girls in the 16- to 19-year-old age group also agreed with this statement. Thirty per cent of the male respondents reported that they would not want to marry a nonvirgin. As the sample was broken down by age, it was found that, with increasing age, fewer of the males condemned nonmarital sexual activity in their future spouse (Sorensen, 1973).

The Sorensen (1973) and Reichelt (1977) findings indicate that the "sexual revolution" is not synonymous with promiscuity and widespread sex in adolescence. Reichelt, in his study of 1190 adolescents in a Detroit Planned Parenthood teen clinic, reported that only 5 per cent of the teens felt that it would be a social disadvantage to be a virgin. What has been called irresistible peer pressure to have sex during adolescence may be an overreaction on the part of adults. Although adolescents are struggling to form their unique sense of self and sexual morality, most adolescents are able to withstand the peer pressure and remain virgins if that is what they wish.

SHARING OF SEXUAL PLEASURE

Same sex exploration is more commonly encountered and reported by adolescents than was previously believed (AASECT[a], 1977; Rosenthal, 1977; Sorensen, 1973). It has been described as a normal part of sexual development that begins in childhood and continues in adolescence. Same sex exploration usually precedes heterosexual experimentation because adolescents at this time in their lives do not possess the necessary social skills to initiate such a heterosexual encounter (Rosenthal, 1977). Homosexual experiences in adolescence seem to be more common among males than females. Eleven per cent of Sorensen's male subjects and 6 per cent of female subjects reported having homosexual experiences. An additional 25 per cent reported being approached for such encounters. Interestingly, those who reported being approached or involved in some homosexual activities reported most often that the activity took place with a peer. Very rarely did such activity take place within the adult-young adolescent pairing that so many believe to be the norm. Support for the myth of adults seducing young adults into homosexual encounters was not evident.

Mutual masturbation is often practiced by adolescents prior to intercourse, and for many it serves as an effective substitute for intercourse. Masturbation was defined earlier as sexual arousal of oneself through stimulation of the sex organs. Mutual masturbation includes two or more individuals stimulating themselves or each other. Oral-genital sex is often included in these mutual masturbatory encounters. Although still technically illegal in many states, oral-genital sex has become more commonly accepted as a normal method of foreplay and/or substitute for intercourse among many couples (Hyde, 1979; Gordon, 1971). "Cunnilingus" is the medical term used to describe activity in which the woman's genitals are stimulated using the partner's mouth. The clitoris is usually the primary site for stimulation, although direct clitoral stimulation can be painful (Masters, 1966). Many women report that they achieve more intense and pleasurable orgasms with this type of stimulation (Hyde, 1979). A commonly used term for cunnilingus is "eating." The counterpart of this activity, one in which the male's penis is stimulated by his partner's mouth is called fellatio, or "sucking," or "blow job." The glans penis and the shaft of the penis may be licked or sucked by the partner, leading to eventual orgasm if the activity is continued. Some couples perform both of these activities (cunnilingus and fellatio) simultaneously. This may be referred to as "sixty-nine," for the position that the partners take to accomplish this. Some individuals become concerned that such sexual behaviors are unsafe because of the potential for infection. No special precautions are necessary other than taking care not to contaminate the vagina with organisms present in the anus.

More unmarried teenagers are having intercourse, and first intercourses are occurring at earlier ages than previous studies had indicated (Miller, 1976; Sorensen, 1973; Zelnick, 1977). In 1973, 71 per cent of the males and 56 per cent of the females had had intercourse at least one time by the age of 15 (Sorensen, 1973). In 1977, Zelnick found that 55 per cent of the combined sample had had intercourse by the age of 19. (This difference can be partially explained by the fact that Zelnick utilized nondirective interviews in which the topic of intercourse would not be covered unless brought up by the adolescent or the parent.) Although adolescents tend to have more partners than in the past and are beginning to have intercourse earlier, the frequency of reported intercourse has not increased (Zelnick, 1977).

Miller (1976) discovered three main motivations for intercourse and three main impediments to intercourse in his female sample. Eighty-five per cent reported that the desire to give pleasure was a positive motivation to have intercourse. Love was identified by 77 per cent as very important in encouraging intercourse. Finally, 77 per cent reported that the desire to receive pleasure was a major incentive for intercourse. (These percentages add up to more than 100 per cent because the women could respond positively to more than one answer.) Deterrents to intercourse include a fear of pregnancy (85%), a desire to avoid intercourse during menstruation (66%), and a lack of interest at the time intercourse was available (54%).

With 85 per cent reporting fear of pregnancy, one would think that contraception would be a major issue for adolescents. In fact, studies have indicated that contraceptive use among adolescents is very low (Miller, 1976; Sorensen, 1973; Zelnick, 1977). It seems that the greater the presumed sexual commitment, the greater the efficacy of initial contraceptive practice. Further information on adolescents and the use of contraception will be covered in the chapter on contraceptives. It has been included here to make the reader aware of the striking implications of increasingly earlier intercourse among adolescents and the low use of contraception in this group.

Males and females differ in their feelings about nonmarital intercourse (Sorensen, 1973). Women often reported feelings of guilt, regret, discomfort, worry, and of being used and disappointed after intercourse. With additional sexual experiences, these feelings decreased. Men, on the other hand, were found to report more positive emotions, including excitement, pleasure, satisfaction, and power following their initial intercourse. The usual pattern for relationships was one of "serial monogamy." In this pattern, adolescents entered into generally monogamous relationships with the intention of being sexually faithful. The relationship was considered to be of uncertain duration. When the relationship ended, most adolescents went into similar relationships with other individuals. The promiscuity and random sexual encounters thought to exist among adolescents were not found.

THE NURSE'S FEELINGS

During their careers, nurses encounter many types of problems that they have not experienced themselves. For example, many medical-surgical nurses have never suffered from the illnesses or undergone the surgery that their clients have experienced. All nurses, however, have gone through adolescence, some with more difficulty than others. In order to effectively deal with adolescents, nurses must first evaluate and settle issues of their own adolescence and must guard against overidentification and the erroneous feeling that they "know" what the adolescent is feeling. The world in which adolescents now live is vastly different from when the nurse was an adolescent. In addition, memory tends to dull some of the agonizing and thrilling experiences of adolescence.

Talking with adolescents may elicit memories in nurses of their own adolescence. They may recall aspects with feelings of regret or guilt for past experiences. Nurses may feel that their own adolescence was too restrictive or that adolescents today are too free in their verbal and behavioral expression. Many nurses may have grown up with the belief that intercourse should be practiced for the purpose of procreation only. The nurse's overall value system may differ drastically from that of the adolescent client. In this situation, as in all other counseling situations, the nurse must respect the individual's right to his or her own beliefs and convictions.

In our society adolescents exist in an ambiguous position. They are not considered adults, and yet they do not fit into the roles of children. The nurse, by treating the adolescent as an equal whose input is valuable and important, can usually win the confidence of the adolescent client. However, because adolescents are not certain of their own values, the nurse's efforts to discuss sexuality may initially be met with hostility. Understanding that the hostility is not a personal attack enables the nurse to deal with it more rationally and calmly.

THE NURSE AS EDUCATOR AND COUNSELOR

The American Association of Sex Educators, Counselors and Therapists (AASECT) has defined and differentiated between sex education, counseling, and therapy (AASECT[a], 1977). All nurses should be adequately prepared to fulfill the overlapping functions of sex educator and sex counselor.

Sex education is defined as the process by which factual information about sexuality is presented in order that individuals can integrate it into their lives and modify their attitudes. Sex counseling goes somewhat further, in that it involves helping the individual to assimilate sexual knowledge into fulfilling life styles and socially responsible behaviors. Both of these functions fall within the range of nurses' abilities. The nurse is often the first health care professional to whom clients and their families turn with their concerns about sexuality. The well educated and sensitive nurse is an excellent resource who has often gone unnoticed in the delivery of sexual health care.

The basic nursing preparation received by nurses does not sufficiently prepare them to become involved in sex therapy. The field is highly specialized, involving in-depth forms of treatment by which individuals are helped to deal with the more serious sexual problems, especially some of the sexual dysfunctions. This role is one that can be fulfilled by nurses who receive additional training and supervision.

In examining the role of the nurse in sex education, the reader should keep in mind that the nurse dealing with adolescents in any setting is a potential resource for sexual health care, education, and counseling. The discussion here will focus briefly on the current situations of sex education programs in the junior and senior high schools, on parents' feelings about sex education programs in the schools, and finally, on specific points for nurses involved in the sexual health care and sexual education and counseling of adolescents.

The volume of sexual information to which adolescents are exposed is enormous. Most schools report some kind of sex education program for adolescents. In many cases only the physiology of reproduction is taught without being related to the psychological aspects of human sexuality (Reichelt, 1977). Some schools still have the stereotypical one-time lecture in gym class, which includes a talk on menstruation for the girls and on venereal disease for the boys. These talks are, of course, sex-segregated (AASECT[b], 1977). These exposures to sexual information should not be considered effective sex education for adolescents. Values clarification, a task of adolescence, is an integral aspect of effective sex education for adolescents as well as adults. Educators must be thoughtful and sensitive in their facilitation of discussion and activity without interference or judgmental attitudes.

In determining the content of sex education programs, whether in the school, church, health care delivery system, or home, the following topics are appropriate for adolescents of junior and senior high school age (AASECT[b], 1977).

1. Customs, values, and standards in dating and boy-girl group relationships, with an emphasis on masculinity and femininity and their current meanings for adolescents.
2. Economic, social, legal, and psychological factors involved in carrying out the responsibilities of adulthood.
3. Consideration of marriage, family planning, infant care, vocational choices, and opportunities.
4. Conflicts confronting young men and women in their social and personal relationships.
5. Divorce, unwed parenthood, masturbation, and homosexuality.

The content area presented displays more concerns than physical sex. Given an open and nonjudgmental educator who possesses the correct information, a sex education program that contains opportunities for values clarification can be one in which the adolescents are actively involved and in which they are encouraged to form their own values.

One of the impediments of effective sex education in the public schools in the past has been the feeling of parents that the schools were not the appropriate setting for sex education. Some felt that only the parents should be involved in this, while others felt that it was the responsibility of religious organizations to teach sex education. According to a 1977 Gallup Poll on birth control and sex education (Digest, 1978), 77 per cent of the parents interviewed reported favorable attitudes toward the teaching of sex education in the schools. This percentage of individuals supporting school-based sex education reflects an increase of 12 per cent over the figure obtained in a 1970 poll. The increase in support regarding the inclusion of contraception in these sex education classes is more striking. In 1970, only 36 per cent of the individuals participating in the poll supported the inclusion of discussions of contraception in the sex education curriculum for adolescents, while in the 1977 poll, 69 per cent supported such discussions. The increase in adolescent pregnancies may in part explain the increasing acceptance of this previously avoided topic.

When asked if they discussed sex and sexuality with their parents, 72 per cent of male and 70 per cent of female subjects (Sorensen, 1973) reported that they did not. Adolescents felt that their parents were out of touch with the way sexuality is experienced by adolescents today. The subjects felt that the parents tended to enforce values on their children that were based on the parents' own experiences. In addition, many felt that their parents were untruthful to themselves about their children and the sexual behavior that occurs in adolescents. The subjects felt that their parents really did not wish to know what their children were doing in the sexual realm.

If adolescents are not getting sexual information from their parents, and if the sexual education received in the school setting is based largely on physiology alone, where are the adolescents receiving their education? Friends and the media account for a great deal of the information that adolescents obtain on the subject of sexuality. These were the primary sources of information for 68 per cent of the females and for 69 per cent of the males (Reichelt, 1975). The information received from both of these sources may be misleading and/or erroneous. Adolescents carry the burden of trying to live up to the mythical image of the sexually sophisticated young person who should not have to ask for more information on sex and, therefore, do not feel free enough to ask (AASECT[b], 1977).

In the absence of adequate communication about sexuality with the parents, some adolescents seek other adults to fulfill the function of parental counselor on sexual matters (Sorensen, 1973). Nurses are ideal people to fulfill such a role. They can correct misinformation in a manner that is nonthreatening to the adolescent, while supporting her or him in striving for independence and a sense of sexual identity.

Thus far, the goals for adolescent sex education have been covered briefly. Goals such as these are not restricted to use in formal sex education programs but can be utilized in a variety of settings by many individuals. Nurses can utilize these objectives as a broad framework for sexual health care of adolescents, regardless of the setting in which the adolescent is encountered (AASECT[b], 1977). The following list summarizes and clarifies these objectives:

1. To provide thorough, accurate, factual information on all aspects of human sexuality and the sexual maturation process.
2. To provide opportunities for increasing self-awareness and self-acceptance of one's own sexuality.
3. To increase understanding of other people, including their needs and values, and to provide the necessary communication skills to enhance interpersonal relationships.
4. To recognize the individuality of sexual behaviors, needs, and preferences, as well as the broad spectrum of sexual variations.

5. To provide opportunities to clarify one's own values about sexuality and to integrate those values into the development of personal standards of behavior and an understanding of one's own decision-making process.
6. To develop an appreciation of human sexuality as an integral and positive part of human life.
7. To provide specific information on special areas of sexual concern and ways of seeking help for sex-related problems.
8. To provide opportunities for increased understanding of masculinity and femininity, broadly defined, and of how humans become boys and girls, men and women. (Note: Individuals of both sexes are becoming more concerned with the implications of the feminist movement on their lives. A careful, unbiased look at the meanings of sex roles in contemporary society is necessary as a part of sex education.)

In addition to the goals stated above, two additional, more future-oriented goals will be mentioned. The development of meaningful sex education should begin prior to adolescence, in order that the child's understanding of human sexuality is a continuous process, coinciding with physical, emotional, and social development. Sexuality information need not be separated from other aspects of the school curriculum. Rather, it should be integrated into the program as it is integrated into the complete human experience.

The second future goal involves sex education efforts directed toward parents, professionals, and other individuals who have contact with adolescents. These individuals need sex education in order that they themselves can become more effective sex educators.

THE NURSE, THE ADOLESCENT, AND THE HEALTH CARE SYSTEM

Although it has been well established and documented that many adolescents are sexually active, in many areas adolescents are still unable to obtain contraceptives, treatment for venereal disease, or counseling about problem pregnancies without written permission from their parents (Woods, 1979). These adolescents may feel that they are alienated from the health care system, and may avoid seeking preventive care. Once again, adolescents may find themselves in the in-between situation of being not quite adults and not quite children. If they do seek sexual health care, they may find that the staff, including the nursing staff, may be less than accepting and supportive. Adolescents may be faced with nurses who force their own morals on them, assuming, for example, that the client is too young to be having sexual intercourse and therefore not supplying the adolescent with information about contraception. Alternatively, medical care workers may force their ideas of the appropriate form of contraception on adolescents, not allowing them to choose personally acceptable methods. Finally, adolescents may be faced with health care workers who, because of their own biases, are completely unaware that adolescents may be experiencing sexual feelings at all, and who, because of this, may omit any reference or discussion of sexuality with the client. Because adolescents are often embarrassed about their lack of knowledge about sexuality, they may not directly ask for the information they want, but may instead present themselves for care for an unrelated problem, hoping that the topic will "come up." The nurse who is not aware that the adolescent experiences sexual feelings will not be sensitive to what the client may not be saying, resulting in inadequate guidance of the adolescent and alienation of the adolescent from the health care system.

Ellen, a 16-year-old adolescent, has been brought to her mother's OB/GYN physician by her mother, with the intent of obtaining contraception. The nurse practitioner who is to see Ellen invites her into her office in order to take a sexual history (see Chapter 2 for a detailed sexual history). The office is private and away from the waiting room. In calling Ellen in, the nurse specifically informs Ellen's mother that it is better if she can obtain the history data alone with Ellen. She assures her that if Ellen wishes, she may be present during the physical examination, which will include a breast examination and a pelvic exam. (The assessment of the genitalia will not be included in this discussion. For an explanation of the role of the nurse as an educator and as the examiner in this situation, please see Chapter 2.)

Once inside the office, the nurse begins by asking Ellen questions about how she learned about her sexuality. Ellen states that her mother told her the "facts of life" prior to the time she experienced menarche. She is not sure exactly how old she was: she thinks about nine. Ellen remembers that her mother told her that only married couples have intercourse. When the nurse asks how Ellen thinks her mother feels about seeing her as a sexual person, Ellen states that she thinks that her mother has "really changed her tune," and that she must think that Ellen is promiscuous. With encouragement from the nurse, Ellen tells her that she is not sexually active, nor does she intend to be, but that her mother "made" her come for this appointment because she had been dating one particular boy. She felt that her mother suspected that they were already "screwing." The nurse assures her that contraceptives will not be forced on her if she does not wish to have them, and explains that this appointment is an excellent opportunity to begin Ellen's gynecologic care in any event. She assures her that the examination will not rupture the hymen. When Ellen seems reassured, the nurse returns to the sexual history, inquiring what, if anything, Ellen has learned about masturbation from her parents. Ellen recalls no discussions of this. She begins to appear nervous, playing with her hands and shifting in her seat more than she had previously. The nurse states, "Many people learn at an early age that touching themselves around their genitals feels very good. Then, when adolescence begins, they feel strong sexual urges that are often very pleasurably relieved by self-stimulation. How old were you when you first began to masturbate?" In response to this question, Ellen becomes decidedly uncomfortable, laughs somewhat, and replies that only oversexed girls masturbate. In fact, she says, masturbation is often the first step to promiscuity, since the person becomes so dependent on sexual stimulation that she is not able to stop when she is with a boy. Ellen also reports that when people masturbate they think of someone of the same sex while masturbating, and they eventually become homosexual and lead unhappy lives.

The misconceptions held by Ellen about masturbation are many. She is aided by the nurse in investigating those feelings. The nurse reassures Ellen that most women masturbate and that no harm can result from masturbation, other than the guilt felt by some people. As the discussion continues, Ellen admits that she has been masturbating to orgasm ("until I come") for several years, although she would "die" if her mother found out about it. Confidentiality is again discussed with her to assure her that what is mentioned between Ellen and the nurse are private matters not to be shared with her mother. Ellen is concerned that she has been masturbating "too much" lately. She has been more intimate with her boyfriend, and has been using masturbation to release her sexual tensions, since she is sure that she does not want to have intercourse. At this point in time, she feels that she wants to remain a virgin until she is married. She admits this with embarrassment, assuming that she is the "only one in the world" who wants this. Statements of the prevalence of this desire seem to surprise and comfort her.

Ellen is also reassured that homosexual fantasies are very common during masturbation, both for men and for women, and that they do not mean that the individual will become an active homosexual. Ellen is reassured that there is no need for guilt over her perceptions of what she thinks are socially unacceptable desires.

Following some additional data collection, Ellen is instructed about what to expect during the physical examination, and states that she does wish to have her mother present for the examination. Following the examination, Ellen tells her mother, with the nurse present, that she has no need or desire for any contraception at this time. Her mother appears surprised at this information and stammers that she just thought that all the kids were having sexual relations these days. After a short discussion in which the nurse helps to educate the mother about adolescent sexuality, the two leave with the understanding that Ellen will contact the nurse when she does need contraception.

The nurse has utilized several important components of counseling during this interview. First, she has provided a private atmosphere in which the client was assured of confidentiality and was given a chance to express her feelings without interruption or judgment by the nurse. Instead of assuming, as her mother had, that Ellen was sexually active, the nurse made no assumptions, allowing Ellen to tell her the facts.

The nurse also provided the client with factual information regarding masturbation, which allowed Ellen to understand that her feelings and behaviors were a natural part of her sexual self. By using statements of universality, the nurse placed the client's behavior within the realm of normal behavior, and allowed for statements of concern about these behaviors.

By allowing Ellen to utilize her own language, the nurse demonstrated further respect and acceptance for Ellen. In this case, the nurse understood the vocabulary utilized by the client. If there had been any misunderstanding or doubt about the use of words, she would have made efforts to clarify them. It is essential that the nurse and the client are using words the same way.

By including the mother in the discussions following the physical examinations, the nurse took the opportunity to educate her on aspects of sexuality and adolescence. It is to be hoped that the open discussion in the office will make future discussions between Ellen and her mother more comfortable. Unfortunately, in this situation little time was available to discuss the effect of the mother's attitude about Ellen's sexual behavior. It was clear that this was upsetting to Ellen, whose friends thought that her mother was really aware of what was going on. Ellen herself took an important step, with the support of the nurse, by telling her mother that she was not sexually active and therefore did not need contraception.

In this situation, the nurse had the primary contact with the client. This is not always the case. However, this does not mean that nurses can only participate in anticipatory guidance, teaching, or counseling if they are the primary care givers. Clinic nurses or office nurses employed in pediatrics can serve the highly useful purpose of educating both parents and children about sexuality. Visiting nurses also have the opportunity for guidance of both parents and children. Of course, the school nurse can have both an informal and a formal role in the sex education of students, as can nurses in family planning clinics.

Nurses in practice may encounter adolescents with serious sexual problems, such as involvements in incestuous relationships, rape, unwanted pregnancies, the aftermath of abortion or adoption, and the full range of sexual dysfunctions. At these or other times, nurses may find that they are not sufficiently prepared to deal with the difficulties of the client. Sex therapy, the intensive form of treatment, may be indicated (AASECT[a], 1977). Nurses must be knowledgeable about outside agencies and professionals to whom they may refer clients. The referral sources must be trusted as competent, trustworthy, and possessing adequate resources to deal with the referral. It is of great importance that nurses explain the reason for referral to the adolescent, who may imagine severe and frightening explanations. It is a part of the respect for the client as an intelligent individual, regardless of age, to inform fully the reasons for referral.

The developmental tasks of adolescence—independence, the development of moral attitudes, the development of a sense of identity, and the developmental capacity for intimacy and commitment—are complex tasks that are often confused by conflicting messages from the media, peers, and formal education. Nurses are in a position to help make this difficult time somewhat easier. They can actively participate in sex education programs, they can provide anticipatory guidance for parents and adolescents, and they can strive to make the health care delivery system more accessible and acceptable to adolescents. Nurses must possess sufficient knowledge, skill, and sensitivity to deal effectively with adolescents. This is a challenge that nursing is ready and able to accept.

References

AASECT(a): *Sex Counseling for Adolescents and Youth.* Washington, D.C., American Association of Sex Educators, Counselors and Therapists, 1977.

AASECT(b): *Sex Education for Adolescents and Youth.* Washington, D.C., American Association of Sex Educators, Counselors and Therapists, 1977.

Chess, Stella, Thomas, Alexander, and Cameron, Martha: "Sexual Attitudes and Behavior Patterns in a Middle-class Adolescent Population." *American Journal of Orthopsychiatry, 46*(4), Oct. 1976.

Crist, Robert, and Hickenlooper, Gale: "Problems in Adolescent Sexuality." *In* Barnard, Martha, Clancy, Barbara, and Krantz, Kermit (Eds.): *Human Sexuality for Health Professionals.* Philadelphia, W. B. Saunders Co., 1978.

Digest: "Large Majority of Americans Favor Legal Abortion, Sex Education and Contraceptive Services for Teens." *Family Planning Perspectives, 10*:3, May/June 1978.

Ehrenreich, Barbara, and English, Dierdre: *Complaints and Disorders: The Sexual Politics of Illness.* Old Westbury, The Feminist Press, 1973.

Gordon, Sol: "What Adolescents Want to Know." *American Journal of Nursing, 71*:3, March 1971.

Hyde, Janet Shibley: *Understanding Human Sexuality.* New York, McGraw-Hill Book Co., 1979.

Kinsey, A. C., Pomeroy, W. B., and Martin, C. E.: *Sexual Behavior in the Human Male.* Philadelphia, W. B. Saunders Co., 1948.

Kolb, Lawrence C.: "Disturbances of Body Image." *In* Ariete, S. (Ed.): *American Handbook of Psychiatry.* New York, Basic Books, 1959.

McCary, James Leslie: *Sexual Myths and Fallacies.* New York, Schocken Books, 1971.

Masters, William H., and Johnson, Virginia E.: *Human Sexual Inadequacy.* Boston, Little, Brown and Co., 1970.

Masters, William H., and Johnson, Virginia E.: *Human Sexual Response.* Boston, Little, Brown and Co., 1966.

Miller, Warren B.: "Sexual and Contraceptive Behavior in Young Unmarried Women." *Primary Care, 3*:3, Sept. 1976.

Reichelt, Paul A.: "The Desirability of Involving Adolescents in Sex Education Planning." *The Journal of School Health, 47*:2, Feb. 1977.

Reichelt, Paul A., and Werley, Harriet H.: "Contraception, Abortion and Venereal Disease: Teenagers' Knowledge and the Effect of Education." *Family Planning Perspectives, 7*:2, March/April 1975.

Rosen, Gerald M., and Ross, Allan O.: "Relationship of Body Image to Self Concept." *Journal of Consulting and Clinical Psychology,* Vol. 32, 1968.

Rosenthal, Miriam B.: "Sexual Counseling and Interviewing of Adolescents." *Primary Care, 4*:2, June 1977.

Secord, P. F., and Jourard, S. M.: "The Appraisal of Body Cathexis: Body Cathexis and the Self." *Journal of Consulting Psychology,* Vol. 17, 1953.

Sorensen, Robert C.: *Adolescent Sexuality in Contemporary America.* New York, World Publishing, 1973.

Tichy, Anna M., and Malasanos, Lois: "The Physiological Role of Hormones in Puberty." *Maternal Child Nursing, 1*:6, Nov./Dec. 1976.

Weideger, Paula: *Menstruation and Menopause: The Physiology and Psychology, The Myth and the Reality.* New York, Alfred A. Knopf, 1976.

Weinberg, Janie Spelton: "The Sexual World of the Adolescent." Address to the Connecticut Nursing Association, 1979.

Whisnant, Lynn, Brett, Elizabeth, and Zegans, Leonard: "Implicit Messages Concerning Menstruation in Commercial Educational Materials Prepared for Young Adolescent Girls." *American Journal of Psychiatry, 138*:8, Aug. 1975.

Woods, Nancy Fugate: *Human Sexuality in Health and Illness*. St. Louis, C. V. Mosby Co., 1979.

Zelnick, Melvin, and Kantner, John F.: "Sexual and Contraceptive Experience of Young, Unmarried Women in the U.S., 1976 and 1971." *Family Planning Perspectives, 9*:2, March/April 1977.

THE YOUNG ADULT

Thus far, discussion of the developmental aspects of human sexuality has been basically straightforward. At adolescence, however, this may be interrupted. When individuals reach adolescence, they make conscious and unconscious choices that will have profound effects on their emerging adult sexuality. For example, the adolescent who becomes pregnant will have to make decisions and accept responsibilities not usually associated with late adolescence or young adulthood.

Because of the increasing number of teenage pregnancies and the greater frequency of nonmarital intercourse among adolescents, this chapter will begin by discussing adolescents who become pregnant. The adolescent female and her partner may have to care for a child before they themselves have completed the necessary developmental tasks that prepare them for adulthood.

The developmental tasks of young adulthood and adulthood will follow. Special attention is devoted to a discussion of sexuality of the pregnant young adult and her partner, since pregnancy is often an integral part of the lives of young adults.

In the section on nursing, the counseling of pregnant adolescents and their partners will be covered in some depth. The nurse has many opportunities for contact with these couples, and anticipatory guidance can be of great help both in avoiding problems and in helping to alleviate them.

LATE ADOLESCENCE

The time when an individual ceases to be an adolescent and becomes a young adult is not clear. The tasks of adolescence are not suddenly met and then forgotten. The older adolescent and the young adult share many of the same concerns, such as becoming independent of parents and striving to establish a viable moral system (Hyde, 1979). Sexual identity must be established. Finally, the adolescent must develop a capacity for establishing an intimate relationship with another person, one that can be sustained.

In later adolescence there is an increase in the amount of shared sexual exploration, both homosexual and heterosexual (AASECT, 1977). The older adolescent has been influenced by peers, parents, and the media. At home, the individual has probably learned that nonmarital chastity is the "correct" behavior. Peers and media, however, give a different message (Anderson, 1978; Crist, 1978; Weinberg, 1979). Sexual behaviors designed to attract members of the opposite sex are stressed in most media advertisements. Romantic love is often portrayed without any of the "how tos" of actual relationships or birth control. Perhaps as a result of these pressures, an increasing number of unmarried teens are having intercourse, often without the benefit of adequate contraception. First sexual activity is occurring at earlier ages, and people are having more sexual partners (Mitchell, 1979; Sorensen, 1973; Zelnick, 1977). Sorensen found that by the age of 15, 71 per cent of the males and 56 per cent of the females were nonvirgins. If the study were to be repeated today, it is likely that even more adolescents would report that they had had sexual intercourse. Sixty-eight per cent of these sexually active teenagers reported that neither partner had used birth control measures (to the best of their knowledge) during their first intercourse.

Adolescent Pregnancy

Approximately 33 per cent of all teenage women giving birth are not married. The pregnant adolescent lacks a primary support that older pregnant women more often have—a husband. In teenage pregnancies, the partner is rarely prepared to support a family or emotionally accept the responsibility of parenthood (Anderson, 1978). When pregnancy occurs in adolescence, the woman and her partner face difficult decisions. They may decide to terminate the pregnancy, to have the baby and give it up for adoption, or to keep the child. Sometimes these choices must be faced by the woman alone.

Because of the irregularity in menstrual cycles in most adolescents, the diagnosis of pregnancy may not be made until the pregnancy has progressed beyond the point at which the adolescent could benefit from safe, early abortion methods, if abortion is her choice in dealing with the pregnancy. Second trimester abortions are more costly and carry greater risks than early abortions. If the young woman has chosen this method, the procedure will usually take place within a hospital. She will experience labor and deliver the fetus. Second trimester abortions are often very difficult for health care workers to deal with, especially when the woman is a teenager. Staff must examine their own feelings and biases before they are able to give the best supportive care that the pregnant adolescent so desperately needs.

Other young mothers elect to complete the pregnancy and then give the baby up for adoption. If this decision has been made, social service agency workers are usually in contact with the woman during her pregnancy as well as after the child is born. In the past, many have felt that it was better for the young mother not to see, touch, or feed her young infant. The rationale for this is that the young mother may become too attached and be unable to give up the infant. However, the more recent trend has been to allow the mother (and father) to see, touch, and generally be alone with the child for a short time. This allows the situation to have a sense of reality to it, and allows the parents to begin what is usually an inevitable grieving process. Whether or not the parents elect to or are allowed to see the infant who is to be put up for adoption, both partners will need tremendous support during this time. The decision to give up a child after experiencing pregnancy and delivery is a difficult one, regardless of the fact that the young adolescent may realize that she is not prepared to care for the child. The nonjudgmental, supportive nurse can be invaluable in this situation. Often just being in the room with the adolescent mother and allowing her to verbalize, if she wishes, can be of great assistance.

The woman who decides to have and keep her baby will experience many difficulties. These problems have been called the "syndrome of failure" (Anderson, 1978). The following problems are included in this description:

1. Failure of the adolescent to fulfill developmental tasks of adolescence.
2. Failure to remain in or return to school.
3. Failure to limit family size.
4. Failure to establish families that are financially self-supporting.
5. Failure to have healthy families.

Developmental Tasks of Adolescence

Some adolescents are able to go through an early pregnancy and successfully deal with the problems. It is a struggle. The pregnant adolescent must meet her own needs as well as those of her unborn child. The needs of the pregnant adolescent are similar to those of all adolescents (Moore, 1978).

1. *Need for acceptance by peers.*
2. *Need for emancipation from parents.* Despite the fact that the pregnant adolescent may need her parents as a support system both during and following her pregnancy, the need for independence persists and must be dealt with. The health care worker who encounters the pregnant teen at a clinic or office with her mother must keep in mind that it is the pregnant teen who is the client.
3. *Need to express feelings to a nonjudgmental, truly interested adult.* Some pregnant adolescents receive the necessary support and "permission" to discuss feelings in group sessions involving other adolescents who are pregnant. Others may prefer not to be involved in group activities. As with any client, the cultural values held by the adolescent will to a large part determine the vehicle through which she is able to express feelings and receive support.
4. *Need to develop a sexual role appropriate to her.* The fact that the adolescent became pregnant does not signify sexual sophistication. The young woman, though soon to be a mother, must develop her own sexual values if she is to be able to define herself sexually.
5. *Need to decide on a vocation.* This task is closely linked to the continuing of education. The pregnant adolescent faces many obstacles if she does decide to return to school following the delivery of her child.

Remaining in or Returning to School

Pregnancy is the single most common cause of school dropout among adolescent women (Mitchell, 1979). Nearly 70 per cent of these women never finish high school. Although the number of women returning to school after delivery has increased in some states, pregnancy is still considered an acceptable reason for the school system to require that the woman leave school. Following long and bitter debates, it has been decided in most states (but not all) that pregnancy is not sufficient cause to dismiss a woman from school. One of the most often cited rationales for excluding pregnant women from regular school classes is that the pregnant woman will be unable, for medical reasons, to carry out the usual school program. Almost all pregnant women, regardless of their age, are encouraged to remain active throughout their pregnancy. Thus this "medical" rationale is false.

A second reason cited for excluding pregnant teenagers from public high school classes is that by allowing them to remain in their classes, the school board may give the impression that it favors or at least condones teenage pregnancy. An underlying fear here is that if peers feel their pregnant friend receives extra attention and the pregnancy seems to carry other benefits, then they too may wish to become pregnant. Adolescents do find peer acceptance of great importance. However, it is the pregnant adolescent who is deviating from the adolescent norm. It is unlikely that she will establish a new norm for her friends.

Finally, the worry has been expressed that the pregnant teenager may not find sympathetic and understanding teachers in a public school. A punitive attitude by a teacher can have a significant effect on the already pressured adolescent. Such behavior should be nonexistent, but must be considered as a possibility in determining what is best for the adolescent.

On the other hand, moving the adolescent to another school may be more difficult for her, since she has already built relationships with teachers and friends. Disturbing peer relations, particularly at a time when the adolescent is vulnerable, is seen as a highly negative factor (Moore, 1978). Requiring students to attend a school for pregnant teens may further alienate the pregnant adolescent, making a return to her normal school following the pregnancy more difficult, and therefore less likely.

The economics of removing a pregnant adolescent from her own school to one designed especially for pregnant adolescents must also be considered. The regular school can offer wider ranges of educational and extracurricular activities than a smaller, less financially secure school for pregnant women. The additional teaching and counseling that the pregnant adolescent needs could be supplied by the health care workers in her regular school.

Limiting Family Size

This does not always become an issue following the birth of the child. Many young women receive their first accurate information on contraception during their hospital stay or at their postpartum visit. While some of these women have repeated pregnancies, many do not. If the adolescent has determined to define herself as a sexually active individual, the likelihood of her successfully using contraception increases greatly.

Establishing Stable Families

In most cases of teenage pregnancy, the father of the baby is unwilling or unable to help support the pregnant adolescent or the baby. Usually, both parents are in school. Several alternatives are available to them. The couple may marry, the husband quitting school and going to work. However, the outlook for these marriages is traditionally very poor. In other instances, the young woman may live with her parents and continue in school, with the grandmother taking on many of the child-rearing and child care responsibilities for the young mother. This arrangement is difficult for both the mother and the grandmother, since the mother of the baby is still trying to become independent of her own mother and may resent her intervention, even if it is for the good of the child. The grandmother in turn may resent her daughter. She may feel that she has already reared her children and may not wish to have the added responsibility that her daughter's baby places upon her. These resentments, and the basic differences between the generations, makes this living arrangement difficult for both the mother and grandmother. A third alternative situation for the new mother and her child involves living on their own. They may or may not be supported financially by the father of the baby. In many cases, the young mother is unskilled and unable to make sufficient money to cover the high costs of day care for her child. As a result, she may be unable to support them both, and may turn to welfare.

Having Healthy Families

The problems of having healthy families begin in the prenatal period and continue into the life of both the mother and her baby. Most adolescents consume an amazing amount of nutritionally poor "junk food." For the nonpregnant adolescent, this poor diet usually does not have serious long term consequences. For the pregnant adolescent, however, diet is far more important. Poor nutritional status in pregnant women has been shown to place the unborn child at greater risk of low birth weight, prematurity, and compromised nutritional status. As a form of denial of the pregnancy, the adolescent may choose to eat junk food rather than the diet recommended. Indeed, many adolescents do not even begin to receive prenatal care until well into the pregnancy. The usual irregularity of the menstrual cycle of the adolescent, combined with the attitude that pregnancy "could never happen to me," may contribute to this prolonged period without necessary prenatal care. Following the birth of the child, the new mother may genuinely not know the proper nutrition and health care measures that she must take to protect herself and her child. The health care professional must realize that often the kind of classes that could prepare the adolescent, such as home economics courses and some of the science courses, may not have been taken by the pregnant adolescent prior to her pregnancy.

In caring for the pregnant adolescent, the health care professional may wish to investigate with the client the role that the father of the baby plans to take, in terms of the pregnancy and after the child is born. Many unmarried teenagers who are having children are deciding to keep the children. If the father of the baby is interested and willing, and if the mother wishes, the father should be included in as much of the prenatal care and teaching as possible. It is not unusual for an adolescent father to attend prepared childbirth classes with the young woman, and then to remain with her as her coach during labor and delivery. The support that he may provide for the young woman is immeasurable and should not be overlooked as a possibility.

THE YOUNG ADULT

The young adult is influenced by a variety of societal and interpersonal issues. As in adolescence, the socially defined developmental task of the young adult is to obtain an education and to choose a vocation. The possible work roles and social roles available to young adults today are far wider than they were in the past, when opportunities for both men and women were rigidly defined. The young adult is faced with choosing a satisfying life role. This freedom to choose can be a burden, since the young adult must weigh between many lifestyles, all of which offer benefits and drawbacks. The new "freedom" is more difficult for some than the restrictive possibilities that existed in the past (Frieze, 1978).

The major developmental task of young adulthood according to Erikson (1963) is to develop intimacy and solidarity versus existing in isolation. The young adult must learn to give and to receive love. In addition, the decision whether or not to marry must be made. Finally, either a marital or sexual partner or partners with whom to share this intimacy must be chosen.

The traditional belief of marriage as the goal of all young adults no longer exists in our society. The image of marriage as an idyllic existence of blissful cohabitation with charming children running around the house is no longer accepted as fact. Increasing divorce rates, the desire of many young women to pursue careers uninterrupted by childrearing, the population concerns of youth, and the general examination of the marriage relationship have led to later marriages and more marriages in which couples have decided against children (Frieze, 1978). Alternatives to the traditional marriage have also become more acceptable. More couples are living together, sharing responsibility for the household without getting married. Couples who decide to have children may choose to each work part time and completely share the childrearing. Communal living and group marriage have become increasingly popular. Couples or individuals live together in a family situation. If children are involved, the responsibilities for them may also be shared. People involved in communal living situations feel that they have combined the benefits of the extended family and a situation in which one is free to "choose" one's family (Frieze, 1978).

Sexual Problems

Nonmarital intercourse is particularly prevalent among young adults. Because of the increased opportunity for sexual activity, the incidence of sexual concerns may increase simply because the young adult has more opportunities to experience sexual difficulties as well as pleasures. Factors that lead to problems in young adults are similar to those encountered in any individual—anxiety, guilt, and lack of accurate information. Some of the more commonly encountered sexual dysfunctions of men of this age include secondary impotence, premature ejaculation, worries about penis size, difficulty in relating eroticism to romantic love, and difficulty in making the transition from masturbation to intercourse.

Secondary impotence and premature ejaculation may result from guilt, anxiety, or lack of accurate information. The young man may experience his early sexual encounters in situations in which rapid ejaculation is valued. Having established this pattern, he may need treatment to overcome this dysfunction. (See Chapter 3.)

Misinformation about penis size and its relationship to the sexual satisfaction of the man's partner can usually be easily corrected by discussion with a sensitive health care professional. If the worries continue, however, the man may find that he has taken on a spectator role, in which his involvement in the sexual act is diminished. This may lead to further dysfunction. Usually, however, reassurance that penis size is not related to sexual pleasure is sufficient to allow the man to relax and enjoy his sexual activities.

Transition from masturbation to intercourse and the difficulties of relating eroticism to romantic love are problems faced by both males and females of this age group. Because of the attention that sex has received in the mass media, young adults may have unrealistic expectations of intercourse, and may feel disappointed that they do not experience an orgasm(s) in which "the earth moves." Replacing the self-centered activity of masturbation with a shared activity is a major readjustment. Both partners may find that they enjoy the sexual stimulation of another person but may be reluctant or too embarrassed to communicate to their partner the techniques that they have found to be successful in solitary sexual stimulation. In early experiences, both partners are likely to find themselves in the spectator role. After hearing so much about sex and the pleasures of sexual activity, they may experience feelings of unreality at first, and may be disappointed to find that sexual relationships that are mutually satisfying take work and the ability to respond in new ways. Worries can be greatly diminished by the nurse who, during the sexual history taking, keeps those concerns in mind and openly discusses them with the client.

Inconsistent orgasm is an often encountered problem of young adult women who are having intercourse. One explanation for this is that the woman may be experiencing guilt over the "double standard" of sexual activity they may have learned as a child. According to this standard, "nice" girls did not engage in nonmarital sexual activities. Perhaps it is the guilt for ignoring this early rule that contributes to inconsistent orgasms. Another possible explanation lies in lack of information. Some women do not know what orgasm is or what it is "supposed" to feel like. They may feel under great pressure to have multiple orgasms with each sexual encounter. This pressure may cause the individual to feel like a spectator during sexual relations, which decreases concentration on the pleasurable aspects of the sexual encounter, and may indeed lead to a decrease in subjective pleasure and consequent inconsistent orgasm.

Because of national campaigns encouraging yearly Pap smears for all women past puberty, most young adult women have visited either a nurse practitioner or a physician for a Pap smear and pelvic examination. During this time, the sexual history information should be collected and the common concerns of this age group discussed. Unfortunately, many males of this age group are "missed" by the health care establishments. Male contraceptives do not require the intervention of a health professional as do female birth control devices such as the IUD, diaphragm, and birth control pills. Because of this lack of contact with the medical world, the young adult male has less opportunity to receive sexual education from health care professionals. Efforts to reach this age group should be made, in order to provide anticipatory guidance.

ADULTHOOD

As individuals mature socially and emotionally, the division between young adulthood and adulthood becomes indistinct. The definition of adulthood often depends on externally measurable events, such as the childbearing and childrearing functions. Adulthood has been defined as that portion of the life cycle that is typically devoted to parenting and to the consolidation of the marital union or a relationship. The developmental task of this age group is generativity versus stagnation and self-absorption (Erikson, 1968). The common interest during this period, according to Erikson, is the establishment and guidance of the next generation. Not all adults are choosing to conform to traditional standards for adult life. Marriage is not one of the "givens" of adults today. Childbearing and childrearing are being carefully re-examined. Erikson's writings may be interpreted as stating that unless individuals go outside of themselves to help in the task of rearing another generation, they are doomed to become selfish, self-centered individuals. This idea can be challenged, however, by individuals who feel that self-knowledge and the enrichment and sharing of the self with another adult is as valuable as the caring of parents for their children. The point is that while generativity is a goal for all individuals, the nurse must be aware that there are many ways that one can define generativity, and must be careful to avoid assuming that any one definition will fit all clients.

Pregnancy and Sexuality

The decision to have a child is a difficult one. The role of parent is the only major adult role that cannot be shed once it has been assumed (Frieze, 1968). For those couples who do not have the opportunity to choose pregnancy, the transition to parent can be even more difficult. Both the father and the mother undergo tremendous changes during the nine months of the pregnancy. The relationship is examined in a new light by both partners, as they try to imagine what life will be like when they must share it with a third person. Often, it is not until the pregnancy has advanced that the couple begins to discuss vital issues, such as child care responsibilities, feelings

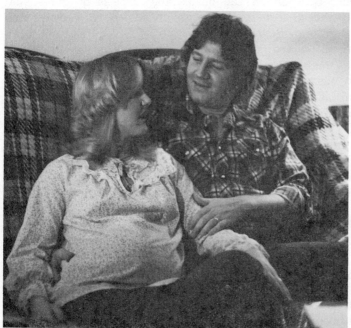

Sexuality during pregnancy is influenced by many factors: the individuals' relationship, their knowledge and attitudes about sexual activity during pregnancy, and physical or medical constraints. The nurse needs to understand these factors in order to help both partners adjust to sexual changes during pregnancy.

Photograph by Jim Tackett

about discipline, and the ways in which they will deal with the additional financial burdens they will experience as the result of having a child. Another, sometimes unanticipated problem that arises as pregnancy is confirmed is the sexual relationship. Much folklore exists about the dangers and pleasures of sex during pregnancy. There have been few studies on sexual activity during pregnancy. Maternity textbooks do not agree about the times when intercourse is without danger and the times when it should be avoided during pregnancy. The reader is often left wondering if it is intercourse itself or the female orgasm which should be avoided in cases in which intercourse is contraindicated.

One explanation for the dearth of information about sexual activity during pregnancy is that physicians represent society's ambivalence about combining the roles of lover and mother. Because the "mother" role is seen as nonsexual, the studying of sexual activity during pregnancy is seen as unnecessary.

Most mammals do not engage in sexual activity when the female is pregnant. Indeed, they have intercourse only at times when it is likely that the female will conceive. Only humans have intercourse at any time during the reproductive cycle of the female. Many observers point to the nonhuman mammals' abstinence from intercourse as the "natural" action that should be followed by humans as well.

A final reason for the lack of studies on sexual relations during pregnancy is that most research on pregnancy and early childbearing periods has been concerned with reducing the mortality and morbidity of both mother and infant (Butler, 1975).

Only recently have sex and pregnancy been accepted as a topic that is proper for study. The data, unfortunately, are not in complete agreement. For example, some couples report that their sexual enjoyment was at a peak during the woman's pregnancy, while others report that neither partner was really interested in sexual contact of any kind throughout the majority of the pregnancy. Some of the differences can be attributed to the misinformation and lack of knowledge possessed by couples during the pregnancy. Many couples fear that intercourse can harm the baby, and may choose to avoid intercourse for that reason. Others may believe that sex is for procreation only and may abstain from intercourse once pregnancy is achieved. Still others may find the pregnant body unattractive, and may wish to discontinue sexual activity until the woman has returned to her prepregnant body figure.

Injunctions to avoid intercourse have been based largely in three danger areas: mechanical, infection, and uterine contractions.

The possible effects of mechanical irritation during intercourse include rupture of the membranes, amnionitis, and placental bleeding. Although these conditions are often given as rationales for abstaining from intercourse at various points of the pregnancy, no firm evidence has been found to support these conclusions (Butler, 1975; Moore, 1978). If a woman is experiencing substantial bleeding, she should be advised to consult her physician and to abstain from sexual activities. It is possible that she may be suffering from a coincidental bleeding problem that might be aggravated by sexual activity. However, it has not been demonstrated that intercourse itself causes such difficulties.

Danger of infection is another rationale for the avoidance of sexual intercourse during pregnancy that has not been proven. In fact, the assumption that a woman is more susceptible to uterine infection during pregnancy is incorrect, since the cervix is tightly closed during most of the pregnancy, and the contents of the uterus are protected from potential sources of infection by a mucous plug. Several exceptions exist, such as cases of incompetent cervix and the transmission of venereal disease. These conditions are covered in the section on negative implications in this chapter.

It is known that uterine contractions occur during female orgasm. The fetal heart beat decreases slightly without apparent effect during female orgasm (Masters, 1966). Orgasm is contraindicated in cases of increased uterine irritability. Women with a history of repeated abortions (miscarriages) and women who are now suffering from or who have suffered from premature labor in past pregnancies are also considered at risk. These women and their partners should be carefully counseled to restrict their sexual activities. It must be stressed that orgasm through any means, including intercourse, oral stimulation, or masturbation, is contraindicated. It is the orgasm, not the intercourse, that is potentially harmful to these women.

Sexual Desire in Pregnancy.   The expression of our sexuality encompasses far more than genital sex. Especially in pregnancy, nurturance needs increase for both partners (Anderson, 1978; Bing, 1977; Zalar, 1976). Pregnancy is a stressful time for the prospective parents. Physical closeness is of great importance. For those women who are without partners during their pregnancy, the needs for nurturance may go unmet, with resultant effects on the mother-child relationship (Rubin, 1970). Mother-child attachment seems slower to develop in mother-infant couples in which the mother has not received the added attention she requires. It is hypothesized that mothers need this additional "taking in" during pregnancy so they are able to give back to the child after birth. Many couples whose sexual relations have been interrupted for some reason during pregnancy find that extra "cuddling" and quiet times together aid them greatly in sharing feelings and thoughts during this time.

The effect of pregnancy on sexual desire is not consistent. An association between the woman's level of sexual interest before pregnancy and the level of her interest during pregnancy has been postulated (Moore, 1978). A woman's interest in sex during pregnancy is probably most closely linked to her level of comfort and well-being (Zalar, 1976).

Some research has indicated that the majority of women experience a progressive linear decline in sexual interest throughout the pregnancy, which is reversed following the birth of the child (Solberg, 1973; Tolor, 1976). Masters' (1966) findings indicated that the desire for and frequency of sexual intercourse generally decreased during the first trimester. The second trimester was found to be one of increased sexual interest and performance, while the third trimester evidenced the most major decrease in sexual interest and activity.

Variations in sexual activity and interest during pregnancy clearly exist. Bing (1977) has graphed the desires for sexual activity reported throughout pregnancy and the postpartum period for her sample. This graph is included on the following page. The general line of sexual interest seems to vary during the pregnancy as different physiological and psychological changes occur.

In the following sections, the changes that occur during the three trimesters of pregnancy and during the postpartum period will be discussed in terms of sexual activity and the sexuality of the pregnant couple. (Note: This discussion assumes that the pregnant woman has a partner throughout her pregnancy. Unfortunately, this is not always true. With or without a

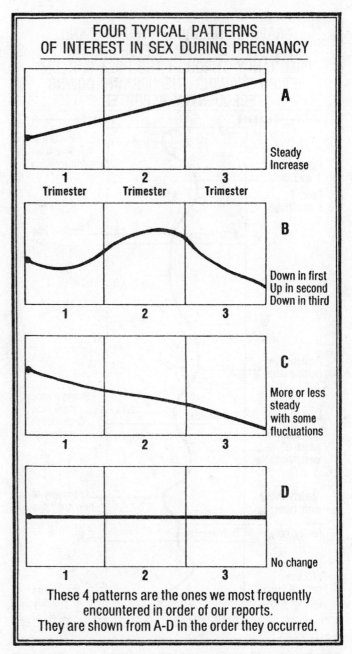

FOUR TYPICAL PATTERNS
OF INTEREST IN SEX DURING PREGNANCY

A

Steady
Increase

1 Trimester   2 Trimester   3 Trimester

B

Down in first
Up in second
Down in third

1   2   3

C

More or less
steady
with some
fluctuations

1   2   3

D

No change

1   2   3

These 4 patterns are the ones we most frequently
encountered in order of our reports.
They are shown from A-D in the order they occurred.

From Bing, E., and Coleman, L.: Making Love during Pregnancy. *Reprinted with permission from Bantam Books, Inc. (Copyright © 1977 by Elizabeth Bing and Libby Coleman. All rights reserved.)*

partner, the pregnant woman has sexual and nurturing needs. Since many pregnant women do have partners, this model has been chosen. It is the personal hope of the author that all pregnant women receive the support and nurturing that will enable them to progress through the difficulties of pregnancy and emerge ready to accept the joys and responsibilities of parenthood.)

First Trimester. A commonly encountered rationale for decreased sexual activity during the first trimester of pregnancy is the extreme fatigue and

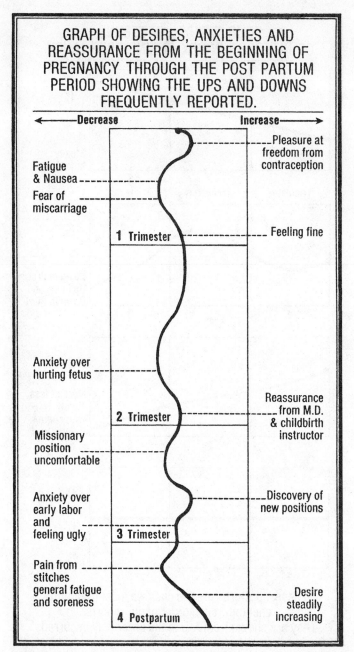

GRAPH OF DESIRES, ANXIETIES AND REASSURANCE FROM THE BEGINNING OF PREGNANCY THROUGH THE POST PARTUM PERIOD SHOWING THE UPS AND DOWNS FREQUENTLY REPORTED.

From Bing, E., and Coleman, L.: Making Love during Pregnancy. *Reprinted with permission from Bantam Books, Inc. (Copyright © 1977 by Elizabeth Bing and Libby Coleman. All rights reserved.)*

lethargy experienced. These usually disappear or significantly decrease by the end of the first trimester. Nausea and vomiting may also inhibit sexual desire during the first trimester. In addition, some women, especially women experiencing their first pregnancy, may experience extreme breast tenderness. Given these conditions, one can easily see how the sexual drive could be affected (Anderson, 1978; Solberg, 1973; Zalar, 1976).

For some men, the physical changes that occur may have a negative effect on their own sexual desire. For example, some couples report that although they had previously enjoyed oral sex (cunnilingus), because of the increase in vaginal discharge and the change in the smell of the discharge, the man was no longer interested in engaging in the previously enjoyed activity (Bing, 1977). The discharge is usually a cloudy white mucus of thicker consistency than normal. It is nonirritating and does not signify that the woman has a vaginal infection.

In addition to the purely physical changes that the pregnant woman experiences, emotional and psychological factors play a part in the sexual life of the pregnant couple. For example, a commonly encountered fear held by both men and women is that intercourse will harm the baby or cause a miscarriage. This fear is present even in cases in which there are no symptoms to indicate the possibility of such events (Bing, 1977; Solberg, 1973).

Some men report that they do not find the pregnant body attractive, and some may feel repulsed by it. As a result, sexual relations may be discontinued. The elimination of sexual activity may be acceptable to both partners. If this is the case, and if the couple continue to be affectionate and meet each other's needs for nurturance and support, then the situation is not one of stress. If, however, only one of the partners feels that sexual activity during pregnancy is unattractive, both partners may need help to understand the situation without guilt or shame. Finally, for those who feel that intercourse is permissible for procreation only, when the woman becomes pregnant, sexual activity may be discontinued, since it would be redundant.

On the other hand, some pregnant women report that their sexual activity increased tremendously during the first trimester of pregnancy. The freedom from having to utilize contraception or from worrying about becoming pregnant leads to far greater enjoyment of intercourse in some cases. The increased engorgement of the genitalia which begins in the first trimester may lead to increased enjoyment of sexual activity. Some women report that they experience their first orgasm during early pregnancy (Anderson, 1973).

Second Trimester. The second trimester is generally the most comfortable period of the pregnancy for making love (Bing, 1977; Masters, 1966; Zalar, 1976). Some reasons for this increased interest in and performance of sexual activity in the second trimester are:
1. Adjustment to the idea of pregnancy.
2. Decreased nausea and vomiting.
3. Decreased risk of miscarriage.
4. Elimination of breast tenderness.
5. The abdomen is not so large as to be in the way during lovemaking.
6. Increased pelvic congestion that may lead to greater desire for sexual activity.

Many women experience their most frequent emotional highs and lows during the second trimester (Bing, 1977). These fluctuations of emotions were found to have an effect on the sexual activity of the couple, but were usually not reported as a problem if the couple had been prepared for these mood swings.

Orgasm is experienced somewhat differently during pregnancy. The increased pelvic congestion may lead to increased or decreased sexual pleasure. In addition, beginning in the second trimester and continuing into the third, the uterine contractions that accompany orgasm may lead to cramping and aching in the lower abdomen or back following orgasm. If this occurs, usually gentle massage will help to alleviate the discomfort. It may, however, lead to a decreased interest in sexual activity on the part of the woman (Anderson, 1978).

Third Trimester.   Traditionally, physicians have advised women to abstain from intercourse for the last six to eight weeks of pregnancy. This injunction against sexual activity during this period of time may in part explain findings that the third trimester is universally represented as the time of most major decrease in sexual activity and interest (Masters, 1966; Moore, 1978; Solberg, 1973; Tolor, 1976). The sheer size of the abdomen of the woman in her third trimester of pregnancy presents problems of position and comfort for intercourse. Most couples who choose to continue to have intercourse find that the side or rear-entry positions for coitus are the most comfortable and possible during this stage of pregnancy (Hyde, 1979). Orgasm, as mentioned earlier, is experienced subjectively differently during the final trimester of pregnancy. Some women experience chronic uterine spasms with orgasm. These uncomfortable (but not painful) spasms may last as long as one minute, and may be upsetting to both partners. Gentle massage of the lower abdomen or back often will relieve discomfort. Because of these spasms, however, many couples decide to eliminate female orgasm. If this is the case, alternatives for sexual expression should be discussed.

There are times during the third trimester when sexual activity is indeed contraindicated. Once the membranes have ruptured, women are advised against intercourse, since the membranes are no longer present to protect the unborn child from potential infection. Intercourse is also contraindicated when labor has begun (Anderson, 1978). Some couples find that intercourse is not comfortable after the infant's head has become engaged in the mother's pelvis. For primiparous women, this may occur several weeks prior to delivery, while for multiparous women, engagement does not usually occur until labor has begun. If a couple finds that intercourse is uncomfortable after the head has engaged, counseling the couple on noncoital activities should be considered. The abdominal discomfort and the anxiety that penetration may cause at this time should be dealt with as quickly as possible by the health professional (Butler, 1975).

Labor and Delivery.   Labor is experienced differently by different women. For some, labor is described as the ultimate expression of feminine sexuality (Anderson, 1978; Bing, 1977). These women often equate the delivery experience with similar sensations they have experienced during orgasm, including the vasoconstriction, pressure, exhilaration, exhaustion, and relief following orgasm (delivery).

Many women do not share these feelings of sensuality during the delivery experience. For them, the experience is recalled as tremendously difficult work that, once over, was essentially forgotten in the excitement of seeing the baby that they had worked so hard to deliver. It is not remembered as physically pleasurable. The parallel between the changes in delivery and sexual arousal do exist. Care must be taken to avoid carrying the parallel to the extreme. Just as the increased engorgement of the genitalia in pregnancy may lead to increased enjoyment of sexual activity for some women, for others the sensitivity is too great and may be perceived as painful. Presenting the delivery experience to women soon to deliver as the "ultimate orgasmic response" is simply not true for many women and can establish unrealistic expectations for the woman and her partner.

Alternatives to Hospital Delivery.   The move to more "natural" delivery has been well documented, and support groups for out of hospital deliveries have increased greatly. Prior to the 1920's the vast majority of deliveries occurred in the home. When the hospital became the preferred location for normal obstetrical delivery and postpartum care, some viewed pregnancy as having undergone a change in which it was treated as an illness rather than a natural event. Medical interventions such as routine episiotomies (stitches), lithotomy position for delivery (woman on her back with her legs in stirrups), routine fetal monitoring, and the routine use of IV's for all patients are seen by some as unnecessary and intrusive interventions (Arms, 1975; Edwards, 1973; Ritchie, 1976; Ward, 1976). For many, delivery has been "taken away" from the family, with the physician usurping the center of attention. They feel that women have been unnecessarily convinced of the need for medical intervention, and they prefer to deliver their babies at home, free of medical rules and regulations. According to Edwards (1973), ". . . they seek more achievement from the act of giving birth and prefer to place their trust in friends who have had many children rather than in skilled strangers in a hospital."

Some of the reasons for out of hospital deliveries are enumerated (Arms, 1975; Ritchie, 1976; Ward, 1976):

1. *The sense of birth as being in harmony with the body, with loved ones, and with the natural order of the world.*

   For those who truly believe that birth is an entirely natural occurrence, any intervention by the medical staff of a hospital is seen as unnecessary.

2. *The influence of the women's movement, which emphasizes sharing between a man and a woman.*

   Until very recently, men were excluded entirely from the birth process, being forced to "wait outside" while their partner delivered (or more accurately, the physician delivered) the child. It is in part due to the pressure of couples to have the father share in the delivery that men are usually allowed in delivery rooms today. However, in some areas the father is still barred from delivery, especially in cases in which cesarean deliveries are performed.

3. *Nostalgia for times past.*

   Many attribute this move to return to more simple times as a major impetus to the move away from hospital delivery.

4. *"Doing things naturally."*

   This is closely linked to the nostalgia move. In addition, though, many feel that there is too much unnecessary medical intervention in the process of childbirth. For instance, they feel that the perineum can stretch without tearing, making the now routine episiotomy unnecessary. Many are also alarmed at the rapidly increasing rate of cesarean deliveries. It is felt that medical intervention that is too early accounts for many cases of unnecessary surgical delivery.

5. *Disenchantment with the impersonal treatment received in hospitals.*

   The experience of the birth and early days of the new infant's life are seen as times that "should" be spent with loved ones and family. Rigid hospital schedules, initially conceived to help prevent the spread of infections, are seen as intrusions. In addition, the staff of hospitals are not intimately involved in the family who has just delivered, and therefore may not share in their joy. This, coupled with inadequate staffing, has led to much displeasure with the hospital care provided for maternity patients.

6. *The desire to save on hospital bills.*

   This concern is becoming more significant for ever larger portions of the population. The hospital bill for a normal delivery with minimal anesthesia and a four day stay for the mother and the infant is now in the thousands of dollars. Medical insurance does not adequately cover these costs in most cases. The family without insurance faces these staggering bills themselves.

7. *Decreased danger of cross infections in the home.*

Despite the precautions taken in nurseries and postpartum units, infections do occur. In a full nursery, infection can potentially spread to all of the children. In the home, however, the new infant is exposed to far fewer people, and the home usually does not contain the microorganisms commonly found in the hospital.

The discontent felt by this growing portion of the population regarding hospital delivery has not been without effect. In fact, hospitals are increasingly examining alternatives that will be acceptable to all potential clients. For example, hospitals are shifting more toward becoming "birthing centers," in which a more homelike environment is provided. The father and often other siblings are allowed to be present during the labor and delivery. The rooms in these birthing centers are usually decorated in a more "homy" fashion than normal institutional rooms. When the woman is about to deliver, she is not rushed from the labor room to a delivery table where she is strapped down for the duration. Some of the birthing rooms are equipped with special labor beds that are also used for delivery. If the woman chooses, she may deliver in different positions, such as squatting or sitting up holding her legs apart. For breech presentations, she may be encouraged to labor in a hands and knees position. (Note that the immediate tendency to decide on a cesarean delivery for breech presentations is not made here [Edwards, 1973].)

In some cases the birthing centers are not directly within the hospital, and may be staffed with specialized staff, such as nurse midwives. Other hospitals may convert traditional labor rooms to "birthing rooms." The benefit of both of these alternatives lies in the ability and accessibility of medical intervention should some emergency situation arise. As family centered maternity care has become more popular, health professionals in maternity have become more involved in the care of the family. This increased involvement, including teaching infant care, sexuality, and so on, carries with it the potential for increasing the satisfaction of both clients and staff regarding hospital maternity care.

The use of anesthesia in hospital delivery has decreased tremendously with increased knowledge of its potential dangers to the unborn child. This move to decreased medication has met with approval from those who feel that birth is a natural process that need not be "tampered" with. As a result of the work of LeBoyer, many couples now request and experience a "gentle birth" in which the baby is delivered in a darkened room slowly and gently. The cord is not cut until it has stopped pulsating in order to allow the lungs to begin their work more slowly. Waiting for the cord to stop pulsating also allows the infant to receive an additional transfusion of blood. Following the cutting of the cord, the infant may be placed in a warm bath for the purpose of accustoming the newborn to the forces of gravity more slowly. Finally, the infant is put to the breast rather than in an infant warmer. The skin-to-skin contact of the mother and infant has been found to be sufficient to keep the temperature appropriately elevated.

The procedure of the gentle birth is based on the premise that birth is a traumatic event for the infant. For the first time the infant is exposed to harsh hospital lights, the shock of the first breath, the noises of the hospital environment, the decreased temperature, the forces of gravity, and all of the other inevitable changes of environment. These abrupt and all-encompassing experiences are made easier for the infant undergoing gentle birth. The techniques are those utilized by midwives and those practicing home delivery. Introduction of such techniques in hospitals assures the couple of the availability of the emergency services of the hospital while they are receiving the natural, unhurried care of the LeBoyer method.

In order to help decrease the cost of hospital delivery, some hospitals have programs for low risk mothers and infants that allow for early discharge (sometimes only a few hours after the delivery) and perinatal home care (Ritchie, 1976). If a couple decides to have a child in their home, attended by a midwife or physician, most insurance companies will not cover the charges.

Despite the changes in the delivery of obstetrical care in this country, many couples are still deciding to have their children at home. These couples still need and should be encouraged to receive proper prenatal care, good nutrition, and attendance at some method of birth training (Edwards, 1973). Unfortunately, in a sometimes punitive move, some physicians refuse prenatal care to women who have decided to deliver their babies at home. This is inappropriate behavior on the part of the physician. If a client is refused treatment, she should be encouraged to seek the necessary prenatal care elsewhere. Some couples who have been refused treatment have gone on to exert great consumer pressure on physicians who display such questionable ethics. The health and safety of the mother, the child, and the father of the child should be foremost in the mind of the health care worker. All possible moves to ensure this safety should be made.

Postpartum Sexuality

Anyone who has seen a vaginal delivery can understand the fear that nearly every couple experiences regarding future sexual relations. Many men and women feel that the vagina cannot possibly return to its predelivery state. They fear permanent damage from the stretching of the vagina during delivery (Zalar, 1976). This fear is sometimes exacerbated by the so-called "extra stitch" in the episiotomy "for the husband." Some health care professionals joke that the physician adds one stitch more than is necessary in repairing the episiotomy so that the woman's vagina will be as tight as it was prior to delivery. Many women then fear the first intercourse, feeling certain that the episiotomy is too tight, and that they will experience great pain with early intercourses following delivery. In fact, the vagina is highly elastic, and does return to its normal size shortly following delivery. The vagina will again expand to accommodate the penis during intercourse as it did prior to delivery, with or without the "husband stitch."

Following pregnancy, the sexual drive usually returns fairly quickly (Hollendar, 1974; Masters, 1966). For some, though, the return of the sex drive may be more prolonged, owing to the fatigue of early parenting, the readjustment of the hormonal levels, and the general adjustment to the role of parent of a newborn.

In the past, couples have been advised to abstain from intercourse until after the six week postpartum checkup. Many couples feel able to and desire to have intercourse well before that time. The rationale for advising abstinence has been primarily to avoid infection. The cervix is essentially closed 24 hours after delivery. The chance for endometrial infection as a result of organisms introduced during intercourse is unlikely. For most women, the episiotomy is healed by seven days. Intercourse actually tends to soften and help the healing of the episiotomy scar (Anderson, 1978).

Recently, couples have been advised to refrain from intercourse only until the lochia has changed to the straw-colored lochia alba. Of course, intercourse should not be attempted until both partners are comfortable with the idea, emotionally as well as physically. The health professional should be aware that many men are just as anxious about resuming intercourse because of the fear of causing pain to their partners as are the women who fear that early intercourse following delivery will be painful.

It is necessary that the nurse talk to the couple before they leave the hospital. If the couple chooses to deliver at home, the nurse or other professional making home visits should include discussion about the resumption of sexual intercourse with the couple. If this is not discussed (other than perhaps warning the couple to abstain until the six week check) and the couple does begin to have intercourse prior to that time, they may experience guilt and fear that their action may have some long-term negative effects. One potential effect of early intercourse following pregnancy is another pregnancy. Many couples are not aware of the fact that a woman can ovulate without having a period in the postpartum period, especially if she is breast-feeding, and can therefore become pregnant. Anticipatory guidance regarding contraception for the early as well as later postpartum period is necessary and indicated.

Breast-feeding can be a source of embarrassment for the breast-feeding mother and her partner. Many women who breast-feed find that they become sexually aroused during nursing (Moore, 1978). For some the arousal and orgasm that may occur during breast-feeding lead to guilt. The possibility of such feelings should be discussed with the woman and her partner prior to the birth of the child. Some men have negative feelings about the arousal of their partners during breast-feeding. The man may feel a kind of possessiveness about the breast, and may feel jealousy that the infant is providing the woman with sexual stimulation. Such feelings are best discussed prior to their occurrence, so that they can be dealt with in a relaxed and nonthreatening atmosphere.

Another potential source of embarrassment for the lactating woman and her partner is the uncontrollable spurt of milk that the woman may lose in response to sexual stimulation (Moore, 1978; Zalar, 1976). If the couple finds this release of milk unappealing, the woman may be advised to wear a bra with absorbent pads during sexual activity. She should not use tissues in the bra, as the tissue fibers may enter the nipple and cause later irritation.

Breast-feeding (and sometimes nonbreast-feeding) women may find that their natural vaginal lubrication seems to be decreased when intercourse is resumed. This lack of adequate lubrication may lead to pain on intercourse. The use of sterile lubricant (such as K-Y jelly) is often sufficient to alleviate the problem. The nurse should be aware that many couples are too embarrassed to mention the decreased lubrication, and should provide the couple with the information that such an occurrence is not unusual. They can then be advised about measures to alleviate the discomfort. For some breast-feeding women, the sterile lubricant may not be sufficient to relieve the discomfort during intercourse. In such cases, a prescription estrogen vaginal cream may be necessary. The creams are almost always effective.

NURSING INTERVENTIONS
Nurse as Teacher

The nurse has many potential areas of contact with the pregnant couple: prenatal clinics, classes for expectant parents, family planning clinics, inpatient maternity units, postpartum clinics, and/or as a visiting nurse for pregnancy and postpartum care. In each of these settings, the role of the nurse is concerned to a great extent with client teaching. The nurse who is committed to providing family centered care should not ignore the pregnant couple's need for shared love and intimacy in planning.

The sexual history should be taken with the rest of the general history, in order to provide a data base for future discussions and to indicate to the client that the area of sexuality is open for discussion between the nurse (or physician) and the client. Language that is understood by clients must be utilized by the professionals. If necessary, clients may be taught some new words that they are comfortable with to describe their anatomy and the changes that are occurring to the body of the pregnant woman. Great care must be taken to avoid forcing the client to adopt the medical terminology with which health care professionals are comfortable. This tactic has the effect of alienating the clients and making them feel embarrassed and inadequate. In short, it hinders rather than facilitates the formation of a trusting relationship. Vocabulary should be understood clearly by the nurse as well as by the clients. If there is any doubt, the nurse must clarify what is meant by the words used by the nurse and by the clients.

In collecting the history data, the nurse should strive to learn what the pregnancy means to the clients. If, for example, a couple reports that the pregnancy represents their shared love, they may expect the pregnancy and the child they will bear to strengthen the relationship. If the pregnancy was initially unplanned and/or unwanted, it may be seen by one or both of the partners as weakening the relationship. The potential for stress in a relationship is increased when pregnancy is not a joint decision, or if pregnancy is utilized as an attempt to "save" a weak marriage (Zalar, 1976).

Eliciting feelings about pregnancy and the changes that it will inevitably cause is not difficult, even in cases in which the motivation for pregnancy may not be what the nurse may view as "right." Recognizing bias is mandatory if the nurse is to effectively care for the client and her partner in a nonjudgmental manner. Nurses are not expected to change their own ideas to conform with those of clients, but neither is it appropriate to inflict biases on the clients.

Some examples of questions that will elicit feelings about the pregnancy are:

1. *How is the baby going to change your lives?*
   This question gives both the client and the nurse a chance to examine whether or not the client's impressions of having a child are realistic. It can give the nurse a good starting point from which to begin teaching during the pregnancy.
2. *How has it changed your lives already?*
   The client's response to this question may open the way for discussion of changes in sexual expression as a result of the pregnancy. In cases of unwanted or unplanned pregnancy, it can give the nurse a view of the support systems that the client is likely to be able to rely on throughout the pregnancy.

3. *What plans do the pregnancy and having a child interrupt?*

Even in cases where pregnancy is completely planned and wanted, there is always a feeling of ambivalence when the pregnancy is confirmed (Rubin, 1970). Since a couple cannot count on becoming pregnant exactly when they wish (in most cases), the pregnancy usually will upset or necessitate some rearrangement of plans. The way in which the client perceives the pregnancy and its effect on plans is significant in determining her feelings about the pregnancy.

4. *How are you going to manage these interruptions?*

Following the preceding question in this way seems natural, but should not be overlooked. The client's coping can be assessed here, as well as the coping of those around her.

Once the data base of the history is collected, the nurse can begin teaching clients about pregnancy and early child care. Physiological and psychological changes that occur as a result of pregnancy should be included. It is most relevant and important to the client to learn what to expect in her current stage of pregnancy and in the stage that is soon to follow. Explaining infant bathing is not going to be salient to the woman experiencing severe nausea and vomiting in the first trimester of pregnancy. She will be far more interested in measures to help her deal with this sickness, and in the fact that in most cases the situation is short-lived. Anticipating difficulties and dealing with them before they occur helps avoid misunderstanding later. Anticipatory guidance should be utilized in dealing with the sexuality of the woman and her partner throughout the pregnancy. As Clark (1974) has stated, "If each couple could receive adequate instruction in foreplay, positions, and other methods of achieving sexual satisfaction in as straightforward a manner as they are instructed about the hospital delivery room, many of their problems might disappear or never develop."

Alternatives to Intercourse

In some instances, intercourse during some portion of the pregnancy may be contraindicated. It is entirely appropriate and desirable that the nurse possess the knowledge and comfort to explore alternatives for sexual arousal and release with the woman and/or her partner (Anderson, 1978; Zalar, 1976). Some of the alternatives include:

1. Solitary masturbation
2. Mutual masturbation
3. Oral–genital sex
4. Anal intercourse
5. Use of alternative sites for intercourse (e.g., groin space between upper thigh and abdomen or between the breasts)

Before nurses can be effective in assisting couples in discussion of the alternatives to intercourse that are available, they must be aware of their own feelings about these alternatives. If the nurse feels that any of these practices are perverse and/or immoral, clients are usually sensitive enough to pick up the nurse's discomfort and will therefore not discuss these activities with the nurse. In addition, the nurse will be reluctant to inform the clients of viable alternatives to intercourse, should these alternatives need to be discussed.

Even in cases where there is no actual contraindication to coitus, clients may benefit from the increased knowledge of sexual options that exist.

Learning (or learning more) about these practices informs clients that these practices are not dangerous and that they are commonly encountered activities. Statements of universality can be useful in such discussions. For example, a broad statement such as, "Many couples find that mutual masturbation becomes more frequent in pregnancy, especially toward the end of the pregnancy when the abdomen makes the traditional positions for intercourse uncomfortable. How have you dealt with this?" can lead to an accepting discussion of alternative modes of sexual expression.

In discussing oral–genital sex with clients, the nurse should explain potential dangers of embolism formation when air is forcefully blown into the vagina. Some individuals blow air into the vagina during cunnilingus. Especially during pregnancy, the woman runs a greater risk of air embolism and potential death (Butler, 1975).

For clients who find anal intercourse acceptable and enjoyable, the nurse should discuss the importance of avoiding contamination of the vagina or urethra. Use of a condom, which is removed after anal intercourse, may be suggested.

Contraindications to Sexual Activity During Pregnancy

Although many of the restrictions on intercourse during pregnancy have been lifted, there are still some situations that will necessitate abstaining from intercourse and/or female orgasm (Anderson, 1978; Zalar, 1976). Perhaps one of the earliest periods when intercourse may be contraindicated is during the first trimester in cases of threatened abortion. If the woman is experiencing this difficulty, she should be counseled to abstain from intercourse until two weeks after the symptoms subside. In addition, she should be warned to avoid any stimulation that could lead to orgasm. Masters (1966) documented the fact that orgasms from oral–genital sex and masturbation are usually more intense than those experienced during intercourse. The woman and her partner should realize that in the case of early threatened abortion it is female orgasm that is contraindicated, not only coitus. If the woman has a history of early miscarriage (abortion), she may be advised to abstain from sexual activity until she has passed the first trimester of pregnancy.

Women whose cervix is not tightly closed, those who have what is called an "incompetent" cervix, do not have the protection afforded by a closed cervix. The risk of premature labor is very real for this small portion of pregnant women; therefore, sexual activity, especially female orgasm, is contraindicated. In most cases labor will begin prematurely with or without orgasm, but it may be hastened by orgasm. If the woman has the cervix sutured closed (cerclage), she is usually advised to wait for two weeks after the cerclage procedure before having intercourse.

Women diagnosed with placenta previa or abruptio placentae are advised to avoid coitus and all sexual stimulation. These conditions are potentially life threatening to both the mother and the child. However, they are rare and must be diagnosed by a professional.

In cases of suspected or known uteroplacental insufficiency, female orgasm may be contraindicated, since orgasm may cause late and variable decelerations in the fetal heart rate. This decrease in the fetal heart rate (discussed earlier) may lead to hypoxia in the already sick infant. This contraindication is not complete, and must be judged on the basis of the specific case.

A history of premature labor may be another case in which the woman may be advised to abstain from orgasm, especially after thirty-two weeks of gestation. In the case of premature rupture of membranes, intercourse is contraindicated because of the increased risk of infection to the infant.

Both the client for whom sexual activity is contraindicated and her partner need support and guidance. If possible, it is desirable to discuss the rationale for the suspension of intercourse (or of female orgasm) with both partners. This can contribute to better knowledge for each of the clients and can prevent any misunderstanding that may occur if the client herself is not sure of the reasons for the prohibition and then relates these reasons in a confused state to her partner.

For some individuals, the prohibition against sexual activity is equated with a cessation of all sensual and nurturing activities. This should be discussed fully, especially in light of the added needs that both partners will experience as a result of the pregnancy. Some couples, regardless of the ability to enjoy sexual relations, may for one reason or another decide that the man will seek his sexual satisfaction with another partner until the pregnancy is over. For some, this alternative may be highly acceptable, whereas others may have more difficulty adapting to it. The nurse can serve as a facilitator in such discussions, provided that sufficient rapport with the clients has been established.

The nurse has many roles during pregnancy, including those of teacher, counselor, and patient advocate. The role of the nurse regarding sexuality during pregnancy is to assist the couple in achieving a satisfactory sexual relationship during the pregnancy that does not cause guilt or worry in either partner. This is the goal toward which nursing care for the sexual health of the couple is aimed.

References

AASECT: *Sex Education for Adolescents and Youth,* Washington, D.C., American Association of Sex Educators, Counselors and Therapists, 1977.

Anderson, C., Clancy, B., and Quirk, B.: "Sexuality During Pregnancy." *In* Barnard, M., Clancy, B., and Krantz, K. (Eds.): *Human Sexuality for Health Professionals.* Philadelphia, W. B. Saunders Co., 1978.

Arms, Suzanne: *Immaculate Deception.* Boston, Houghton Mifflin Book Co., 1975.

Bing, Elisabeth, and Colman, Libby: *Making Love During Pregnancy.* New York, Bantam Books, 1977.

Butler, J. C., and Wagner, N. N.: "Sexuality During Pregnancy and Postpartum." *In* Green, Richard (Ed.): *Human Sexuality: A Health Practitioner's Text.* Baltimore, Williams & Wilkins Co., 1975.

Clark, A. L., and Hale, R. W.: "Sex During and After Pregnancy." *American Journal of Nursing, 74*:8, Aug. 1974.

Edwards, Margot E.: "Unattended Home Birth." *American Journal of Nursing, 73*:8, Aug. 1973.

Erikson, Erik H.: *Childhood and Society.* New York, W. W. Norton and Co., 1963.

Frieze, I., and Sales, E.: "Making Life Decisions." *In* Frieze, I. H., Parsons, J. E., Johnson, P. B., Ruble, D. N., and Zellman, G. L. (Eds.): *Women and Sex Roles: A Social Psychological Perspective.* New York, W. W. Norton and Co., 1978.

Hyde, Janet Shibley: *Understanding Human Sexuality.* New York, McGraw-Hill Book Co., 1979.

Masters, William H., and Johnson, Virginia E.: *Human Sexual Response.* Boston, Little, Brown and Co., 1966.

Mitchell, Jack: "Teen Pregnancy—How to Cope." *Parade,* June 10, 1979.

Moore, Mary Lou: *Realities in Childbearing.* Philadelphia, W. B. Saunders Co., 1978.

Ritchie, C., Swanson, Ann H., and Lee, Ann B.: "Childbirth Outside the Hospital—

the Resurgence of Home and Clinic Deliveries." *Maternal Child Nursing, 1*:6, Nov./Dec. 1976.

Rubin, Reva: "Cognitive Style in Pregnancy." *American Journal of Nursing, 70*, March 1970.

Solberg, D. A., Butler, J., and Wagner, N.: "Sexual Behavior in Pregnancy." *New England Journal of Medicine, 228*:1098–1103, 1973.

Sorensen, Robert C.: *Adolescent Sexuality in Contemporary America*. New York, World Publishing, 1973.

Tolor, Alexander, and DeGrazia, Paul V.: "Sexual Attitudes and Behavior Patterns During and Following Pregnancy." *Archives of Sexual Behavior, 5*:6, 1976.

Ward, Charlotte, and Ward, Fred: *The Home Birth Book*. Washington, D.C., Inscape Publishers, 1976.

Wood, Nancy Fugate: *Human Sexuality in Health and Illness*. St. Louis, The C. V. Mosby Company, 1979.

Zalar, Marianne K.: "Sexual Counseling for Pregnant Couples." *Maternal Child Nursing, 1*:3, May/June 1976.

7

SEXUAL REALITIES IN AGING

Ours is a society that has been called "youth oriented" and "throw away." Youth and all of its advantages are stressed in the media, by peers, and by people in the medical field. Until very recently, aging and the changes that accompany it were viewed as illnesses, to be dealt with through sometimes very aggressive medical means. Over the past years, with the growing number of elderly who have become vocal in our society, the view of aging as a disease is slowly beginning to change. One area in which the change is very slow is that of sexuality. Although it is being recognized that older people have much to offer to the young in terms of history, wisdom, and love, the rights to sexual fulfillment of the elderly are often denied or repressed.

    The purpose of this chapter is to discuss sexuality in the aging adult, including both the myths and the realities. Much time will be spent on the discussion of the prevailing myths, since they form the basis of a great deal of misinformation that exists regarding the sexual activities of the elderly. These myths will be refuted and discussed in the light of current knowledge in the field of human sexuality.

    Following the discussion of myths, the changes that occur in the human sexual response cycle of the older person will be covered. Included in the sexual response area will be a discussion of menopause and the effects of the commonly encountered stresses of the middle years on both men and women.

    Nursing implications are discussed last in the chapter, although the reader can easily see their application throughout. They have been left to the end of the chapter, however, so that the reader is able to apply these implications to suggested problems with a firm base of knowledge of sexuality in aging. General information relating to counseling relationships is reviewed with applications to the problems of the elderly. The important roles of the nurse as teacher and as patient advocate are also discussed at some length. The overall theme presented is the importance of respect for other individuals, regardless of their situation. The nurse is shown to occupy a unique position with the capacity to help change the harmful myths that surround aging and sexuality. In addition, the nurse has the knowledge and skills to provide a warm, accepting atmosphere in which aging clients can work through and come to a positive resolution of their feelings about sexuality and how their sexuality has been affected by the aging process.

COMMON MYTHS AND MISCONCEPTIONS ABOUT SEXUALITY AND AGING

The number of myths about sexuality in older people that exist in the minds of both young and old people in our society is astounding considering the relatively short time that has passed since sexuality in the aging has been considered acceptable for discussion in "polite" circles. The misconceptions exist partly from lack of knowledge and partly because so-called knowledgeable sources have been misinformed or have, unaware of their own personal biases, passed on such information through lay publications or other media. Seven commonly encountered myths, as well as factual information regarding these beliefs, will be discussed here:

1. Sex does not matter in old age. The later years are supposed to be (and usually are) sexless.
2. Interest in sex is abnormal in older poeple.
3. Remarriage after the loss of a spouse should be discouraged.
4. It is all right for old men to seek younger women as sex partners, but it is ridiculous for older women to be sexually involved with younger men.
5. Old people in institutions should be separated by sex to avoid problems for the staff and criticism by families and the community.
6. Emission of semen through any kind of sexual activity weakens one and therefore should be avoided in old age.
7. Masturbation is a "childish" activity confined to youngsters and adolescents.

Myth 1: *Sex doesn't matter in old age. The later years are supposed to be (and usually are) sexless.*

This is perhaps the most commonly encountered myth regarding sexual activity and the aging population. The mere prevalence of this myth may serve as a self-fulfilling prophecy. It is well known that successful sexual functioning depends on attitudes and beliefs as well as physiological potential (Masters and Johnson, 1966; Rubin, 1965). We sometimes forget that the elderly client or relative with whom we are dealing was also once young and also heard and repeated the ideas that sex in old age was more a thing of fond memories than of ongoing pleasure. It is considered improper somehow to even think of an older person as sexual. Consider elderly individuals who grew up with the notion that sexual activity is "supposed" to stop with advancing years. Suppose that they still feel sexual urges at 60 or 65. How can they come to terms with these feelings? Individuals may feel a tremendous amount of guilt and shame at being "oversexed" and exceptions to the more orderly rule of a neuter old age. A real sense of isolation may be experienced, along with fears of discussing this with others, since such disclosures of feelings are expected to be met with outright rejection. Lacking the proper support and education, then, elderly individuals may force themselves into a sexless and unhappy old age.

What are the sources for this myth and its remarkable "staying power" in the face of information that clearly refutes it? Three factors seem to be consistently relevant to the continuation of this myth. First, the youth orientation of our culture perpetuates the idea of a sexless old age. Youth, including smooth skin, shapely bodies, and firm muscles, is highly valued in our society. In a culture that stresses youthful appearance and vigor, it is hard for some (especially when they are young) to believe that someone who no longer possesses the prized youthful appearance can possibly be considered sexually attractive by another person. Therefore, it follows that it is difficult, if not impossible, to picture the older person as being sexually active.

The second factor is somewhat more emotionally deep than the emphasis on youth. The denial of sexual activity of the aged in our culture may be a carryover from the Victorian idea that sex was acceptable for procreation only. Sex for other than procreational purposes was considered sinful at that time. The older person is obviously past the reproductive years, and sexual relations can no longer be justified by the promise of procreation. Many of the older people alive today were brought up during or soon after this sexually repressive period of time. For example, the 82-year-old woman now entering a nursing home learned her sexual values in the early 1900's. She may have been taught that the only acceptable reason for sexual intercourse was to "be fruitful and multiply."

Finally, the incest taboo seems to offer the most deep-rooted explanation for the general discomfort expressed by most people about the sexual expression of the elderly. Many people who deal with the elderly in different capacities (social workers, physicians, nurses, nursing home administrators, nursing aides) tend to identify elderly people with their own parents. Because of the incest taboo, they feel distinctly uncomfortable even thinking about these elderly people being sexually active. The basis of the incest taboo includes the forbidden nature of sexual relations with parents and other close relatives. To achieve this, society exerts strong negative sanctions, extending to the point that to even contemplate such activity is extremely uncomfortable for the individual (Weideger, 1976). It is hypothesized, therefore, that the lack of objective, nonjudgmental treatment of older individuals as sexual beings results from strong reactions to the incest taboo. This may be one reason why family members may allow or even encourage the segregation of their aging parents from members of the opposite sex in institutional settings. Nursing home administrators report that children are often so unable to handle thoughts of their own parents' sexuality that they actively campaign to discourage the administration from making sexual release available (McKinley and Drew, 1977).

Margaret Kuhn, the well-known and outspoken organizer of the Gray Panther movement, has urged people to view old age in its positive aspects and strengths and to escape from the tyranny of this myth of old age as a sexless time (Kuhn, 1976). As Ms. Kuhn states, the elderly approach the sexual act, and indeed their entire sexuality, with unique strengths not possible for those still in their youth. The older individual can bring to the sexual relationship unique experiences, memories, and views of sexuality as a source of power and joy. Kuhn views the older couple as having the ability to take the time and effort to achieve a tenderness that can lead to a deeper form of sexual expression. The interaction of sexuality in older persons is seen as a type of communication that would have been impossible in the younger, more hurried years. The older person is described as free to explore many more forms of expressing and finding intimacy, warmth, and closeness with members of the same or the opposite sex. Finally, Kuhn states that sexual activity may actually be physically beneficial in that it decreases psychological tension and tends to increase the adrenal gland's output of cortisone, a steroid useful in the treatment of arthritis.

The attitudes toward aging and sex in the myth and in Kuhn's rebuttal are strikingly different. The latter presents sexuality in its rightful sphere, as an integral part of the human being and essential to his or her well-being, while the former classifies the expression of sexuality in older individuals as abnormal, deviant behavior.

Myth 2: *Interest in sex is abnormal for old people.*

Although closely related to the previous myth, this idea places the presence of sexual feelings into the area of pathology. It is included here to provide another opportunity to stress that sexual desire in the elderly is completely normal and usually continues throughout life, given certain prerequisites that will be discussed in the section of human sexual response in the aging adult.

Many of the elderly in our population have grown up under the influence of Victorian attitudes of sex, and may themselves view any sexual interest as abnormal. It is necessary, and of great importance, that these elderly people be encouraged to value their bodies, emotions, and spirit, and that they be encouraged to appreciate their own experiences and wisdom. To deny the normal sexual urges of older adults is to force them to lose their self-esteem and their sense of self.

Myth 3: *Remarriage after the loss of a spouse should be discouraged.*

It is a fact that in our society women live longer than men, and thus in the older years, far outnumber men. As a result of their greater longevity, most women experience loss of a spouse. For women who have been happily married and who have been enjoying a happy and fulfilling sex life with the spouse, widowhood can be a true social crisis. For many older women in our society, status and roles are defined by husband and by children. The widow may be suddenly forced into an acute identity crisis, and may find widowhood to be unusually traumatic and bitter. If she is able to emerge from this stressful time and find another person with whom she would like to spend the remainder of her life, her proposed remarriage is often met with great resistance by their adult children. It may be met with a sense of embarrassment; with the feeling that "Mother should be old enough to know better." Finally, the idea of remarriage for older individuals has been given psychiatric explanations. It may be seen as a kind of "last fling" for aging men and women who "deny" their age and cannot bear to think that youth (and therefore sexual expression) is over. In women, it is often attributed to menopausal phenomena, traceable to some glandular dysfunction. It may be further described as regressive behavior or a kind of escape (Rubin, 1965).

Once again, the shock and shame experienced by adult children at the idea that their aging parent may wish to remarry can be attributed to their discomfort at viewing their aging parent as a sexual being. A sense of "loyalty" to the dead parent may also contribute to the strong feelings of the children. They may view the coming marriage of their still living parent as somehow "disloyal" to the memory of the deceased parent. This feeling of having to protect the memory of the parent who is unable to defend himself or herself is a very significant block to open communication between the parent still living and the children.

Myth 4: *It is all right for old men to seek younger women as sex partners, but it is ridiculous for old women to be sexually involved with younger men.*

The double standards of sexual activities for men and women in our society do not end when couples marry. The more restrictive view held by society about women and their sexual activities continues throughout life, well into old age. Think, for example, of the number of books, movies, and other stories, romantically told, of the so-called "May-December romances." How often have these romances included the older woman with the younger man? This phenomenon, although it would seem an obvious solution to the increasing numbers of women in the older age brackets, is not considered acceptable behavior for women. The general reaction to women who do find a relationship with a younger man is often one of contempt, both for the woman and her new partner. The woman may be considered foolish to think that a young man could consider her sexually attractive, while the man may be accused of "using" the older woman for some reason, often financial security. Although the situation of the older man—younger woman couple is better accepted in our society, they too are subject to social pressures. The man may be advised that he too is being "used" and should "come to his senses" and "behave appropriately." Once again, the positive valuation of the elderly individual is essential to overcome the judgments of an overcritical society. All people have the right to happiness and fulfillment, regardless of their ages.

Myth 5: *Old people in institutions should be separated by sex to avoid problems for the staff and criticism by families and the community.*

This myth can be seen as something of an extension of the concept that old age is a sexless time, and that older people who do experience sexual feelings are abnormal. Expressions of sexuality by older people, especially those in nursing homes, have been viewed as manifestations of confusion or acting-out behavior. To prevent these "problems," the elderly in institutions have been segregated by sex. As some nursing home administrators have become more open and more knowledgeable about sexuality in the elderly, they have met a tremendous amount of resistance from family members regarding the sexual expression needs of elderly parents. The adult children of the elderly sometimes have great difficulty in dealing with the reality that their parents are still sexual beings (Butler, 1977; Chapman, 1976; McKinley and Drew, 1977; Moran, 1977). A more detailed discussion of the elderly in nursing homes follows later in this chapter and therefore will not be pursued at great length here. Kuhn (1976) has called for the organization of residents and their families for the purpose of pushing for policy changes in nursing homes and other institutions. She demands an affirmation of the rights of patients and residents to privacy and to the opportunity to fully express their sexuality. Resistance to this type of organization is strong, both from the residents and from the families of residents. Viewing the aged person as a valuable human being with legitimate needs and strengths is an essential first step to the policy changes that are so necessary.

Myth 6: *Emission of semen through any kind of sexual activity weakens one and therefore should be avoided in old age.*

This false concept can be found amazingly far back in our history. Stories about avoiding sexual activity before strenuous tasks can be found in writings from the ancient Greeks and the ancient Chinese (Rubin, 1965). More recent support for this myth can be found in locker rooms in many areas at the present time. There is often still an injunction to avoid "breaking training" (which, of course, will include avoiding sexual activity), especially before an important athletic event. The idea is that sexual activity will sap the strength of even the most virile young man. Imagine then, the risk of such a decrease in strength in an older man! Older men are often discouraged from sexual relations because of their age-related "weaker" state. That this myth is defeating and discouraging to the elderly who wish to remain sexually active is clear. Less clear is the fact that it is completely untrue, both for the young man and the old (Masters and Johnson, 1966).

It is possible that this myth's origin lies in the belief that masturbation is dangerous and should be avoided.

Myth 7: *Masturbation is a "childish" activity confined to youngsters and adolescents.*

This rather accepting statement on masturbation, though restrictive, does not consider the attitudes of some of the elderly. The teachings that the elderly received in their youth regarding sexuality in general and masturbation in particular are of particular importance. Victorian views on masturbation are extremely harsh. Masturbation was considered the root of severe physical and mental disabilities. It was thought to cause permanent nervous afflictions, blindness, and insanity. Masturbation was called by some in this Victorian era the most terrible of all vices, destructive to the mind, body, and soul of the individual and to the best interests in humanity. In addition, it was viewed as the cause of many of the "female complaints," including uterine hemorrhage, vaginal discharge, cancer of the uterus, cystocele, and less life-threatening haggard features and general debility (Ehrenreich, 1973; Rubin, 1965). In light of present knowledge, it is difficult to take these warnings seriously, but, indeed, at that time they were taken very seriously. For example, masturbation was considered an affliction in women that was often "cured" by surgical removal of the clitoris!

The beliefs that masturbation will lead to such serious problems as those stated above have been proven wrong, although fear still exists, especially in the minds of those who were taught of such dangers in their youth. It is a fact that masturbation is prevalent among practically all people, regardless of their age or marital status (Kinsey, 1953; Masters and Johnson, 1966, 1970). Rubin (1965) has viewed masturbation within marriage in a very nonjudgmental light in his statement, ". . . After marriage, masturbation often serves a useful and constructive purpose as a supplement to intercourse in balancing out unevenness in the sex needs of the partners. . . . It is a positive safeguard to the happiness of the marriage and is entirely harmless when done without guilty feelings." For many, though, the guilty feelings are difficult to overcome.

It has been found by Masters and Johnson (1970) that masturbation seems to increase in older women after menopause. Unmarried women, or women who have never been married, were found to continue with their previous patterns of masturbation. Women who no longer had a sexual partner, owing to illness, death, divorce, or social isolation, were responsible for the increased incidence of masturbation in this age group. The activity is not viewed as deviant. In fact, it is seen as a natural and adaptive behavior, given the fact that sexual urges continue well into old age.

SEX RESEARCH AND THE ELDERLY

One of the activities that can be pursued in order to help eliminate the damaging myths that still abound regarding the sexuality of older persons is research into this topic. Unfortunately, although sex research has proliferated tremendously in the last 10 to 20 years, research on the elderly and their specific strengths and problems has been largely neglected. Some reasons for this include the discomfort of the researchers with their own sexuality; the fact that physicians (who presumably would carry out such research) receive little training in sexuality; and, of course, the fact that physicians find it especially difficult to deal with the sex lives of patients of their parents' generation (Chapman, 1976).

Studies that have been carried out have been done primarily by three groups of researchers: Kinsey and his associates (1953); Masters and Johnson (1966, 1970); and Pfeiffer and his associates (1968, 1972). For the purpose of this discussion, Kinsey's and Masters and Johnson's findings will be combined. It must be noted that these findings are based on a very small sample in both cases, since it was not the primary intention of either research team to examine the sexuality of the aged population. Some generalities have been found, however, and can serve as a basis for this discussion and for further research.

Kinsey (1948, 1953) and Masters and Johnson (1966, 1970) found that many men and women can and do have satisfying sex lives well past middle age. Several necessary conditions were found to be common in both populations of men and women studied. The stronger the sexual urge in youth, it was found, the greater the likelihood of continued sexual activity in later life. This finding is contrary to a popular belief that one can prolong sex life by being inactive in earlier years and less active in older years. The rationale for such an idea is that a person possesses a finite amount of sexual energy, and that once that limit is reached, sexual activity must cease. The findings clearly refute such an idea (Chapman, 1976; Rubin, 1965).

A second condition found to be necessary for sexual activity to continue among the aging population was the availability of a sex partner. This has been found to be crucial for both men and women. Even if sexual activity is interrupted for a few months, it may be difficult or impossible to resume (Masters and Johnson, 1978). In fact, some counselors are advising self-stimulation (masturbation) to some of their elderly clients if an illness that precludes sexual activity with their partner exists (Chapman, 1976).

The final condition found necessary for sexual enjoyment concerns early sexual experiences. It was determined that individuals who had enjoyable sexual experiences in their youth were more likely to find sex satisfying in their older years than those had had not. In fact, it was found that those who did not have what they would define as a "good sex life" in their youth were more likely to use age as a justification for ending their sex life.

Pfeiffer and his associates, in several longitudinal studies using structured interviews and self-administered questionnaires, found support for the notion that sexual activity does, indeed, continue well into old age. Although he did find a trend to decreasing sexual activity in advancing age (over 78 years old), a significant portion of the sample over the years showed an actual rise in the patterns of sexual activity and sexual interest. The most commonly given reason for stopping intercourse was death of the spouse. There was also a highly significant finding that in cases where both spouses were living and intercourse had been discontinued, the stopping of intercourse was almost always attributed to the man, by both male and female subjects. Many more factors influencing sexual activity were found for men than for women. The factors for men included age, present health status, social class, use of antihypertensive drugs, present life situation, physical function rating (by subject), and concern over the physical findings of the examination. The levels of sexual interest and activity for women were principally reflected in the availability of a socially sanctioned, sexually capable partner. Past sexual enjoyment was most highly correlated with continuing sexual functioning for women. Martial status was a powerful determining factor in the female subjects' sexual behavior (Pfeiffer, 1968, 1972).

MEANINGS OF SEXUAL ACTIVITY FOR MIDDLE AGED AND OLDER ADULTS

Prior to discussing changes in the sexual response cycle in the older individual, it is important to examine the importance and subjective meaning of the sex act for the elderly individual. In fact, we should examine at what age individuals are considered in middle age and at what age they are considered to be elderly. In the past, with the shorter life spans in our society, middle age had been defined as being at around 35 to 40 years of age. With the increased longevity of both men and women, middle age, the middle portion of the life span, may actually begin at 50. An individual is redefined as old at 70 rather than at 50, as was previously accepted. If we accept 50 as middle aged, we can soon see that in our society this age is practically synonymous with depression. Eriksons' developmental task for this period in life is that of self-esteem versus despair. The middle aged man is usually at the height of his competitive career, and is, as such, under a tremendous amount of pressure outside of the home. The woman approaching middle age is usually also experiencing the menopause, as well as the stresses of children leaving the home. In the past, depression has been attributed to menopause itself, but more attention has been devoted to the idea that the depression may stem from the role changes that occur in this age rather than from the physiological changes. Women who have been employed outside of the home may be feeling similar pressures as those experienced by their husbands. Women who do not work outside of the home are subjected to the radical role changes that accompany children leaving home. If a woman has defined herself largely as mother and this role no longer exists, she will have difficulty in adjusting. In addition, the husband-wife unit must now change to a relationship that it has not occupied for many years—that of two marital partners without children present. This change too will be a significant stress on the marital relationship. With this in mind, we will examine the meaning of sexual activity for the middle aged and older adult.

More and more in our society the sexual relationship is being recognized as an important, vital aspect of human relations. It is viewed as a vehicle through which couples share deep intimacies. Continued sexual relationships are seen as providing an extremely important source of psychological reinforcement. The desires for intimacy, companionship, love, and affection make up an integral aspect of the individual's self-esteem. With advancing age, there is a definite change in the body image. For some individuals, this change is as traumatic as the body image changes that accompany adolescence. Other parallels with adolescence also exist. Often older and middle aged people are experiencing acute role identity crises. This, combined with

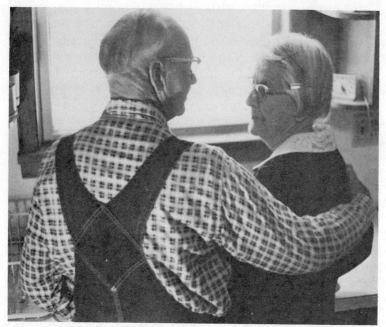

Photograph by Jim Tackett

The needs for intimate touch, for affection, and for sexual contact continue throughout life. The behaviors that express these needs may change as the body ages, but the needs continue.

their changing sense of sexuality, leads to a very fragile self-esteem, much as we see in adolescents. This is not to imply that the problems are the same, nor is it an attempt to oversimplify the undeniable problems faced by the aging adult. The parallel is drawn solely to demonstrate that aging, particularly in the middle and older years, can be seen as potentially as stressful to the individual as adolescence.

What are some of the additional meanings of sexual activity for the aging adult? Companionship is surely a very important factor. The value of the intimacy and communication in sexual relations has already been discussed. Touch is another very important part of sexual activity. The gentle tenderness and concern that are part of the sexual relationship serve as powerful reinforcers to individuals that they are worthwhile and physically attractive. The sense of love and belonging are essential for the continued self-esteem of all individuals, including the aging people in our society (Glover, 1977; Gress, 1978; Moran, 1977; Rubin, 1965).

CHANGES IN THE HUMAN SEXUAL RESPONSE CYCLE IN AGING

The changes that occur in old age regarding sexual functioning are obviously not sudden or dramatic, but reflect slow changes that begin in middle age and continue. For women, sexual potency has been found to remain at its more or less maximum level until the age of 55 to 60. In fact, the decreased inhibitions that accompany aging may even lead to an increased interest in sexual activities. (This may in part explain Pfeiffer's findings discussed earlier.) In order to follow the general format begun in the chapter on human sexual response, the changes through the four phases of sexual response suggested by Masters and Johnson (1966) will be traced. Younger women will be defined as those who are 20 to 40 years old, while older women will be defined as those 50 to 70 years old. Please keep in mind that the changes described are generally slow, and may go unnoticed for quite some time.

Excitement Phase—Women. Younger women, during the excitement phase, will evidence vaginal lubrication as a result of any form of effective sexual stimulation within 15 to 30 seconds. Older women may require from one to five minutes of undemanding sexual play before any vaginal lubrication can be noted.

Plateau Phase—Women. The marked uterine elevation and skin color changes in the labia of older women during the plateau phase are less marked than in younger women. In addition, the clitoral hood and the fatty tissues of the mons decrease with age. Despite these obvious changes, no loss in subjective pleasure has been reported to result.

Orgasmic Phase—Women. This phase is shortened with advancing age. The vaginal contractions occur at 0.8 second intervals, but they occur only four to five times, as compared with the eight to twelve contractions in younger women. The uterine contractions found during this phase are also reduced in most cases, one to two for older women as opposed to three to five for younger women. Occasionally, the uterine contractions in the orgasmic phase are found to increase tremendously, leading to uterine spasms that may last as long as one or more minutes. Women who report such spasms usually experience them subjectively as lower abdominal pain that radiates into the vagina and labia majora, or even as far as into the legs. Except occasionally during pregnancy, this type of uterine spasm is rarely reported in premenopausal women.

Resolution Phase—Women. Continuing with the pattern of a shortened sexual response cycle, the resolution phase is more rapid in the older woman than in the younger woman, with the labia returning to its normal color very quickly and the uterus returning to its pelvic position very rapidly after the orgasmic phase.

In addition to the changes described above in the sexual response cycle in women, certain other physiological changes occur with aging. As women age, and as their estrogen levels decrease, some fairly predictable changes in the genitalia occur. The tissues of the vulva and vagina atrophy to some degree and become thinner and more susceptible to trauma. This condition, sometimes called "senile" atrophy, may cause some women to discontinue their normal sexual activity owing to pain in intercourse (dyspareunia). Often, though many older people are not aware of this, the simple use of a water soluble lubricant (such as K-Y Jelly) on these tissues can completely remedy the situation. For more persistent problems, estrogen creams have been found to be very successful in treatment, without the risk of the systemic effects of oral estrogen replacement.

Another change in the genitourinary system of the aging female is the finding of increased bladder and urethral irritability after sexual intercourse, often resulting in increased urgency to urinate immediately after intercourse. The increased sensitivity of these structures to the force of penile contact is due to the thinning mucosal linings, which had previously served as anatomic cushions to protect the urethra and bladder from mechanical irritation

(Masters and Johnson, 1970). Estrogen replacement therapy is sometimes prescribed for this condition, and will be discussed in more detail later. The decreased ability of the older man to achieve erections that are as hard as those of his youth may be an asset, considering the woman's increased susceptibility to painful intercourse due to mechanical irritation. Many women find various types of tactile stimulation more likely to facilitate orgasm throughout life than direct penile-vaginal contact. The incidence of masturbation does increase during the older years. Masters and Johnson, in *Human Sexual Inadequacy,* have strongly stated their encouragement to men and women to continue with their sexual activity in old age in the following statement, "To a significant degree, regularity of sexual exposure will overcome the influence of sex-steroid inadequacy in the female pelvis."

The physiologic changes that occur in the sexual response cycle in men parallel those observed in women. Again, the stages of the response cycle will be utilized as a guide, and young men will be defined as 20 to 40 years old, and old men as 50 to 70 years old.

Excitement Phase—Men.   As men age, there is some delay in achieving erection. When the erection is achieved, it may not be as full or as hard as it was during youth. A man who always had what he considered to be an "instant" erection may fear impotence when this no longer occurs. If he has not been educated to understand that this is a normal occurrence, he may become impotent (Chapman, 1976; Masters and Johnson, 1966).

Plateau Phase—Men.   During the plateau phase, the young man has a larger amount of testicular elevation and scrotal sac vasocongestion than the older man. In addition, the older man may notice a decrease in the amount, or complete absence, of pre-ejaculation emission. The older man is better able to control and prolong the plateau period than is the younger man. This prolonged period is one of thorough enjoyment of elevated sexual tension for the man, and can serve as a means of satisfying a female partner more fully than could be achieved during intercourse in youth.

Orgasmic Phase—Men.   In men, the orgasmic phase is divided into two stages: ejaculatory inevitability and ejaculation. Ejaculatory inevitability is the stage at which the young man is no longer able to hold back his ejaculation. It usually lasts from 2 to 4 seconds. The subjective feelings are caused by regular contractions of the prostate at about 0.8 second intervals and continuing through both stages. The subjective report of the ejaculation stage is "one of a flow of a volume of warm fluid under pressure and the emission of seminal fluid bolus in ejaculatory spurts with pressure sufficient to expel the fluid content 12–24 inches beyond the urinary meatus" (Masters and Johnson, 1970). In older men, as in older women, the orgasmic phase is decreased in length. There may be a decrease in or absence of the ejaculatory inevitability stage. There is a corresponding decrease in the prostatic contractions to only one or two, and a decrease in the expulsive force to 3 to 12 inches. In older men, there is also a gradual decrease in the amount of seminal fluid production in the orgasmic phase. These changes, as well as the changes discussed for women, do not detract from the reported subjective enjoyment of the sexual act. Problems seem to occur primarily when men do not understand the physiological appropriateness of their altered sexual response changes and begin to have performance fears. Occasionally in the orgasmic phase in older men, ejaculatory inevitability is prolonged as the result of spastic contractions of the prostate. This may be subjectively evaluated as painful.

Resolution Phase—Men. The resolution phase of the sexual response cycle in older men is more rapid that it is in younger men. The older man may lose his erection very rapidly after ejaculation, and may find that he has an increased refractory period. This increase in the amount of time needed before the man can return to full erection under the influence of effective stimulation can be quite alarming to the man who is not aware that this is a normal change and does not affect his potency. As in women, it has been found that a consistent pattern of sexual expression helps to maintain the sexuality (Butler, 1977).

Masters and Johnson (1966) found that for women the most important factor in determining sexual activity was an acceptable and able sexual partner. They have outlined five commonly encountered reasons for decrease in male responsiveness with aging:
1. Monotony of a repetitious sexual relationship
2. Male concern with economic pursuit
3. Mental or physical fatigue
4. Overindulgence in food and drink
5. Physical and mental infirmities

Boredom with the partner is described as the most constant factor in the loss of interest in sexual activity in men. Two reasons for this are postulated by Masters and Johnson. The first is that in patriarchal societies prevailing attitudes view males as naturally polygamous. The man may be "programmed" in his youth to expect variety in his sexual partners. This attitude is considered to contribute to the sexual restlessness and the search for new partners, even in cases where the new partner is a less effective sexual partner than the established partner. It is the newness that is exciting. A second explanation is that both partners may become less attentive to each other's outside pressures. The apparent lack of concern can be very upsetting to an individual already sensitive about sexual performance in middle age.

Male concern with economic pursuits has already been touched on earlier. The man between 40 and 60 years old is at the competitive height in his occupation. His preoccupation with his career and economic problems may lead to a decrease in sexual desire.

Although physical fatigue is certainly a stress that may lead to a decrease in sexual activity, mental fatigue is seen as a much greater deterrent to sexual functioning. Depression is especially linked with a decreased sex drive.

At times throughout the life cycle, individuals may overindulge in food or alcohol as a response to stressful situations. This overindulgence, especially with alcohol, can lead to greatly diminished abilities as well as sexual desires in the man. Alcohol is a known central nervous system depressant that has definite depressing effects on the ability of a man to achieve and maintain an erection. Even one sexual failure in a man already feeling the effects of depression and stress may lead to secondary impotence. Chronic abuse of alcohol is another aspect of this problem, but one that will not be discussed here, since it is a disease process in itself.

Physical and mental infirmities clearly have a potentially inhibiting effect on sexual performance. Particularly in cases of chronic metabolic diseases, such as diabetes, sexual functioning may be altered, and this must be understood. This will be covered in the chapter on medical conditions. In considering the effect of physical and mental infirmities on the older male, one must keep in mind that the regular partner may be the one with the infirmity. If this is the case, masturbation may be the most acceptable form of sexual release available, and may be encouraged by professionals caring for the ill partner. Regularity of sexual expression is the key to sexual responsiveness for the aging male.

The final factor to be discussed is the fear of failure. This fear is often the root cause of secondary impotence. It serves as a self-fulfilling prophecy that can be most damaging. An awareness of the normal changes to expect in aging may be sufficient to prevent performance fears.

MENOPAUSE

Although the term menopause technically refers to the cessation of menstruation in women, it has come to signify a stage in the lives of both women and men. If this broad definition of a stage of life, usually occurring at around 50 years of age, is accepted, then the period can be used to define "male menopause" and "female menopause." Before discussing menopause in men and women, however, some of the stresses and losses that are common to both men and women during this phase will be enumerated. They should be taken into consideration as a backdrop to any problems encountered by the aging adult, including those with sexual implications. It is foolish for professionals to think that sexual problems exist in a vacuum, separate from the influences of the rest of the world. Sexual functioning must be viewed in the context of the whole life situation. Some of the losses common to members of this age group are as follows (Berman, 1976):

1. Loss, caused by death, relocation, or simply withdrawal, of people around them who give meaning to their lives (spouse, children, relatives, etc.).
2. Loss of role and status following retirement, with concomitant loss of income.
3. Some loss of cognitive function. (This is less likely with adequate nutrition and stimulation in the absence of severe illness.)
4. Loss of physical power or physical health.

Menopause—Female

Physiological menopause, the cessation of menstruation for at least 12 consecutive months, usually begins between the ages of 48 and 52. The process lasts approximately two years. Biological changes that accompany the cessation of menses include a decrease in the production of estrogen and progesterone. At menopause, the ovaries become less responsive to the pituitary hormones FSH and LH, with a resulting decrease in the production of estrogen and progesterone and the cessation of ovulation. (The cessation of ovulation is actually a more gradual process than is commonly believed, since although women continue to have menstrual periods throughout their childbearing years, some of these cycles are anovulatory.) Because the ovaries are not responding to the levels of FSH and LH commonly present, the pituitary releases more of these hormones. This is, however, ineffective to stimulate ovulation but does result in a hormone imbalance in the woman.

The most commonly encountered response of the body to this hormone imbalance is the "hot flash," or "hot flush" as it is sometimes called. The flash is experienced as a sudden sensation of heat in the upper body, and is sometimes accompanied by a red, blotchy appearance of the skin of the upper body. The flash may last for several seconds to several minutes. Some women sweat heavily during the flashes, while others report a subjective feeling of heat without sweating. Often, following the flash, the woman will feel quite chilled. Flashes occur during the day and night. If they occur during sleep, they often awaken the woman, thus disturbing her normal sleep patterns. The actual cause for the flashes is not known, although it is thought to be related to the aforementioned hormone imbalance and the body's attempt to readjust itself to a decreased level of estrogen.

A decrease in vaginal moisture and elasticity is also associated with the menopause in women. Because of the general atrophy of the vagina, women may experience dyspareunia, which can often be completely eliminated by the use of an artificial lubricant. The vaginal atrophy and decrease in lubrication make the woman more susceptible to vaginal infections, which may also lead to dyspareunia. The infections, which generally are collectively called atrophic vaginitis, respond to treatment and can often be completely eliminated as a source of difficulty if the woman will seek the appropriate medical care and receives humane, thoughtful treatment as an active sexual being.

Some other symptoms associated with the menopause in women include swelling of the extremities, especially the ankles and feet (dependent edema), palpitations, dizziness, sleeplessness, headaches, decreased energy, and fatigue. The last symptoms, sleeplessness, headaches, and fatigue, may be secondary to hot flashes, which may be disturbing the sleep.

The actual cause or causes for these symptoms and the other symptoms discussed above are not known conclusively at this time (Boston Woman's Health Collective, 1976). There are two prevailing theories. The first has been discussed already—the estrogen deficiency theory. This idea seems to have come from the finding that treatment with estrogens can alleviate many of the symptoms associated with menopause. The second explanation offered for menopausal symptoms is a theory of cultural origin. It is hypothesized that the aging process itself is extremely stressful in our youth-oriented society. Menopause reminds the woman quite clearly that she is aging. She may then respond to the cultural bias that presupposes that all women will experience menopausal symptoms. It has been found that the woman for whom the mother role has been very important is the most likely to suffer at the loss of her reproductive capacity at a time when the children are leaving home (Hyde, 1979). Such an explanation, although it may contribute to an explanation of why some women experience symptoms while others do not, does not satisfactorily explain all cases of menopausal symptoms. Speaking to this cultural expectation of menopausal symptoms, it is interesting to note that, although at least 50 per cent of all women suffer some uncomfortable symptoms, only about 10 per cent of these are severely affected, to the degree that they will seek medical care (Hyde, 1979; Weideger, 1976).

Treatment of menopausal symptoms should be considered only when the symptoms significantly interfere with the normal activities of daily living. The woman may not be aware of the potential side effects of the treatment, which can be formidable. In order to educate clients on this topic, nurses must become knowledgeable themselves.

The major form of accepted medical treatment for menopausal symptoms utilized at present is estrogen replacement therapy (ERT). The practitioner who prescribes estrogen for the treatment of menopause is, by definition, treating an estrogen deficiency disease; that is, menopause is defined by the practitioner as a disease state rather than as a normal phase in a woman's life. Estrogen, usually in the form of the commonly prescribed drug Premarin, may be administered continuously or cyclically. It has been thought that the cyclic use of estrogens would avoid the potential for long term harmful effects of uninterrupted hormone replacement therapy. The data on these long term effects are confusing to the professional and may be nearly impossible to decipher for the lay person. Retrospective correlational studies have been performed on women with endometrial cancers. That is, studies have been performed on these women for a multitude of factors in order to determine what, if anything, these women have in common thay may predispose them to endometrial cancer. A common significant link is long term use of estrogen replacement therapy. When considering the findings from correlational studies, one must be careful not to read more into them than actually exists. A cause-and-effect relationship cannot be inferred. There may be any number of variables other than the use of estrogen replacement therapy that could account for the incidence of endometrial cancer, such as genetic makeup, diet, emotional makeup, or other factors. For some women though, the knowledge of the above-mentioned data is sufficient to convince them to avoid estrogen therapy. They should be given the opportunity to use estrogen creams, which are applied directly to the vaginal tissues, as an alternative to oral replacement estrogens with their systemic effects. The creams are effective in decreasing the vaginal symptoms that occur at menopause. Only when the symptoms significantly interfere with the client's activities of daily living should estrogen replacement therapy be considered. At that point, it may be determined that the benefit of such treatment outweighs the risks.

Not all women are good candidates for estrogen replacement therapy. Women with a history of cancer, recurrent cysts, or blood clots should not be so treated. In addition, women with kidney disease, liver disease, endometriosis, or fibroids should use estrogen replacement therapy only under very close medical observation.

The risks and potential side effects of estrogen replacement therapy are very similar to those of birth control pills. Increased susceptibility to blood clots and increased risk of hypertension are two of the most serious potential side effects of estrogen replacement therapy. In addition, women may experience nausea, breast tenderness, fluid retention, and an increase in breast size. Breakthrough bleeding, another commonly encountered side effect of hormone therapy, is more dangerous in menopausal and postmenopausal women, since it may serve to mask more serious disorders if it is dimissed as a withdrawal bleeding caused by insufficient hormone effects. To avoid this problem, most physicians prescribe a combination type pill, used cyclically, so that they will be quickly alerted to any abnormal bleeding.

The major benefit of estrogen replacement therapy is a reduction in menopausal symptoms. For many women the symptoms are completely alleviated. Estrogen replacement therapy may also be responsible for a decrease in osteoporosis. However, this effect lasts only three to nine months and the rate of osteoporosis may actually increase after this time (Boston Woman's Health Collective, 1976).

The stereotypical image of the menopausal woman is not an attractive one. She is seen as ". . . exhausted, irritable, unsexy, hard to live with, irrationally depressed, and unwillingly suffering a 'change' that marks the end of her active (re)productive [sic] life" (Boston Woman's Health Collective, 1976). As with old age, myths about menopause abound (Rubin, 1965; Butler, 1977; Weideger, 1976). Some of the more commonly encountered myths that are specific to menopausal women are noted (Butler, 1977; Rubin, 1965):

1. There is a loss of attractiveness and the development of masculine features after menopause.
2. Insanity often accompanies menopause.
3. Menopause is a terrible ordeal, with symptoms that will persist indefinitely.
4. Cancer is more likely at menopause than at any other time.
5. After menopause a woman loses her sexual desire and is less capable of sexual functioning than before menopause.

Myths 1 and 5 can be discussed together. Masculinization at menopause does not occur. Fear of losing attractiveness may certainly contribute negatively to a woman's sexual desire, as surely as fear of failure to attain an erection can be a deterrent to a man's sexual functioning. The commonly described physiological changes do not necessarily signify decreased ability of a woman to function sexually, provided she has access to proper counseling and information.

Fears of insanity at menopause spring from the tremendous publicity that the involutional psychoses have received. True psychosis at menopause is very rare. Only 10 per cent of all women suffer from menopausal disturbances that are severe enough to prompt them to seek medical treatment. The number of women who develop psychosis is infinitely smaller than this 10 per cent figure. The fear of insanity may be aggravated in some women when they experience depression, mood swings, or other commonly encountered symptoms associated with role changes. They may interpret these new symptoms as the first step toward eventual insanity. Their anxiety may magnify these symptoms, causing the depression to inadvertently worsen. Supportive care, coupled with information about the exceedingly rare incidence of psychosis as a result of menopause, can help to decrease unnecessary and unfounded fears.

The fear of cancer developing at menopause is more difficult to soothe. It is true that the incidences of some types of cancer, such as breast cancer and cervical and uterine cancer, do seem to increase in postmenopausal women, but an examination of the incidence of cancer in women illustrates the fact that it is distributed fairly evenly throughout the life cycle (Rubin, 1965).

The fact that only a small proportion of women experience severe menopausal symptoms has already been discussed at some length. The widespread fear of severe symptoms, however, can be seen as support for the cultural theory of the origin of menopausal symptoms.

Do the attitudes of women reflect these myths? Several researchers have investigated this question (Neugarten, 1963; Rubin, 1966; Weideger, 1976), and findings seem to confirm that women who have not yet experienced menopause tend to have the most negative and fearful attitudes toward it. Middle aged women had a more positive view, feeling that menopause would not create a major discontinuity in their lives. Older women, women who were currently experiencing menopause or who had already finished menopause, seemed to be the most positive toward it, perhaps because they had been through it and had found that their worst fears had not been realized. Some older women were found to recognize menopause as a type of "recovery." They reported that they felt better, more confident, calmer, and freer than before menopause. Often women reported that they enjoyed the freedom from the menstrual period, which they saw as an inconvenience once their child-bearing years were over. The freedom from fear of pregnancy was an important factor in reported increases in sexual desires and enjoyment in the later years.

The changes in attitudes of women toward menopause that seem to exist at different ages are quite interesting and somewhat unexpected. Logic would seem to indicate an increased anxiety with impending menopause rather than the decrease in these fears that was actually reported by women in these samples. Perhaps the subjects were not a random sampling, or perhaps the myths are dying out, slowly but surely. Whichever is the case, it is of great importance to the psychological well-being of women and their partners to be aware of the realities of sexuality during and after menopause. Lack of information can contribute to an increase in anxiety and a consequent decrease in sexual expression where no decrease is indicated.

Menopause—Male

There is no real male complement to female menopause. There is, however, a gradual decrease in testosterone and sperm production in aging men. As a result of the decreased output of sex hormones, some men exhibit nervous symptoms such as are commonly associated with the female menopause—irritability, insomnia, depression, and sometimes even hot flashes. The condition may strike professionals and friends as funny; thus, a man experiencing the symptoms is not as likely to receive support for his feelings and may isolate himself to avoid the joking he may encounter as a result of these symptoms (especially hot flashes). There is also an increased incidence of prostate enlargement in men as they grow older. It is estimated that 10 per cent of men at the age of 40 have enlarged prostates, while 50 per cent of 80-year-old men have this problem. An enlarged prostate can cause urinary problems as well as performance fears (Hyde, 1979).

More important to our discussion of role changes at this time of life is the typical "career crisis" experienced by many men in this age group. Often further advancement within their careers is unlikely. Rather than feeling appreciated for this years of experience, they may feel that they are seen as rigid and old fashioned. In fact, their fears in this regard may be justified.

At this point, the man may realize that some of the dreams he has held throughout his adult life will never be fulfilled. This realization may lead to depression and contribute to an already faltering sense of self-esteem.

Because of the decreasing speed of erection and the difficulty some men experience in maintaining erections, virility fears may become very real and disturbing to men in this age group. This may lead to a fear of failure during intercourse. This is often the period in life in which previously monogamous men may have extramarital affairs. These affairs, though often upsetting, can be viewed at least partially as a move toward reaffirmation of the man's sexuality and sense of control over his life and his destiny. Masters and Johnson have found that sometimes if a man has been impotent with his usual sex partner, he may avoid further sexual activities with her out of a fear of failure. He may then seek and be successful with another partner. The success may lead him to believe that his impotence is limited to his usual sexual partner. His fears of performance failure may make this another self-defeating and self-fulfilling prophecy. Knowledge of the normal nature of his decreased speed in attaining an erection can do much to allay the fears of the aging man.

Menopause can be a difficult time for both women and men. Given the appropriate guidance and teaching, however, this developmental crisis has the potential for growth and a positive resolution.

NURSING IMPLICATIONS

Introduction

Thus far in this chapter we have confined discussion to the aging client and to society's attitude toward the older person. We will now turn our attention to the nurse and her unique role in dealing with the sexual changes in the elderly.

In order to review and illustrate the four components required in the establishment of a therapeutic relationship, a commonly encountered situation will be presented. These components, which were discussed in Chapter 1, are as follows (Benjamin, 1969; Lief, 1976):

1. Sensitivity of nurses to their own attitudes, values, and feelings
2. Sensitivity of nurses to their patients' attitudes, values, and feelings
3. Assurance of confidentiality
4. Development of trust

Ellen is a young nurse who graduated several months ago. Mr. Bell is well known to the nursing staff, having been admitted many times before. He is 72 years old and usually docile. At times, however, he had been known to be very sexually aggressive with the nurses, especially the younger ones, patting them and grabbing for various parts of their bodies. His behavior has been punished by tying his hands down to the geri-chair in which he sat. At report, Ellen learned that she was assigned to work with and take care of the unit's "dirty old man." Since Ellen was new to the unit, she questioned the staff on the general behavior of Mr. Bell and was assured that she would "find out soon enough."

Thus far, Ellen was in the first stage of understanding. All that she understood about Mr. Bell was that he had been joked about and generally avoided by the nursing staff. At this point Ellen felt a definite sense of anxiety about dealing with Mr. Bell.

After report, Ellen visited her patients briefly, including Mr. Bell. He was in bed and she remained at the foot of the bed. However, he was not able to hear her so she had to move closer to him. As she approached the bed, he grabbed out for her and pinched her on the abdomen. Ellen's first reaction was that of anger. She pulled

away roughly and told Mr. Bell that the behavior was inappropriate. After she admonished him, Mr. Bell seemed to behave better and Ellen then continued on her rounds.

Once Ellen was out of the room she attempted to figure out what caused Mr. Bell's advance. She was certain that she felt it to be degrading to her, but she wasn't ready to understand it from Mr. Bell's point of view. After thinking about the situation for some time, Ellen decided that she would view Mr. Bell's inappropriate behavior as the testing behavior that is normally seen in the beginning phases of a relationship. Feeling this to be the case, Ellen was more able to deal with Mr. Bell without feeling as angry. She decided that she would set limits on his behavior but would not avoid him. as was her initial response to the situation. Ellen was in the second stage of understanding here. She had called on her own knowledge and had come up with a very plausible explanation for Mr. Bell's inappropriate behavior. It is important to note here that Ellen was able to separate herself from the situation. She did not take the behavior exhibited toward her personally, but recognized that it served some purpose for Mr. Bell.

As the day continued, Ellen tried to determine how she would feel in Mr. Bell's situation. He was alone in the hospital, with a wife who lived several hours from the hospital. She was able to visit him only once a week when she was able to find a ride to the hospital. Even though he had been in the hospital before, Ellen recognized that Mr. Bell must have been suffering from feelings of impotence in such a strange and threatening atmosphere. While in the hospital, Mr. Bell was not treated as an individual of worth, but rather as a geriatric patient, and a troublesome one at that. Ellen spent some time during the day talking to Mr. Bell, who seemed to respond very well to her limit setting. She found out from him that in his youth he had worked in building construction and had been extremely strong. However, he reported that since he had aged, all that was now behind him. Ellen began to see what a strain it must be on such a man to become old, with the inevitable physical changes that accompany aging. She then began to see his behavior as

an attempt to try to maintain his self-image as a strong masculine and virile man, despite his dependency at the moment.

Ellen had proceeded more into the third stage of understanding here. She was beginning to understand how Mr. Bell felt in his situation. Her discussion with him indicated a real interest in Mr. Bell, to which he responded very favorably. By the end of the day, the previously "helpless" Mr. Bell was actively participating in his own care, and the inappropriate behaviors with Ellen had significantly decreased. Ellen reasoned, and correctly so, that Mr. Bell's self-confidence had been improved as a result of the respect and understanding she had shown him. A trusting relationship between the two of them had begun to develop because of Ellen's interest, understanding, and openness. Mr. Bell felt comfortable that Ellen would disclose only that information necessary to enable the staff to better understand his situation.

Ellen's behavior with Mr. Bell demonstrated sensitivity to her own feelings and a sensitivity to Mr. Bell's feelings. The so-called "dirty old man" syndrome is cited repeatedly in the literature (Blazer, 1977; Fox, 1977; Peace, 1974). Most often, the behavior is not sexual but is a result of anxiety on the part of the patient. The appropriate treatment is to respond to the client with respect and to provide positive feedback rather than avoiding and labeling. Limit setting is clearly necessary at the beginning stages of the relationship, but it has been found that if the individual is given increased responsibilities and chances for success, the self-confidence will improve. This improved self-confidence is almost surely to be followed by a decrease in the inappropriate behaviors. To behave as Ellen did in this situation is not easy, especially in light of the information and sanctions she received from her peers to avoid Mr. Bell as much as possible. She behaved in an appropriate and professional manner, and received rewards for her efforts.

It should not be assumed that it is only men who express their frustration by sexually inappropriate behavior. Women too feel threatened with a loss of power and femininity in some situations and may react in much the same way. Again, the same type of interaction is necessary—one of support and firm guidance.

THE NURSING HISTORY WITH AGING ADULTS

In order for nurses to function properly as teachers of the elderly regarding sexuality, and as counselors for this group, they must have at their disposal some baseline of data from which to proceed. The sexual history is an important and essential tool for nurses to utilize to identify problems and strengths and to then formulate a mutually acceptable plan of care for the client. It is in the area of obtaining the information on the sexual history that many nurses become nervous and somewhat reluctant to proceed. They fear that they are "prying" and that the clients will not provide them with the necessary information, or that the clients will tell them that it is none of their business. However, as Pfeiffer (1968) found, "It is nevertheless the experience of long-term investigators in this field . . . that people are reasonably open about the sexual behavior when it is inquired into by an objective observer who is thoroughly comfortable with the subject of inquiry."

An outline for the sexual history data that are relevant to the elderly population is presented here. This history is taken from Masters and Johnson (1970). The nurse may or may not need to use this form completely. The situation will have to dictate that information which is seen as necessary. This particular format has been utilized, since it is the most complete form that the author has yet encountered, and because it conforms to some of the necessary rules for eliciting sexual information.

History: Aging Population

(These questions should be used in addition to general material; they are designed to provide a point of interrogative departure *only*.)
  1. What is the current state of the marriage?
     a. What are your "feelings" for your partner?
     b. What is your partner's response to you?
     c. What in your marriage is of mutual interest?
     d. Do you spend leisure time together?
  2. How have your sexual attitudes altered in recent years?
     a. Those of your partner?
     b. Those of your friends?
  3. How have your sexual patterns altered?
     a. Frequency of intercourse?
     b. Difficulties with intercourse?
     c. Responsivity with intercourse?
     d. Your partner's responsivity or difficulties with intercourse?
  4. How have your social attitudes changed?
     a. Residual "double standard" concepts?
     b. Your religious viewpoints?
     c. Your political viewpoints?
     d. Your partner's social attitudes?
  5. *(Husband)* Are you regularly employed?
     a. Nature of employment?
     b. Fulltime? If not, describe.
     c. What other professional interests?
  6. *(Wife)* What are your interests outside the home?
     a. Are you employed? If so, describe.
     b. What percentage of your time is spent outside the home?
  7. What are your family commitments?
     a. Children still living at home? Describe level of time demand.
     b. Relatives that demand share of time? Describe.
  8. What is your state of physical health?
     a. Describe generally.
     b. Any specific difficulties? Describe.
     c. Previous surgery? Describe. Pelvic surgery (male or female)?
     d. *(Wife)* Menopausal symptoms?
        (1) How much distress? Describe symptoms.
        (2) Sex hormone replacement? If so, describe.
     e. Maintenance dosage of any form of medication? If so, describe.
     f. Partner on maintenance medication? If so, describe.
  9. What hobbies or other areas of interest?
     a. Those of your partner?
     b. Do these outside interests enhance or substitute for marital communion?
     c. Your partner's opinion?

10. What are the specific interests that bring you to treatment at this time?
    a. Did you or your partner initiate treatment demand?
    b. What changes would successful treatment make in your marriage?
    c. What changes in you as a personality?
    d. What changes in your partner as a personality?

General Material

(The following material should be developed with chronologic significance within this interrogative framework as indicated by content of answers to questions and general demeanor of patient at the time question is answered.)
  1. Major environmental changes, nature and effect.
  2. People: attitudinal influence, contributing to social and sexual value systems.
  3. People: sexual influence, contributing to sexual value system.
  4. Random events of sexual significance.
  5. Events of sexual orientation, outside life-cycle expectations:
     a. Incest
     b. Illegitimate pregnancy
     c. Abortion
     d. Rape
     e. Infidelity
     f. Homosexuality
     g. Random (other)

This form is a continuation of the sexual history form presented in the second chapter of this book. The format is general in nature and should be tailored to the individual needs of the client.

Often during sexual history taking, areas of concern will arise. These concerns can be alleviated at that time with appropriate knowledgeable and supportive teaching by the nurse.

The setting for the interview is very important to the ultimate success of the history taking. The nurse should provide a relaxed atmosphere in which external distractions and interruptions are minimized as much as possible. Privacy must be provided, and assurances of confidentiality are necessary. Particularly when dealing with older people, in taking the sexual history the nurse should avoid the use of patronizing language. Calling a person "Granddad" or "Grandma" rather than by his or her name places the person in a group-defined role that generally denies him or her individuality and sexuality. Respect for the individual is of great significance.

In determining the amount of sexual activity, the nurse should avoid direct questions, which can be seen as very threatening. Asking elderly clients whether or not they are having their usual amount of sexual activity at the present time gives them many more possible ways to answer. Assumptions are avoided by the use of such statements.

One area not included in the general guidelines for the history provided earlier is the determination of the drugs, if any, that elderly clients are currently taking. Many of the drugs prescribed by physicians for the treatment of the chronic diseases that are common to elderly people have the side effect of decreasing libido; that is, they decrease the sex drive. Some of the more common drugs that have this as a potential side effect follow (Glover, 1977):

Drugs Often Used by Elderly that Tend to Suppress Libido

Antispasmodics-Anticholinergics	*Sedatives*
Diphenhydramine	Barbiturates
Propantheline bromide	Antiasthmatics
Atropine	Alcohol
Trihexyphenidyl	Flurazepam

Narcotics
    Codeine
    Meperidine
    Oxycodone
    Heroin

Stimulants
    Epinephrine
    Amphetamines
    Caffeine (small amounts)
    Anorexic agents
    Methylphenidate
    Ephedrine

Antihypertensives
    Chlorothiazide
    Guanethidine
    Hydralazine
    Rauwolfia alkaloids
    Pargyline
    Methyldopa

Antianxiety Agents (in large doses causing CNS depression)
    Meprobamate
    Diazepam
    Chlordiazepoxide
    Oxazepam
    Clorazepate dipotassium

Antidepressants
    Tricyclics
    Monoamine oxidase inhibitors
    (MAOI)

Tranquilizers
    Phenothiazines
    Thioxanthenes
    Butyrophenones
    Dihydroindolones
    Haloperidol

If it is determined that the elderly client being interviewed is taking any of these drugs, more careful questioning into his or her sexual activities following this drug regimen should be considered. The client should be educated by the nurse that the possibility of decreased libido does exist as a result of the drug therapy. If this is distressing to the client, the nurse should encourage the client to discuss with the physician the possibility of alternative treatments to reduce or eliminate the undesirable side effects. Often, just the knowledge that medication is the cause of the dysfunction or lack of interest can greatly support the client, who may have been imagining far worse causes for the problem.

After the nurse gathers the sexual history data, a problem and strength list can be generated. Often the nurse will find large areas of misinformation and doubt that will require a great deal of teaching. The role of nurse as teacher is both necessary and appropriate. The primary goal of the well-educated and informed nurse is to share with clients knowledge of the effects of aging on sexuality. Counseling should be available for the aging adult regarding vaginitis, dyspareunia, impotence, and the effects of disease on the sexuality of the aging individual (Burnside, 1975). In addition, the nurse is in a position to encourage regular physical examinations as a preventive form of health care.

The importance of masturbation, especially when sexual partners are unavailable, is another area in which the nurse can serve the function of teacher. Masturbation serves some valuable functions. The practice of regular sexual release, including masturbation, helps to preserve potency in men and sexual functioning in women. Masturbation offers release of sexual tension and may bring about an increased sexual appetite. Overall, masturbation leads to the general well-being of the individual (Butler, 1977).

The Nurse as Educator

The goal of education about sexuality of the aging is to establish the right of older people to express their sexuality freely and without guilt (Rubin, 1965). Part of the educational responsibility of the nurse is to work to clear away the mental obstacles that in our society prevent the fullest and most creative expressions of sexuality. Nurses must emphasize the need for society to recognize that sexuality in older people is normal. As Kuhn has encouraged, the elderly should be viewed in relation to their positive aspects, including the positive value of their sexuality.

The Nurse as Patient Advocate

The role of nurse as patient advocate encompasses the roles of counselor and teacher but is viewed separately here to include discussion of care of the elderly in nursing homes and institutions. The nursing home has been seen as primarily responsible for neutering the elderly in our society (Moran, 1977). It has been, and continues to be, common to segregate patients in nursing homes by sex. This separation of men and women is even enforced in cases where married couples enter the nursing home together (Butler, 1977; Chapman, 1976; McKinley and Drew, 1977; Moran, 1977). It would appear that expression of sexuality within the nursing home is considered taboo. Any violation of this institutional taboo is likely to be met with punishment in the form of ridicule, bed checks, medication to curb the "inappropriate" behavior, and/or threats of discharge. Privacy is practically unheard of, despite the fact that many of the individuals living in nursing and convalescent homes are not seriously ill. Conjugal visits between married couples are rarely provided for and for couples who are not married they are nonexistent. Group activities planned for the elderly in the nursing home seem to be geared to a juvenile level, without regard or provision for distinct male or female preferences. This total denial of the sexuality of the older resident of the nursing home can be devastating. If, to compensate for the lack of sexual release with a partner, elderly residents decide to masturbate, they risk the censure of the staff if they are "caught." Masturbation, which is common in institutions, seems to be a source of great discomfort to many professional staffs.

Some older residents of nursing homes have reported that they feel they have been reduced by the staff to the status of infants (McKinley and Drew, 1977). They complain that they are constantly surrounded by sexually attractive young staff people. If the resident should reach out to touch any of these younger people, the touch is likely to be met with intense disgust and the individual labeled a dirty old man or a confused and foolish old woman. In addition to being exposed daily to these attractive staff members, the individual is expected to undress in front of them without displaying any sign of sexual excitement. This is obviously more difficult for the male patient, whose sexual excitement is more difficult to disguise. As a result of this treatment, they may become very resentful of the "neuter" status into which they have been forced.

What is the role of the nurse in all of this? Education is of great importance here. Nursing homes must include in-service education in sexuality of the aging adult as part of the curriculum. Discussion of sexuality openly with staff, peers, and students is required so that problems can surface and be discussed and handled with common sense and honesty while avoiding embarrassment. The staff of the nursing home can be taught to use each other as resources in dealing with sexual situations. The legitimate role of the aged individual as a sexual being must be recognized.

Given an educated staff, the role of the nurse as patient advocate is more easily understood. Nurses are in an excellent position to intervene on behalf of the aged in matters of sexuality. Their professional status may allow them to demand more attention to the problems, and their calm acceptance of sexuality in the elderly can be an excellent starting point in the education of the families of the elderly regarding sexual expression in their parents.

Some issues to be confronted regarding the sexual expression of residents include segregation of residents by sex, privacy, social permissiveness, and creation of an environment in which the individual is supported and respected. To start, when elderly couples are admitted to a facility, nurses should push for the careful frequent assessment of the needs of both individuals. Double beds should be provided for couples. It must be remembered that the act of merely sleeping in the same bed with another individual, even without sexual relations, can be an important lifelong pattern that can cause great anxiety if disturbed.

Privacy for all residents is crucial. The practice of a quick knock before entering a room is not sufficient. Staff must be encouraged and even required to refrain from entering a room unless given permission by the client. (This is not possible, of course, when the elderly person is so ill as to require close observation, but can be carried out in almost all other situations.) The staff should realize that sexual activity, in order to be enjoyable to both parties, cannot exist with the constant threat of interruption.

Most of the foregoing discussion concerned the married couple in the nursing home. There are many more women than men in the older age brackets. Attraction to a new partner, perhaps one met in the nursing home, is not uncommon. These new couples, if not ridiculed and separated, have the potential to develop deep and meaningful relationships, which may include sexual activity. The nursing home staff must come to terms with their prejudices about sexual activities among the elderly in general, and then must learn to deal with sexual activity between people who are not married. Sexual expression remains a need throughout life, regardless of marital status.

The basic idea in this discussion of sexual expression in the elderly in nursing homes is to push for an attitude of permissiveness to expressions of sexuality. Sexuality should be encouraged in the elderly. Masturbation can be recommended to the elderly client if this appears to be the only available outlet. Indeed, masturbation can be encouraged within the context of a continuing relationship to help make up for differences in sexual drive.

SUMMARY AND CONCLUSIONS

In this chapter have been discussed the common myths concerning sexuality in older people and the ways in which these myths can be eliminated. The facts about the changes in human sexual response cycle of the aging man and woman have been covered. Menopause in both women and men has been described. Finally, the role of the nurse in dealing with the sexuality of the elderly has been discussed.

Nursing is in a position of great importance regarding the field of sexuality. Nurses are educating themselves and others on this topic, and are learning to have the time commitment and skills to ensure the sexual expression of their clients. The goal of holistic care, caring for the whole individual, is closer to being met now that nurses are dealing with the sexual realities of their clients.

References

Benjamin, Alfred: *The Helping Interview*. Boston, Houghton Mifflin Company, 1969.

Berman, Ellen, and Lief, Harold: "Sex and the Aging Process." *In* Oakes, Wilbur, Melchiode, Gerald, and Fischer, Ilda (Eds.): *Sex and The Life Cycle*. New York, Grune and Stratton, 1976.

Blaser, Dan: "Adding Life to Years: Late Life Sexuality and Patient Care." *Nursing Care, 10*:28–29, July, 1977.

Boston Woman's Health Collective: *Our Bodies, Ourselves*. New York, Simon and Schuster, 1976.

Burnside, Irene: "Sexuality and Aging." *In* Burnside, Irene (Ed): *Sexuality and Aging*. Los Angeles, The University of Southern California Press, 1975.

Burnside, Irene: "Sexuality and the Older Adult: Implications for Nursing." *In* Burnside, Irene (Ed): *Sexuality and Aging*. Los Angeles, The University of Southern California Press, 1975.

Butler, Robert N., and Lewis, Myrna: *Aging and Mental Health*. St. Louis, C V. Mosby, 1977

Chapman, Ruth: "No Longer at Risk: Sex Among the Elderly." *Family Planning Perspectives, 8*(5):253, September/October, 1976.

Ehrenreich, Barbara, and Enflish, Deirdre: *Complaints and Disorders: The Sexual Politics of Sickness*. Old Westbury, The Feminist Press, 1973.

Fox, Nancy L.: "Speak Out for the Double Bed." *Journal of Practical Nursing. 27 (8)*:22–23, August, 1977.

Glover, Benjamin H.: "Sex Counseling of the Elderly." *Hospital Practice. 12*:101–113, June, 1977.

Gress, Lucille.: "Human Sexuality and Aging." *In* Barnard, Martha, Clancy, Barbara, and Krantz, Kermit (Eds.): *Human Sexuality for Health Professionals*. Philadelphia, W. B. Saunders Company, 1978.

Hyde, Janet S.: *Understanding Human Sexuality*. New York, McGraw-Hill Book Co., 1979.

Kinsey, A., Pomeroy, W., and Martin, C.: *Sexual Behavior in the Human Male*. Philadelphia, W. B. Saunders Co., 1948.

Kinsey, A., Pomeroy, W., Martin, C., and Gebhard, P.: *Sexual Behavior in the Human Female*. Philadelphia, W. B. Saunders Co., 1953.

Kuhn, Margaret E.: "Sexual Myths Surrounding the Aging." *In* Oakes, Wilbur, Melchiode, Gerald, and Ficher, Ilda (Eds.): *Sex and the Life Cycle*. New York, Grune and Stratton, 1976.

Lief, Harold, and Berman, Ellen: "Sexual Interviewing of the Individual Patient Through the Life Cycle." *In* Oakes, Wilbur, Melchiode, Gerald, and Ficher, Ilda (Eds.): *Sex and the Life Cycle*. New York, Grune and Stratton, 1976.

Masters, William: "Geriatric Sexuality." *Reproductive Biology Research Institute*, unpublished. Boston, 1978.

Masters, William, and Johnson, Virginia: *Human Sexual Inadequacy*. Boston, Little, Brown and Co., 1970.

Masters, William, and Johnson, Virginia: *Human Sexual Response*. Boston, Little, Brown and Co., 1966.

McKinley, Hedi, and Drew, Belle: "The Nursing Home: Death of Sexual Expression." *Health and Social Work. 2*:180–187, August, 1977.

Moran, Joyce: "Sexuality After Sixty." *Association of Rehabilitation Nursing*. July/ August, 1977, pp. 19–20.

Neugarten, Bernice L., and Kraines, Ruth: "Women's Attitudes Toward the Menopause." *Vita Humana. 6*:140–151, 1963.

Pease, Ruth A.: "Female Professional Students and Sexuality in the Aging Male." *Gerontologist*. April, 1974, pp. 153–157.

Pfeiffer, Eric, Werwoerdt, Adriaan, and Wang, Hsioh-Shan: "Sexual Behavior in Aged Men and Women." *Archives of General Pyschiatry. 19*:753–758, December, 1968.

Pfeiffer, Eric, and Davis, Glenn: "Determinants of Sexual Behavior in Middle and Old Age." *Journal of the American Geriatrics Society. 20* (4):151–158, April, 1972.

Rubin, Isadore.: *Sexual Life After Sixty.* New York, Basic Books, Inc., 1965.

Semmens, James, and Semmens, Jane: "The Sexual History and Physical Examination." *In* Barnard, Martha, Clancy, Barbara, and Krantz, Kermit (Eds.): *Human Sexuality for Health Professionals.* Philadelphia, W. B. Saunders Co., 1978.

Weideger, Paula: *Menstruation and Menopause: The Physiology and Psychology, the Myth and the Reality.* New York, Alfred A. Knopf, 1976.

Woods, Nancy F.: *Human Sexuality in Health and Illness.* St. Louis, C. V. Mosby Co., 1975.

Issues in Sexuality

CONTRACEPTION

INTRODUCTION

The wish to control the reproductive process has been expressed in various forms throughout history. Today's widespread availability of contraception has been won only through great effort.

In recent times, the terms "family planning" and "contraception" have been used almost synonymously. This usage is not appropriate, as it takes away from the separate meanings of both phrases. The term "contraception" literally means "against conception" and includes all measures taken to avoid pregnancy. No judgment is made as to whether the individual or couple wishes to postpone or completely avoid pregnancy. The term "contraception" is unacceptable for many who view reproduction as an essential part of the lives of all adults. Partly in response to negative reactions to the word "contraception" and partly in an effort to be more precise about the goals of birth control measures, the term "family planning" evolved. In "family planning" there is an implicit acceptance that the individual or couple plan to have children at some time in the future but for some reason want to postpone their family for an undetermined period. Alternately, the term "family planning" can signify a method by which children can be spaced according to the desires of the parents. In either case, "family" is an essential part of the concept of "family planning."

This chapter has been entitled "Contraception" purposely. It is not within the scope of this chapter to discuss the decisions involved in family planning. Rather, the focus lies in the actual contraceptive behaviors, counseling, and history, as well as in the nursing interventions utilized in these areas.

The first section briefly covers the history of contraception. The reader can gain some perspective of the difficulties and successes that have accompanied the so-called "birth control movement," especially in this country. Legal aspects of contraception are discussed in the second section, including the issue of contraceptive use among minors and the issue of informed consent. The third section deals with studies on contraceptive behavior. The fourth and final section is devoted to nursing and deals at some length with the factors necessary to help clients determine what types of contraception, if any, are acceptable to them. In this section, the available methods will be reviewed. Specific situations that are likely to be encountered in nursing practice, such as postpartum contraception, sterilization, and the difficult contraceptive client, will be addressed in this final section.

HISTORICAL PERSPECTIVES

Judeo-Christian Views

In the ancient Judaic culture, any contraceptive that did not interfere with the process of "correct" heterosexual intercourse was permitted. Any interference with the physical act was not "correct." For example, the use of a condom would place a barrier between the man and the woman and was therefore considered unnatural and "incorrect." Similarly, withdrawal was condemned, since it called for an interruption in the process of intercourse (Gordon, 1976). In the Old Testament, one can find references to the prohibition of the practice of withdrawal.

In the ancient Judaic civilization, the family was of great spiritual value and was the ideal toward which individuals would strive. The responsibility for propagation was placed upon the man. Although the family was (and continues to be) important in the Jewish culture, population expansion was not a religious priority or an economic necessity for the ancient Jews.

In early Christianity, a total condemnation of birth control evolved. Sexual pleasure was rejected as the most evil of many evil pleasures. Although, according to St. Paul, sexual pleasure was acceptable within marriage, birth control was viewed as giving license for sexual indulgence, and was therefore forbidden.

About four centuries after St. Paul, Augustine strengthened the prohibition on sexual pleasure even further, mandating that sexual intercourse was to be engaged in only for procreation. The sexual drive itself was described as an evil burden that had been placed upon man as a result of the Fall. Birth control, especially the rhythm method, was considered to be a mortal sin (Gordon, 1976).

By the thirteenth century, Thomas Aquinas codified the prohibitions on sexual pleasure to the point that every act of intercourse even within marriage came to be seen as a sin unless it was performed with "reproductive intent."

Nineteenth Century Views on Contraception

Despite the opposition to the use of contraception from the powerful Catholic church, many individuals and couples decided to use the birth control measures that were available to them during the nineteenth century. These methods included withdrawal, douching, and/or the use of intravaginal sponges or cloths. In comparison with our current level of sophistication in the field of contraception, these methods appear poor at best, but they were all that were available at the time. The vulcanization of rubber (around 1840), which led to the development of the latex condom and the diaphragm, was among the first major breakthroughs in contraceptive technology.

Even after more effective means of contraception became possible, individuals wishing to utilize these methods often had difficulty in obtaining them. As of 1873, birth control devices could not be sent legally through the mail. They fell under the dictates of the Comstock laws, federal legislation prohibiting the mailing or importing of "obscene, lewd, or lascivious" materials. Anthony Comstock, secretary and leader of the influential Society for the Prevention of Vice, detailed a specific portion of this legislation, stating that "all information and devices pertaining to the prevention of conception" fell under this law (Sharpe, 1977). The American medical establishment supported the so-called Comstock laws during the nineteenth century. In fact, it was not until 1912 that a physician, Dr. Abraham Jocobi, then president of the American Medical Association, recognized publicly the possibility that family limitation might be advisable (Pickett, 1971).

Twentieth Century Contraception

Opposition to the use of contraception was often based on the fear of "race suicide." During his presidency (1904–1908), Theodore Roosevelt was very vocal regarding the dangers of race suicide. According to Roosevelt, upper and middle class people were not providing sufficient numbers of children to "build the national strength." It was reasoned that if the upper and middle classes chose to limit family size, the lower classes and immigrant populations, with their inferior genes, would soon take over the nation. The "worst evil," according to Roosevelt, was the possibility that the "old native American stock" would become, or had become, less fertile than the immigrant population. The upper classes had to maintain their power and therefore were "duty-bound" to avoid limiting family size (Sharpe, 1977).

The American view of the large family as the ideal continued in this country even after Europeans became more aware of the dangers of overpopulation. The ideas of Malthus were accepted in Europe far earlier than in the United States, partly because the United States' economic and social development was largely isolated from that of the European world, and partly because until around 1890, the United States was considered a nation of expansion in which the larger family had a practical value (Pickett, 1971). Malthus is responsible for our current understanding of the mathematics of overpopulation. He demonstrated that population growth is geometric rather than additive; that is, if a family had three children who each had three children, the net gain in population would be nine in one generation. If each of these nine children had three children, the gain would be 27. The progression illustrated for population growth is geometric—$3 \times 3 \times 3$. This view, figured on the basis of whole populations, led Malthus to predict severe overpopulation in a much shorter time than had been generally believed.

In the early 1900's, Margaret Sanger began her work in the United States, educating women about birth control. In her early writings, Sanger was quite radical. For instance, in *The Woman Rebel*, which she wrote and printed, she damned religion, the Rockefellers, and marriage. In addition, she published a pamphlet discussing the contraceptive techniques that she had learned of in her travels in Europe. In 1914, charges were brought against Sanger and her paper for violation of the Comstock laws. She left the United States to avoid imprisonment.

While Sanger was in exile in Europe, the National Birth Control League was formed in the United States. It was made up primarily of upper class women who shared some of Sanger's beliefs about the rights of women to control their reproductive capacities.

Sanger returned to the United States in 1916 after receiving a pardon. At that time, she opened the first American birth control clinic in New York. Both Sanger and her partner and sister, Ethel Byrne, were later arrested, tried, convicted, and jailed, again under the Comstock laws. The clinic was closed.

Following her release, Sanger joined the National Birth Control League and became its leader. The name of the organization was later changed to the American Birth Control League (ABCL).

By the 1920's the ABCL had 37,000 members, mostly white, middle class, native born Protestant women, who saw birth control as the means to protect American society from the immigrant masses and the unfit. Note that the League at this point was aiming its contraceptive learning toward the lower classes to prevent their overpopulation. Birth control was not yet seen as a step toward the better health and emancipation of women.

In 1923, Margaret Sanger began the Clinical Research Bureau. This was to be a center for the medically supervised study of contraceptive devices. The bureau was isolated from the medical profession, which still generally chose to support the notion that birth control was not necessary. One woman physician made up most of the medical support of the clinic.

In the late 1920's and early 1930's, people's views on contraception began to change. Contraception became acceptable in two cases: for those with very large families and when pregnancy would present a grave danger to the health of the woman. The desire to prevent unwanted children was not considered an acceptable rationale for the use of birth control.

In 1930, the Comstock laws were essentially reversed by a federal court decision allowing "advertisement and shipment of contraceptive devices intended for legal use . . . for the prevention of disease." Interestingly, although the first vulcanization of rubber occurred in the 1840's, it was not until the late 1920's that the vulcanization method was in wide enough use to make latex rubber condoms and diaphragms available to the public.

In 1937, the American Medical Association issued a cautious statement endorsing birth control clinics under strict medical supervision. To achieve this end, the American Birth Control League and the Clinical Research Bureau merged to form the Planned Parenthood Federation of America. The new board, unlike the largely woman-controlled American Birth Control League, was controlled by male physicians.

The advent of America's participation in World War II led to further support for the birth control movement. As men were needed overseas, the need for women in industry led to a push by the United States Public Health Service for states to provide birth control for women in war industry. The use of contraception for these women came to be seen as a patriotic move. In addition, there was a growing awareness of the need for contraception in the poorer countries of the world. Research for newer and more effective methods of contraception began in earnest.

In 1959, Oppenheimer released the first reports of a successful intrauterine device (IUD), and in 1960 the first oral contraceptive, Enovid, was introduced in the United States after clinical trials with Puerto Rican and Haitian women. Nicknamed "the pill," Enovid, manufactured by the Ortho Pharmaceutical Company, contained 10 to 15 mg of estrogen in each daily dose. In comparison with the 30 to 50 μg doses now in use in oral contraceptives, it can be seen as a distant relative of current oral contraceptives.

The 1960's saw further policy changes in the birth control movement. In 1962, the Planned Parenthood Federation of America merged with the World Population Emergency Fund to become Planned Parenthood-World Population. In 1963, the combined PP-WP began a major public push for significant federal involvement in birth control programs, both foreign and domestic.

In 1965, the Office of Economic Opportunity, an agency dealing primarily with the poor, was the first federal agency to make a direct grant for birth control services for the poor. The Maternal and Child Health and Mental Retardation Amendment to the Social Security Act also provided money for prenatal care and later increased emphasis on birth control. In 1967, Congress enacted legislation requiring states to provide family planning services in their public health programs and for women on welfare. Finally, in July of 1969, President Nixon made the first presidential address ever to be directed to the "problem of population growth." In his address, the president proposed the adoption of a national goal to provide birth control services to all women in the United States who wanted them.

The emphasis on birth control and the birth control movement in the 1970's has changed to an even more liberal view. The official view of PP-WP now stresses family planning as a right for the health and welfare of mothers and children. The local officiates may choose other emphases if they wish. The 1970's saw another beginning split with the views that birth control should be available to all. Some political groups who oppose abortion had begun, at the end of the 1970's, to oppose some forms of birth control. These groups, notably the Right to Life organization, propose to ban the use of birth control pills and IUDs because of their potential as abortifacients.

LEGAL ASPECTS

Minors and Contraception

In order to ensure that contraceptive devices would be available to all who wished to use them, a test case was brought before the Supreme Court (381 U.S. 479 [1965]). In the 1965 ruling, the Supreme Court held that the fundamental constitutional right of privacy included the right to the access to contraceptives. However, this right was not extended to minors. In fact, in order to prevent minors from obtaining over-the-counter forms of contraception, many of these contraceptives were removed from public display. In order to obtain these devices, the individual had to ask for them. Minors would be refused.

In 1977, the Supreme Court (431 U.S. 678 [1977]) ruled that minors had the right of access to contraceptives under the same right of privacy act. This ruling did not apply to the use of prescription methods of contraception such as the pill, IUD, or diaphragm. As of this writing, no case in the Supreme Court has been decided in favor of restricting the right of minors to obtain contraceptives of any type (Paul, 1979).

The paucity of court decisions on the question of contraceptives for minors does not mean the area is free of debate. Many adults feel that parental consent should be required before an adolescent is given contraception. In light of the current increase in teenage pregnancy and teenage births, the general consensus seems to be to allow minors access to contraception in the hope of reducing the rate of teenage pregnancy (Digest, 1978).

Informed Consent

In recent years there has been a trend toward the use of consent forms for clients considering the use of contraceptive devices. This move has been brought about by several factors: the increased concern for the right of individuals to make informed decisions about their health and about their lives; the increased number and scope of malpractice suits brought against physicians; anxiety about the potential hazards of the various methods of contraception; and political pressures (Paul, 1979).

In 1969 and 1970, two Food and Drug Administration commissioners and the Secretary of Health, Education, and Welfare affirmed that every woman taking birth control pills had the right to be informed of the potential benefits and risks of this treatment. At that time, detailed labeling was devised. When this labeling was presented to the American Medical Association for approval, it was rejected on the grounds that such information could "needlessly" frighten women. A compromise was reached, which led to a brief warning that the physician dispensed. The small pamphlet, entitled "What You Should Know About the Pill," contained a question and answer format between a woman and her physician. The questions most often revolved around how to take the pill, and had very little reference to the potential hazards of birth control pills (Seaman, 1977).

In July of 1977, the Department of Health, Education and Welfare released its "Program Guidelines for Project Grants for Family Planning Services." These guidelines mandated that all federally funded projects that provided family planning were required to receive signed informed consent from each patient. No specific language was mandated for the consent forms (Paul, 1979).

Finally, the FDA regulations (21 C.F.R. 310.501-310.502) required that women using birth control pills or IUDs receive a manufacturer's insert describing all risks and benefits associated with the message with each package. Again, specific wording was not ordered, although the content to be included was more specifically stated. It was left to the manufacturers to design the warnings, which were to be approved by the FDA. The resulting warnings tended to be lengthy and complicated, and have been judged by some to be highly fear-producing. Most subjects will deny or forget information that is highly fear-producing, perceiving it to be too threatening. Thus, there may be some question as to whether or not the required inserts are actually helping to achieve informed consent.

The notion of informed consent is somewhat confusing legally. The signing of an informed consent form should be the culmination of an educational process during which the needs of the patient, the risks and benefits of all available treatment alternatives, the patient's responsibilities for self-observation for signs of method failure, and the proper treatment method have been explained and are understood (Paul, 1979). One method that has been designed to achieve this goal is the BRAIDED method. Each of the letters stands for one of the components of informed consent:

*B*enefits of treatment
*R*isks of treatment
*A*lternatives to treatment
*I*nquiries about the treatment are encouraged
*D*ecisions to withdraw from the use of a method are all right
*E*xplanation of what to expect from the treatment and how to use the method
*D*ocumentation of the above (usually the client is asked to sign a form that restates the above)

In order for clients to successfully sue a physician on the grounds that informed consent was not given, they must establish that they would not have taken the treatment if they had understood the risks involved and that they were not properly informed of these risks. The physician is not required to provide complete disclosure in the following cases (Paul, 1979):
1. In cases of emergency when informed consent is impossible
2. When complete and candid disclosure might have a detrimental effect on the physical or psychological well-being of the patient
3. When the patient has specifically requested not to be informed

As health care consumers become more knowledgeable and sophisticated about health care, informed consent may be one way to decrease the distance between physicians and clients. Currently, it is tacitly understood that part of the so-called "professional autonomy" of the medical profession is the notion that the physician possesses skills and knowledge so esoteric that they cannot be understood by the average person (Freidson, 1970). This has often been the rationale given to avoid informing clients of their treatment. However, the trend now seems to be toward demystifying and simplifying medical terminology so clients can indeed be fully informed about their treatments. In many cases, it is the nurses who are simplifying the material for clients. Their role in this area is extremely important and will be covered later in this chapter.

CONTRACEPTIVE BEHAVIOR

Studies

Despite the fact that effective contraception is now available to virtually all individuals who wish to use it, expected declines in the birth rate have not materialized. It must be concluded then that availability is not the only factor that determines the use or nonuse of contraception.

Because of the dramatic increase in the teenage pregnancy rates in the United States, many studies have been conducted to investigate why teenagers are not utilizing the available methods of contraception. Reichelt (1975) and Burbach (1980) found that adolescents on the whole were poorly informed in most areas regarding birth control. Twenty-five per cent of the female sample were unable to state when the fertile time in their cycle occurred. Subjects were found to be better informed about abortion and the availability of contraception than they were about birth control itself.

Overall, the findings tend to support Goldstein (1976) in his assertion that individuals who show a capacity to plan ahead, who feel they have control over their futures, and who feel morally free to enjoy sexual intercourse for reasons other than procreation were most likely to be successful in the use of birth control methods. Conversely, women who did not accept the responsibility of intercourse sufficiently to plan for it were generally found to be poor contraceptive risks.

Miller (1976), in a study of 52 single, never previously pregnant 17- to 26-year-old women, discovered some interesting communication patterns between the partners. The average age for first intercourse in this sample was 18. Most women reported that they allowed the first intercourse to occur only when they felt themselves to be in a safe period of their cycle. In this particular sample, only 40 per cent of the women were correctly able to identify the "safe" periods. In addition, the men were often reported to have utilized withdrawal during this first intercourse, without prior discussion with their partner. During the first few months of the relationship, minimal or no explicit communication regarding birth control was reported until one or the other of the partners became anxious enough to discuss the topic while not having intercourse. All of the subjects reported that they had internalized the prohibition on premarital intercourse, and all reported that they felt poorly informed regarding contraceptive methods. Finally, all subjects reported that they were largely ignorant about the nature of sexual experiences in general. Interestingly, an equal number of men and women avoided the use of birth control completely because they wanted pregnancy to occur, since they felt it would lead to marriage.

From this data, Miller created what he called the "Sexual Career Development" of contraceptive usage. In Stage I, couples experienced either unprotected or poorly protected intercourse. This stage usually lasted from one to six months. During this time, there was usually a delayed menstrual period, most often not due to pregnancy. During this stage, clients reported diffuse anxiety, not specifically related to fears of pregnancy.

Stage II, "peer prescription," begins after the client has had a "near miss." The couples were more likely to become moderately anxious regarding the possibility of pregnancy, and at this point many sought information about birth control from peers and parents. After the near-miss experience, however, some of the couples decided that, to avoid the repetition of the fearful situation, they would not have intercourse again. Because of this decision, they reasoned, they would not need contraception. The majority of these couples *did* return to having intercourse, and they essentially returned to Stage I.

The final stage involved the seeking of professional help to determine an acceptable form of contraception that both partners agreed upon. Only after intercourse was accepted as a definite possibility were the contraceptive steps to take effect.

In another series of studies (Zelnick, 1971; Zelnick, 1977), it was found that the use of birth control pills in adolescents had doubled. The use of the IUD had also greatly increased, while the use of condoms, withdrawal, and douching, the most popularly reported methods in the 1971 study, had all decreased significantly. Whereas only 45 per cent of those in the 1971 study reported that they had used contraception during their most recent intercourse, 63 per cent of those in the 1977 study reported using contraception at their most recent intercourse. From the data, Zelnick concluded that the older a woman is at the time of her first intercourse, the more likely she is to use contraception from her first intercourse. In this sample, 55 per cent had had intercourse by the age of 19.

Although the data from the Zelnick studies are encouraging, population statistics continue to show dramatic increases in the teenage pregnancy rates, while birth rates across all other age groups are decreasing. Further investigation is needed to determine what prevents individuals from utilizing effective contraception and what can be done to help prevent unwanted pregnancy in all age groups.

Contraceptive Use

In examining why individuals choose to use contraception, a general list of reasons can easily be generated (Hyde, 1975):
1. To avoid pregnancy among unmarried couples
2. To avoid having unwanted children
3. To avoid having children with birth defects/genetic diseases
4. To avoid health risks to the mother (e.g., diabetes)
5. To improve early marital adjustment
6. To space out pregnancies
7. To curb population growth
8. To permit more self-actualization for women
   Certainly the reader can add to this list.
   While many people share the same general reasons for the use or non-use of birth control, all individuals have their own more private reasons that must be respected. The health care professional must respect the right of the client to choose for or against the use of contraception.
   The decision to use contraception is one that involves many factors from the individual's past as well as current situation. Factors to be discussed here include:
1. Religious attitudes
2. Which partner will accept responsibility for contraception
3. Frequency of intercourse
4. Modesty
5. Cost
6. Availability
7. Effects of method on physical safety and psychological fulfillment
   In terms of religious attitudes, for example, the Catholic who has been taught that any act of intercourse must be opened to procreation may find that the use of oral contraceptives, the IUD, the diaphragm, or condoms is unacceptable.
   Another factor in the choice of birth control methods concerns determining the partner who can most happily and efficiently accept the responsibility for using contraception. The subject of the responsibility for contraception is a potentially loaded one. For some, the responsibility is perceived as belonging to the woman, since it is she who will become pregnant in the event of unprotected intercourse. In fact, many women feel that the use of contraception is not only their responsibility but is also their right in order that they may control their own reproductive functioning. Conversely, there are those who feel that the responsibility for contraception, like the pleasure of intercourse, should be shared. As anyone familiar with the currently available methods of contraception can easily note, most contraception in use today is directed toward the woman. Vasectomy, permanent sterilization of the male, is not acceptable to many men, who may wish to have children in the future. Virtually the only other methods in which the male participates are natural family planning, condoms, and withdrawal. The man may participate in the use of traditionally female contraceptive methods by either helping with the insertion and removal of the diaphragm or, in the case of the other methods, by offering his support for the diligent use of the chosen contraceptive. Many people, both men and women, feel there should be an added push to discover contraception that is safe and effective for men.
   Ideally, both partners are involved in the decision to use contraception. Often, however, one of the partners may decide that the other will use a form

of contraception that the other partner may find unacceptable. For example, the man may tell his partner she must take birth control pills. She may not wish to do so but may feel forced to utilize this method, since her partner may be uncooperative in the use of any other alternative.

A third factor involved in the choice of a contraceptive method is the frequency of intercourse. Some couples may see each other only infrequently or may have the opportunity for intercourse rarely. For these couples, methods such as oral contraceptives, the IUD, or natural family planning may be unacceptable, offering either too much protection, in which the risks outweigh the potential benefits, or too little protection, where the woman's cycle may not coincide with the opportunities for intercourse. For couples having intercourse only rarely, foam and condoms or the diaphragm may be the method of choice. Again, the choice must be made by the couple, taking into account the feelings of each partner.

Modesty may be a strong factor in determining the form of contraception to be used; for example, the woman who is uncomfortable touching her genitals may be a poor candidate for the diaphragm. Lack of privacy and fear of discovery by a parent is often a rationale for refusal to use the pill, the diaphragm, or foam.

Cost and availability are additional factors that must be considered when choosing a form of contraception. Obviously, if a method is too costly it will not be considered for many individuals, regardless of how effective it may be. Also, if a method is not readily available to all potential users it will not be widely used.

The effects of the method upon the physical safety and psychological fulfillment of the couple must also be considered. If one or both of the partners fears that a given method may be harmful, the resulting anxiety can greatly reduce the sexual pleasure. The couple must examine their feelings about the relative safety of any method they consider for contraceptive use.

Despite the fact that highly effective contraception is available to virtually all who seek it out, many people do not use any birth control. Five major reasons for this that have been encountered in the literature and in clinical practice with potential contraceptive users will be discussed. Each of the areas represents one type of deterrent to contraceptive use. Any or all of these factors may be at work in preventing a given individual or couple from effectively utilizing contraception:

1. Misconceptions and myths about contraception
2. Denial
3. Guilt
4. Loss of spontaneity
5. Wish to become pregnant

Myths and misconceptions surrounding conception and contraception continue to flourish, despite the best efforts of educators to correct such misinformation. Perhaps the most common misconception is that women have intercourse only during the "safe" times of their cycles. Few women actually know when the "safe" periods occur. Many men and women also believe it is impossible to become pregnant after only one act of intercourse or if the couple have intercourse only rarely. Obviously, this is untrue, but these notions are difficult to change. Another commonly encountered myth is that young women just past puberty are infertile. The dramatic increase in the teenage pregnancy rate clearly disproves this myth.

As in any dynamic of human life, denial occurs frequently in regard to the use or nonuse of contraception. In order for a person to seek out contraception, the potential for intercourse must be admitted. For a variety of reasons, many people are simply not able to admit this possibility. By denying that intercourse is a possibility, the individuals may be able to avoid facing the fact that they are sexual people.

Closely related to the concept of denial in terms of contraceptive use is the notion of guilt. For example, individuals who feel that intercourse outside of marriage is wrong may avoid planning ahead for intercourse. If contraception is not used during intercourse, the guilt may be decreased by accepting the possible risk of pregnancy. In other words, the individual or couple may be accepting the fact that they may be "punished" for their "bad" behavior by becoming pregnant.

Another aspect of guilt is the reluctance of individuals to utilize methods of contraception that may be found or seen by others. The individual may be embarrassed to have another person find the contraceptive paraphernalia, since that other person would then know or at least surmise that the individual is sexually active. This fear of discovery may be sufficient to dissuade an individual from utilizing effective and otherwise acceptable forms of contraception.

Loss of spontaneity is an often cited rationale for nonuse of contraception, especially regarding the sex-dependent methods such as foam, condom, diaphragm, and natural family planning. The need for spontaneity can be seen, at least in part, as related to denial that intercourse will occur. By requiring that intercourse be fully unplanned, individuals absolve themselves from the responsibility for planning for it. It is true, however, that some of the available methods of contraception are sex dependent and can potentially interfere with foreplay. The condom, for example, must be placed on the erect penis prior to insertion of the penis into the vagina. Foam too must be inserted into the vagina prior to intercourse. For some couples, this interruption may be distracting and unacceptable. For others, however, the application of the condom and the foam may be successfully integrated into the foreplay, and may even enhance pleasure of the partners through this shared responsibility.

Finally, some couples or individuals choose not to utilize contraception because they wish to become pregnant. This wish may be expressed within an ongoing relationship in which the couple agrees to begin a family, or may occur when only one of the partners wishes to have pregnancy result from the intercourse. The reasons for desiring pregnancy are as many and as varied as those for avoiding pregnancy. Some young adolescents see pregnancy as a way out of what they perceive as an unhappy family situation. Others may just wish to have a baby who will love them, somewhat like a doll. Regardless of the motivation, the desire to become pregnant must be considered as a possibility when clients refuse to utilize contraception.

NURSING IMPLICATIONS—CONTRACEPTIVE HEALTH CARE

Factors to Present to Help Client

Because nurses are perceived as approachable, and because they often act as patient advocates, clients seek out nurses with their questions and concerns about contraception. Many clients see nurse practitioners for their contraceptive needs and counseling. The nurse is a person to whom the client can look for factual, unbiased information about contraception. The goal of the nurse in contraceptive teaching and counseling is to help the client to arrive at a decision as to what type (if any) of contraception will be best for that individual. With this in mind, the factors that nurses should have at their disposal will be listed and discussed:

1. Acceptability
2. Accessibility
3. Effectiveness
4. Cost
5. Reversibility
6. Side effects
7. Contraindications
8. Ease of use
9. Mechanism of action

Acceptability.   The best method of contraception is one that the individual is comfortable with and one that will in fact be used. In their attempts to guide clients toward contraceptive methods that are most likely to be successful, health care professionals may lose sight of the client's preferences and comfort. No matter how effective a method is, if the clients are not happy with it, it will not be used. If it is not used, it will not be effective.

Accessibility.   It has been noted that effective forms of contraceptives are available to virtually every individual who wishes to use them. While this is true, it does not mean that every person has access to every method of contraception. For example, some physicians will not dispense contraception to teenagers as a matter of policy. Sexually active teenagers who have been denied contraception by a physician have several alternatives. Certainly, one would hope that they would seek out some other facility, such as Planned Parenthood, for contraception. If this is not possible, they could purchase over-the-counter types of contraceptives such as foam or condoms, which can be very effective.

In various clinics and private offices certain policies have evolved concerning specific forms of contraception. For example, a facility may decide to stop inserting IUDs in women who have never had a pregnancy, since they believe there is, or may have been, a greater expulsion rate in women who have never been pregnant. To avoid the difficulties involved in such situations, a policy may have been made that will prevent a client who is seeking an IUD from receiving one from that facility. In addition, contraindications that exist will by necessity affect the accessibility of certain methods for some individuals.

Effectiveness.   In recent literature, much has been said about the effectiveness of the various forms of contraception. There has been considerable confusion between the statistics quoted for each individual method and for the methods when they are compared with one another. Nurses must be careful to explain the differences between theoretical and user effectiveness to clients.

Theoretical effectiveness is the effectiveness of a method when that method is used perfectly, without error, and exactly according to the instructions (Hatcher, 1978). It is the figure that represents the maximum effectiveness of a method. In determining the *user effectiveness,* all users of a given method are taken into consideration, including those who use the method correctly and those who are careless. User effectiveness, then, is the average enjoyed by a method that accounts for user error (Hatcher, 1978). Confusion arises when various methods are listed by effectiveness, without a statement as to whether the effectiveness is theoretical or user effectiveness. To complicate matters further, in a single listing some methods may be listed according to their theoretical effectiveness, while others are listed according to their user effectiveness. The result of such listings leads to very unfavorable comparisons. For example, comparing the theoretical effectiveness of the birth control pill with the user effectiveness of foam and condoms combined makes the foam and condoms appear far less effective than the pill, when in fact the two are very close in terms of theoretical effectiveness. In the portion of the chapter that deals with the effectiveness of the methods, theoretical effectiveness will be quoted for all methods.

Foam and condoms, the diaphragm, natural family planning, vaginal suppositories, and withdrawal are all immediately reversible. That is, the woman is fertile immediately after the contraception is discontinued. Women taking birth control pills are usually advised to discontinue the pill three to six months prior to becoming pregnant. For some, the menstrual period will return at the regular time after the pill is discontinued. However, for others, secondary amenorrhea may occur. The woman may not have a normal return of her menses for many months or even years.

Women with progesterone and copper IUDs are also being advised to wait at least one month after the removal of the device before attemping to become pregnant. Women with the older plastic IUDs are not usually counseled to delay pregnancy following removal. For them, the IUD is immediately reversible.

At this point in our technology, sterilization is considered to be irreversible, although attempts to devise reversible methods of sterilization are being continually investigated.

The question of reversibility is often a significant one in the initial choice of a contraceptive method. Many couples, faced with the knowledge that they will have to use another form of contraception after discontinuing their preferred form, may choose a less effective but immediately reversible form. It is the right of the client to be informed of the potential risks in regard to return of fertility following discontinuation of various methods of contraception.

Cost. The cost of the various methods will vary from place to place and according to the product. The following prices are estimates and should be utilized as such. The birth control pill costs about $60.00 per year. Foam and condoms cost approximately $50.00 per year ($25.00 for each). IUDs cost about $60.00 per year (note that the IUD is not changed every year). Using the diaphragm with contraceptive cream or jelly will cost about $60.00 per year, and a vacuum abortion can be obtained for about $150.00 (Hatcher, 1978).

In addition to the yearly cost, the amount that must be paid at one time is a consideration. Although the cost for the diaphragm is the same over the period of a year as the IUD, the client may choose to use the diaphragm, since the expense is spread out over the span of the year rather than concentrated in one payment as it would be with the IUD.

Side Effects. Situations that may occur as the result of some treatment or use of some form of medication are usually divided into two categories—

nuisance and dangerous. For example, the discharge that follows use of the diaphragm is considered to be a nuisance side effect, as is the possible nausea that may accompany pill use. In labeling such effects as only nuisance, it should be recognized that being continually nauseated may very well be a firm reason for a client to discontinue the use of birth control pills in favor of a method that would avoid this effect. "Nuisance" should not be thought of by health care professionals as unimportant or insignificant.

Dangerous side effects are those that may be life threatening. For instance, some women develop significant hypertension while taking birth control pills. This hypertension places them at significantly greater risk of cerebrovascular incidents. It has been found that hypertension induced by the birth control pill is almost immediately reversible when the pill is discontinued. This side effect would necessitate discontinuing the birth control pill.

Clients must not only be informed of the potential nuisance effects but must also be made aware of the potentially dangerous effects of any contraceptive they are considering. Clients are thinking individuals responsible for themselves. They, as well as health care professionals, have a role in weighing the dangers of any treatment against the potential benefits of that treatment.

Contraindications. In some cases, a form of contraception may be too dangerous to a client to warrant the risk of its use. For example, women with a history of reproductive cancer have an absolute contraindication to oral contraceptives. Like side effects, contraindications are generally divided into two categories—absolute and relative.

Severe dysmenorrhea is generally listed as a relative contraindication to the use of the IUD. The client should be informed that women who have severe menstrual cramps have been shown to be more likely either to have increased cramps or to be more likely to expel the device. Given this relative contraindication, the woman may make a more fully informed choice and decide whether to risk this procedure.

Ease of Use. The proper method of use for any type of contraceptive must be fully explained to every client. The health care professional must avoid the temptation to think that "everyone knows how to ...". In fact, many people become pregnant because of improper use of a contraceptive method.

Ease of use has already been discussed in terms of sex dependent or sex independent methods. For many couples, this alone can eliminate some forms of contraception. Taking a pill each day may not be possible for some women, who may find their schedule too erratic or may find that they forget to take medications. For them, the pill may not be a good, easy-to-use method.

The IUD is listed by some as the easiest method to use, since after insertion it can be left in place for long periods of time. In addition, it is wholly sex independent. All that the client must do with the IUD is periodically check the device to ensure that it is properly in place. If the client is unable to feel the string, she should be instructed to use some other form of contraception and to see a practitioner to determine if the device has been expelled.

The nurse must guard against making assumptions in this case as in all areas. What may seem to the counselor to be a very easy method may seem quite complex and unacceptable to the client. Allowing for individual differences is essential in helping a client come to a decision as to which, if any, type of contraception will be acceptable.

Mechanism of Action. In explaining how a method of contraception actually works, the nurse may become quite alarmed and disillusioned at the client's lack of knowledge of reproduction. In order to explain the mechanism of action of the various methods, the counselor may be in the position of teaching the client a great deal of simple anatomy and physiology. It is an essential right of the client to have an adequate understanding of the mechanisms of action of all contraceptives, and the nurse is the appropriate individual to teach such information. Time for such teaching should be allowed and encouraged before asking a client to decide on a form of contraception.

The Methods

An in-depth discussion of the various methods of contraception will not be presented here, since it is beyond the scope of this chapter and because it is well covered in other texts. A brief discussion of the methods will be presented, followed by a summary chart of each method.

Birth Control Pills. The first birth control pills were approved by the FDA in the United States in 1960. The pill, Enovid, received its approval based on a clinical study of 132 women. Clinical testing took place in Haiti and Puerto Rico. It was discovered in a 1963 Senate investigation that the sample population consisted of only 132 women who took the pill continuously for more than one year. Of this sample, three women died. No autopsies were performed to determine the cause of death (Seaman, 1977). Since that time, many studies have been performed to investigate the effects of pill use. Long-term studies are now being conducted. Some groups object to the "use" of women as "guinea pigs," but many women choose to risk the unknowns associated with the use of birth control pills.

Recently, much attention has been given to women who are cigarette smokers who take birth control pills (Greenwood, 1979; Hatcher, 1978; Ory, 1980). Light smokers (one pack a day or less) have been found to be at 3.4 times more risk of myocardial infarction than are nonsmokers who take the pill. Women who smoke more than one pack per day and who take the pill are seven times more likely to suffer a myocardial infarction than are nonsmokers who take the pill. The situation for women over 35 years old is even more bleak. Heavy smokers in this group who use oral contraceptives were found to have 39 times greater risk of myocardial infarction than women who neither smoked nor used oral contraceptives. Many practitioners now refuse to prescribe oral contraceptives to women who smoke more than one pack of cigarettes per day. The reasons for this should be explained to the patient, and some other acceptable form of contraception must be offered.

In teaching clients about the proper use of birth control pills, the inclination of many health care workers is to assume that the women know how to take the pill correctly. This assumption is not founded on fact, and can lead to unnecessary unwanted pregnancies. Depending on the type of pill and the method of administration, taking the pill is not exactly the same for each woman. When starting to take the pill, many women like to use what is called the "Sunday" method: The woman will take the first pill of her new pill cycle on a Sunday, regardless of her own cycle at this point. She will be instructed to take one pill each day during the cycle, which lasts for either 21 or 28 days. If she is on a 21 day cycle, her last pill will fall on a Saturday. She will begin her menstrual period several days after this, and will start the next package of pills on the following Sunday. The woman on the 28 day pills will take one pill each day, ending with the placebo pills at the end of the cycle. She too will have her period several days after finishing the birth control pills while she is taking the placebo pills. The reason this method of administration is favored by many women is that it frees them from having their periods on the weekends. Women beginning the pill using this Sunday method should be warned to utilize another form of contraception for at least the first two weeks of the first cycle of the pill.

Another method commonly utilized for beginning a woman on birth control pills uses the woman's own cycle to determine when to begin the pills. The woman is instructed to begin her pills on day five of her cycle. She is taught that the first day of menstrual bleeding is day one of her cycle. After she takes her last pill in the cycle, she skips seven days, or takes the placebo pills, and then begins a new cycle.

Many women notice that their periods become much lighter while on birth control pills. It is not uncommon to have women skip periods completely. If the pills are taken correctly, the chances of pregnancy are minimal. Usually the woman will get her next period without any difficulty. However, if she has not taken the pills every day, and there is a chance of pregnancy, she should not continue the next package. Any woman who misses two consecutive periods should be evaluated for the possibility of pregnancy.

Teaching clients the possible danger signs that may be encountered and for which the clients should be alert is very important. These danger signs should be reported immediately to a physician or nurse practitioner. These warning signs, listed at the end of this chapter, may indicate gallbladder disease, hepatic adenoma, blood clots, or hypertension. Each client should be able to accurately state these warning signs before leaving the office of the practitioner.

Finally, before the client leaves with her new prescription for birth control pills, the woman's own evaluation of her likelihood for proper use of the pill should be discussed (Miller, 1976). Since the taking of the pill is separate from sexual behavior, many people tend to think that the motivation to take the pill daily is not related to the client's feelings regarding sexual activity. In fact, however, in order to effectively utilize the pill, the woman must have a low enough degree of guilt about sexual activity to be able to plan for her future sexual behavior. In addition, if the client is worried about the pills being discovered by another family member, her effectiveness as a pill-taker may be diminished. It is not appropriate for the health care worker to inflict personal views on clients. All factors should be discussed and presented so that the client is free to make an informed choice. Clients should be given an appointment for a followup visit several months after starting the pill to check her progress and discuss any side effects she may be experiencing.

IUD. Use of the IUD became popular in the United States in the early 1960s. The first widely used IUDs were the Lippes Loops and the Saf-T Coils. These devices were made of plastic in various shapes. Early successes with the IUD seemed to be confirmed almost exclusively to women who had already had children. In an attempt to cater to the group of women who had never had children but who wished to utilize this effective method of contraception, newer, smaller IUDs were designed, including the Dalkon Shield, the small Lippes Loop, the small Saf-T Coil, and later, the medicated IUDs, including the Cu7, the Copper T, and the Progestasert.

Each of the IUDs had one or two strings attached to them. These protruded into the vagina when the device was in the uterus. In this way, the woman could easily check to determine that the device was still in place.

Decisions regarding removal or retention of the device in the event of. pregnancy with the device in place have been mixed. In 1974, the Dalkon Shield was removed from the market as a result of septic abortions suffered by women who had become pregnant while the Dalkon Shield was in place. It was determined that the polyfilament string of the Dalkon Shield had acted as a wick to allow organisms to migrate up the string into the uterus, causing infection. Following the intense furor caused by the abortions and the deaths of some of the women involved, the medical community began to look more closely at the potential dangers of leaving an IUD in place if pregnancy should occur. It is not uncommon at this time for therapeutic abortion to be recommended for a woman who conceives with an IUD in place (Hatcher, 1978). Feelings are quite strong that medicated IUDs should be removed in case of pregnancy, since the effects of the medication on the fetus have not yet been determined.

Whether or not the IUD is removed when pregnancy is discovered, these pregnancies seem to have a very high rate of spontaneous abortions. In one study (Huxall, 1978), a 53 per cent rate of spontaneous abortion occurred when the IUD was left in place, while a 48.7 per cent abortion rate was found in cases in which the IUD was removed. Most women today are advised to have the IUD removed if they become pregnant.

The IUD has increased in popularity among younger women, partly because of the increase in the number and type of IUDs available for women who have never had their uterus stretched by pregnancy, and partly because of the growing disenchantment expressed by many women and their partners about the use of oral contraceptives (Jones, 1980). It is the second most popular method of contraception currently used by young women.

Health care professionals must become better educated about the use and potential side effects of IUDs. For many young women, the method is highly acceptable, since no action is necessary to prevent conception other than the initial insertion and the periodic checking of the string to be sure the device is in place. Despite the advances in technology of IUDs, it is not uncommon to hear of women who have not yet had a baby being counseled away from IUDs.

The use of the IUD does require that the woman take the responsibility for contraception and that she admit to herself that she will indeed be sexually active. Coming to terms with this inevitability of sexual activity is difficult for some women and may be a good reason to avoid the IUD.

Although dysmenorrhea is a relative contraindication to the use of the IUD, this does not mean the client should be counseled away from the devices. Some of the smaller devices, especially Progestasert, are designed to reduce the problems of dysmenorrhea that accompanied the earlier IUDs.

Diaphragm.   The diaphragm is a thin latex dome stretched over a flexible metal ring. The dome is designed to fit over the cervix. When used properly with a contraceptive cream or jelly, the device acts as a mechanical barrier that helps to hold the spermicide at the cervix. The diaphragm does not form a seal over the cervix as was previously thought.

A physician or nurse practitioner can fit women wishing to utilize the diaphragm with one of several types of springs. Once the woman has been fitted, it is essential that she receive intensive teaching in order to help her learn to use the device correctly (Gara, 1981). The practitioner who fits the client and sends her home to "try it out" is doing her a great disservice. Studies have found that the diaphragm, with contraceptive cream or jelly, can be a highly effective method of contraception when clients have been taught the proper use of the device (Hatcher, 1978).

Often, the woman must be taught the basics of her own anatomy. She must be taught to locate the cervix, in order to check if the diaphragm is in place after she has inserted it. During her first visit, the client should be shown how to insert and remove the diaphragm, and should then be given time to practice the procedure herself. The practitioner should check the client's insertion to be sure the diaphragm is in place correctly.

By the time the client leaves the education session accompanying her diaphragm fitting, she should be able to insert the device and remove it correctly, and state to the practitioner the proper use and care of the diaphragm, including that it must be used with contraceptive cream or jelly; that it may be inserted up to two hours before intercourse; that it must remain in place for 6 to 8 hours following intercourse; that an applicator full of cream or jelly should be introduced into the vagina if intercourse is to be repeated within the 6 to 8 hours following the first intercourse; and that the device should remain in place an additional 6 to 8 hours after the second intercourse. The client should be instructed to wear the diaphragm for 6 to 8 hours within the next few days, without having intercourse, to be sure that the device is comfortable for that length of wearing time. Finally, she should be instructed to have a recheck appointment, at which time she should be instructed to insert the diaphragm prior to the appointment so the practitioner can check both the fit and the insertion of the diaphragm.

Obviously, a great deal of teaching is suggested for the client interested in the diaphragm. However, this is necessary in order for the client to enjoy the greatest effectiveness of her chosen method of contraception. In most cases, a 30-minute appointment is sufficient to cover all the information, including the fitting of the diaphragm itself.

Some clients may wish their partners to be present at the fitting and teaching of diaphragm use. In order to make the use of contraceptives a shared event, some couples decide to integrate the insertion of the diaphragm into sexual foreplay. It may be the partner who inserts the diaphragm into the woman's vagina. The practitioner should be open to this type of alternative and should make such an experience available whenever possible.

The Cervical Cap. The cervical cap, not marketed in the United States, has long been used in Europe. The cervical cap is a small barrier type of device that fits over the cervix. It can be filled with a spermicidal agent and left in place for up to seven days without further treatment, provided that the spermicide is retained in the cap (Canavan, 1981). Effectiveness reporting varies, usually between 85 to 95 per cent combined theoretical and use effectiveness. With the increasing trend toward nonhormonal and noninvasive contraceptive methods, the cervical cap may gain a great deal of popularity in the United States in the near future.

Foam and Condoms. Foam and condoms used together are a highly effective form of contraception. Unfortunately, few couples are aware of this.

If a couple decides on this form of contraception, both partners must be highly motivated toward consistent and correct usage. The condom must be applied to the erect penis before any penile–vaginal contact is made. It has been found that there is sperm in the lubrication experienced by most men prior to ejaculation. In addition, a space must be left at the end of the condom to catch the ejaculate. The foam may be inserted as long as 30 minutes prior to intercourse. Following the insertion, however, the woman should be instructed to avoid walking around prior to intercourse, since this may cause expulsion of the foam. A new condom and an additional applicator of foam must be used with each successive intercourse.

Following intercourse, the couple should be instructed to have the man withdraw his penis while still erect. One of the partners should hold the top of the condom at the base of the penis while the penis is being removed to avoid the condom slipping off into the woman's vagina. Should this occur, the woman should be instructed to insert an additional applicator of foam immediately (Greenwald, 1977).

Natural Family Planning.   The term "natural family planning" has become more and more popular in recent years. For the purposes of this text, the term is utilized to identify the combination of three types of "natural" contraception: the calendar method (rhythm), the basal body temperature charting method, and the cervical mucus evaluation method.

In the calendar method, the woman records the intervals between the first days of each period for about 12 cycles. Having done this, she can figure out roughly her fertile periods. The woman is instructed to subtract 18 days from the length of her shortest cycle, and 11 days from her longest cycle. These two remaining days represent the earliest and latest fertile days. The woman is then instructed to refrain from intercourse between these days. For example, if a woman's shortest cycle is 24 days and her longest is 30 days, her fertile period would be between day six and day 19. She would be advised to abstain from at least day six until day 19. This long period of abstinence is sometimes lengthened to increase the safety margin. Because young women and postpartum women have very irregular cycles, most of these clients are advised to use the calendar method in conjunction with some other method, such as basal body charting.

Women utilizing the basal body charting method learn to evaluate the point during their cycle when they have ovulated. They do not learn from this method alone the unsafe period prior to ovulation. The woman takes her temperature each day in the morning before getting out of bed, using a specially calibrated basal body thermometer. This thermometer, unlike the traditional ones, is calibrated from only 96° to 99° F, to allow the client to observe smaller changes in temperature. The daily temperature is recorded on a chart. After several months, the woman can begin to recognize a pattern in which her temperature decreases somewhat (around 0.2° F), followed in 24 to 72 hours by a significant increase in temperature, which continues until the woman begins her period. Ovulation occurs during the drop immediately before the rise in temperature.

A difficulty in the basal body temperature charting method is the susceptibility of the woman to external influences. For example, if the woman has a cold, her temperature is likely to be somewhat elevated. In the same fashion, drinking alcohol, taking medication, or even using electric blankets the night before can have an effect on the morning's temperature.

The third of the methods combined to make up "natural family planning" involves evaluation of the cervix and cervical mucus for the changes that accompany each cycle. During ovulation, the normal cervical mucus, which usually appears yellow and thick, becomes sticky and clear. During ovulation the mucus appears similar to a raw egg white and can be stretched into a thin strand, called spinnbarkeit; the maximum length usually coincides with the time of ovulation. In addition, the cervical opening, the os, may appear slightly opened at the time of ovulation.

Many women prefer not to utilize a speculum in order to visualize the cervix, but to note the vaginal discharge throughout the cycle. Difficulties may be encountered, however, when vaginal infection occurs. Semen in the vagina can also alter the appearance of the vaginal secretions, as can lubricants and spermicides.

In addition to observation of the cervical mucus, many women experience feelings around the time of ovulation that they can be taught to identify. It is not uncommon for women to report "heavy" feelings before ovulation or actual pain on one side or the other just before ovulation.

As with the basal body temperature method, cervical secretion observations are measures that will tell the woman she has ovulated. In order for the method to be most effective, she may be advised to abstain during every cycle until after she has ovulated.

Natural family planning is currently the only method of contraception accepted by the Roman Catholic Church. With the newer refinements, such as the observations of the cervical mucus and the basal body temperature charting, very high success rates have been reported. However, because of its newness, no reliable statistics on the combined use of all the aforementioned forms of natural family planning could be found.

The periodic abstinence required by this method can be very difficult for some couples. The health care worker should discuss with all couples alternative forms of sexual expression that do not include penile-vaginal contact. Often the act of mentioning these alternatives to the couple is sufficient "permission" from an authority figure to enable the couple to greatly expand their sexual repertoires without guilt.

Vaginal Suppositories.   One of the newest forms of contraception to be placed on the market is the Encare Oval. This vaginal suppository is inserted in the woman's vagina 10 minutes prior to intercourse. The heat and moistness of her tissues cause the suppository to effervesce and melt, forming a barrier over the cervical os. The active spermicidal agent in the Encare Oval is the same as is found in many of the commonly encountered foams. It is available without a prescription, is immediately reversible, and is somewhat effective. Early reports of effectiveness tended to be quite high and generally were reports of the theoretical effectiveness only. The user effectiveness has been found to vary, but is generally around 88 per cent (Hatcher, 1978). Like the contraceptive foams, if applied prior to oral sex, the male may complain that the taste is unpleasant. Some women find that the effervescing action produces an unpleasant heat, and some will find they have an allergic reaction to the suppository.

Withdrawal (Coitus Interruptus).   Withdrawal has not been included for discussion with the more effective forms of contraception, since it is clearly not very effective. In withdrawal, the man withdraws his penis from his partner's vagina prior to ejaculation. This method, although widely used by young couples, is especially difficult for this group, since it requires a great deal of control for the man at the point in his life when his control is weakest (Lieberman, 1978). Withdrawal, when utilized over a prolonged period of time, has been found to be a risk factor in the development of premature ejaculation, a sexual dysfunction (Greenwald, 1977; Masters, 1953).

Women who object to the use of withdrawal as a form of contraception often do so on the grounds that the anxiety regarding her partner's control can overshadow the pleasure of the sexual encounter. The woman in this situation is, after all, totally dependent on the man's control over his ejaculation. In order to be comfortable with this method, the woman must trust her partner completely (Greenwald, 1977).

The theoretical effectiveness of withdrawal is 85 per cent (Hatcher, 1978). Use effectiveness has been listed between 75 and 80 per cent. This low success rate is due at least in part to the fact that even before the man ejaculates, some of the fluid deposited in the vagina (the pre-ejaculate) contains sperm. The woman can become pregnant from this pre-ejaculate, even if the man withdraws his penis prior to ejaculation.

For some couples, withdrawal may be the only acceptable form of contraception. If this is the case, the couple should be taught how to properly use the method. Some couples may be willing to utilize other sexual pleasuring methods during periods of fertility in the woman. Using these alternatives during the "unsafe" periods can increase the effectiveness of the withdrawal method. No couple should be advised not to use this method if it is the only acceptable one for them. The only case in which the withdrawal method cannot be used is that in which the man is a premature ejaculator and might accidentally impregnate his partner.

Postcoital Contraception.   In some cases, contraceptive measures are not utilized either before or during intercourse. In this situation, especially during the fertile period, women who have had only one unprotected intercourse have the option of a postcoital contraceptive.

The best known of the postcoital methods is the "morning after pill." This method utilizes a very high dosage of oral or injected estrogens, which are administered within 72 hours of the unprotected intercourse. High doses of estrogens interfere with the transport of ovum; they decrease the secretion of progesterone by the corpus luteum; and, it is thought, they disturb the implantation process itself (Huxall, 1978; Hatcher, 1978). Most women who have used this rather extreme method complain of side effects from the medication, notably severe nausea and vomiting. Less obvious is the danger inherent in the administration of high levels of estrogen. The client is at greater risk of blood clots and heart attacks. However, for some, especially rape victims, the medication risk may seem small when compared with the risk of unwanted pregnancy.

Menstrual extraction is another form of postcoital contraception and is utilized by a great number of women. Immediately prior to menstruation, the contents of the uterus are removed with a suction procedure that does not require dilation of the cervix. If the woman has conceived during the month, the products of the conception are removed without the woman's knowledge of the pregnancy. For those who are unsure of their feelings about abortion, the method offers the advantage of not knowing whether there was indeed a pregnancy.

Menstrual extraction gained a great deal of popularity, especially in the late 1970s, among women's groups who supported a method that would also free women from the burdens of a monthly period. The popularity seems to have decreased for several reasons. First, some pregnancies can be missed by this procedure, since the embryo is so small at this time. Despite the procedure, the embryo may remain viable. Secondly, there is some controversy about the long-term effects of repeated emptying on the uterus. It has been postulated that these women may become more prone to the development of malignant growths. Others fear that future pregnancies of a woman who has repeatedly undergone this procedure may end in spontaneous abortions. The controversy continues, but the practice of menstrual extraction seems to be diminishing, especially among women who wish to have children in the future.

Other methods of postcoital contraception include insertion of an IUD after an unprotected intercourse and the use of therapeutic abortion. IUD insertion is usually contraindicated in cases of rape or in women who have multiple partners, since the risk of venereal disease places the woman at greater risk than normal for pelvic inflammatory disease (PID). Abortion, an option chosen by many women, will be discussed in a later chapter.

Postpartum Contraception

Until quite recently, postpartum women were advised by their physicians to avoid intercourse until their six-week postpartum checkup. (Indeed, some physicians continue this practice today. Some women heed this advice, while others do not.) Because the physician assumed that the advice to abstain would be followed, most women were not given contraceptive information prior to the postpartum visit. Owing to the lack of information about the possibilities of pregnancy occurring immediately following the delivery of a child, many women undoubtedly became pregnant. Realistically, most women find they are comfortable enough and willing to have intercourse about two weeks following delivery. For most, the first intercourse may be difficult, primarily because of anxiety about the pain on the part of the woman and fear of hurting the woman on the part of the man. However, many will overcome these fears and have intercourse.

The current attitude toward this early postpartum intercourse is that it is essentially inevitable and may have beneficial consequences. For example, intercourse may soften the episiotomy scar, aiding in healing (Bing, 1977). Many clients are now told to avoid intercourse only until the lochia is no longer red, and until they are comfortable. The question of contraception for these women then becomes an issue.

Lactating women are usually advised against oral contraceptives, since some practitioners feel that the pills cause a decrease in the milk supply. Also, although the amount is small, some of the hormones are transmitted through the milk to the infant. The effects of this are not known.

Since women who are breastfeeding may experience a decrease in vaginal lubrication because of their altered hormonal state, foam and condoms may be an acceptable alternative until the child is weaned. The lubricated condoms, in conjunction with the lubrication afforded by the contraceptive foam, make for much more comfortable and enjoyable intercourse for the couple who may have avoided this method in the past.

Women desiring an IUD following pregnancy are usually advised to wait for at least 8 to 12 weeks postpartum. The reason for this is that the uterus is softer and more susceptible to perforation during the process of involution. Waiting the additional time adds a needed safety factor for the woman.

Because of the changes experienced by the vagina during vaginal delivery, women who have used the diaphragm prior to pregnancy are advised to wait until six to eight weeks postpartum to have their diaphragm rechecked. The vagina is thought to return almost completely to its final shape by the six week check. At that time, the woman may have to be refit for another size diaphragm.

It is essential that all clients be prepared for the possibility of pregnancy in the immediate postpartum period. Few women realize that they can conceive even before they have another period. Many still believe that breastfeeding is an effective method of birth control. (Note: most of the studies on this topic find that in order for breastfeeding to have a contraceptive effect, it is necessary that the mother give the infant absolutely no supplemental bottles or solid food. Even with this restriction, breastfeeding alone does not approach the effectiveness levels of other available methods of contraception.)

For many couples, foam and condoms are the best answer. Some choose to avoid intercourse until the six week checkup in order to avoid the possibility of pregnancy. This is, of course, their decision. The responsibility of the nurse is to present the client with all of the alternatives available to her and her partner.

Sterilization

Clients who decide not to have any children, or who decide that the number of children they have is sufficient, may wish to discuss sterilization. In counseling clients about sterilization, the permanence of such a procedure must be stressed. As medical technology stands currently, the chances of returning fertility to individuals who have undergone surgical sterilization are still very low. Individuals who are uncertain that they wish to be permanently sterile should be made aware that the likelihood of reversal is very slight.

In both male and female sterilization methods, some portion of the reproductive anatomy is removed, making it essentially impossible for the egg and sperm to unite. Although most people consider sterilization to be 100 per cent effective, there are occasional failures. Clients must be informed of this risk prior to the procedure.

Currently, there are no legal restrictions that require consent of the client's spouse for sterilization. Clients receiving sterilization under federally funded programs must be at least 21 years old. There is no requirement for a specific number of children prior to allowing sterilization. Clients who are young and have decided against parenthood may face some opposition from physicians who do not wish to perform an essentially irreversible procedure in young persons, but there is no legal restriction.

As with all of the aforementioned contraceptive methods, obtaining informed consent for sterilization is essential. Clients must be fully informed so that they can make an intelligent choice. This is especially crucial when the procedure is permanent.

The Difficult Contraceptor

The reproductive health care worker does not always have an easy job with clients who wish contraception. Susan, for example, presents a difficult case, and will be discussed to illustrate the complexity of determining an appropriate form of contraception.

History. Susan is a 27 year old, white, slightly obese woman. She has been receiving thyroid medication for the last year for a hypothyroid condition. Early in her sexual life, Susan depended largely on the rhythm method for contraception but found this unacceptable because of the anxiety it produced. She then began to take birth control pills. She took a variety of pills, with minor side effects. After about one year on the pill, she developed a chronic cervical irritation that finally caused her to discontinue the pill. She then had a Cu7 IUD inserted. She was very happy with this method, which produced essentially no side effects, until two years ago, when it was discovered that she was pregnant with the IUD in place. Susan decided to undergo a therapeutic abortion, since she and her husband were not ready to have children at that time. Six weeks after the abortion, Susan had another IUD inserted. This time, the device became embedded in the uterine lining, causing pain and bleeding. The device was removed after one month. Susan decided to return to the birth control pills, and has been taking them for the last 1½ years. Her cervical erosion has returned and seems to be worsening. In addition, she has experienced some skin changes, especially on her face (chloasma). She has come to the clinic, wishing an alternative method of contraception. She is certain that she wishes to avoid sterilization, since she still plans to have children within the next few years. Following discussion of all the available methods of contraception, Susan will decide on a method most acceptable to her.

Nursing Interventions
1. Discuss each contraceptive method in terms of the requirements for informed consent (outlined earlier).
2. Answer Susan's questions about contraception.
3. Use broad, open statements to help Susan examine her own feelings about contraception.
4. Support Susan in her decision, assuring her that she can change her mind if the method she chooses no longer fits her needs at a later date.

Evaluation. Following discussion, Susan did decide on a method of contraception that was acceptable to her. She decided to remain on birth control pills, despite the cervical erosion and chloasma. She felt that the trauma of the abortion she had undergone was too difficult to face again, and that only with the pill would she feel safe. Foam and condoms were rejected by Susan, who stated that they had tried this method and found that the foam (she tried a variety of brands) was irritating to her. The diaphragm was considered too ineffective for the couple at the time.

Susan's case is not unusual. Most health care workers recognize the inescapable fact that the currently available forms of contraception are not perfect, nor are they foolproof. Each client brings a unique history, feelings and ideas to the situation, which all must be weighed in the evaluation of data.

If Susan had developed one of the absolute contraindications to the pill, such as thrombophlebitis, she would not have been given the choice of this medication again. Her "nuisance effects," as they would be called, do not require medical intervention, however.

In this case, the nurse had difficulty in dealing with the client in a nonjudgmental way. The nurse felt that Susan should try the diaphragm, adding condoms during her fertile periods. With the combination of methods, the nurse felt that Susan and her husband could nearly approximate the effectiveness enjoyed by use of the pill, while avoiding the undesirable side effects of the pill. The possibility of this was discussed with Susan, who rejected it completely. It was difficult for the nurse to avoid becoming exasperated with Susan, since she felt that her suggestion was best for Susan. It is necessary to remain nonjudgmental in such situations as this. The nurse was able to recognize that her annoyance with Susan was caused by her own

Text continued on page 182

Birth Control Pills

Mechanism of Action

Combination pill-
1. Estrogen
   Ovulation inhibited by suppression of FSH and LH
   Acceleration of ovum transport
   May inhibit implantation
2. Progestin
   Cervical mucus becomes hostile to sperm
   Capacitation inhibited (interferes with activation of enzymes needed to help sperm penetrate wall of ovum)
   May inhibit implantation
   May decelerate ovum transport

Effectiveness

Theoretical — 99.9%
User: — 90–93%

Relative Contraindications

1. Severe vascular or migraine headaches
2. Hypertension with resting diastolic of greater than 110
3. Diabetes, prediabetes, or strong family history of diabetes
4. Gallbladder disease
5. Undiagnosed abnormal vaginal bleeding
6. Elective surgery planned in next 4 weeks
7. Fibrocystic breast disease and breast fibroadenomas
8. History of heavy cigarette smoking

Ease of Use

1. Sex independent
2. One pill taken daily for 21- or 28-day cycle

Absolute Contraindications

1. Thromboembolic disorder
2. Cerebrovascular incident (or history)
3. Impaired liver function
4. Coronary artery disease
5. Hepatic adenoma or history
6. Malignancy of breast or reproductive system or history
7. Pregnancy — known or suspected

Danger Signs

1. Severe abdominal pains
2. Severe chest pain or shortness of breath
3. Severe headaches
4. Eye problems (blur, flashing lights, blindness)
5. Severe pain in calf or thigh

Side Effects

1. Decreased dysmenorrhea
2. Decreased menstrual flow
3. Regular cycles
4. Decreased mid-cycle symptoms
5. Decreased iron deficiency anemia
6. Decreased premenstrual tension
7. Improvement in acne
8. Increased breast size
9. Decreased endometriosis
10. Nausea and vomiting
11. Fluid retention
12. Headaches
13. Breast tenderness
14. Chloasma
15. Leukorrhea
16. Spotting between periods
17. Missed periods
18. Increased susceptibility to yeast infections
19. Fatigue
20. Blood clots
21. Heart attacks
22. Increased cervical erosion

Adapted from Goldstein, 1976; Greenwood, 1979; Hatcher, 1978; Huxall, 1978; and Seaman, 1977.

Contraceptive Foam with Condoms

Mechanism of Action	Relative Contraindications	Absolute Contraindications	Side Effects
Mechanical barrier that prevents sperm from entering cervix, spermicidal action of the foam	1. Woman who is uncomfortable with handling own genitals 2. Male partner unwilling to use condoms	1. Allergy to latex 2. Allergy to foam	1. Protection from some VD 2. Discharge of foam following intercourse 3. Irritation from foam 4. Decreased sensation for male or female partner from decreased friction 5. May be useful in cases of premature ejaculation 6. Taste of foam may be unpleasant

Effectiveness	Ease of Use	Danger Signs
Theoretical — 99% User — 95%	1. Messy to insert 2. May interrupt sex act 3. No need for prescription 4. Need both partners' cooperation 5. Sex dependent	None

Adapted from Hatcher, 1978; Huxall, 1978; Lieberman, 1978; and Woods, 1979.

Diaphragm (with Spermicidal Cream or Jelly)

Mechanism of Action

Mechanical barrier that prevents sperm from entering cervix combined with the spermicidal action of the creams or jellies

Effectiveness

Theoretical — 97%
User — 83%

Relative Contraindications

1. Woman who is uncomfortable with handling own genitals
2. Uterine prolapse
3. Cystocele
4. Rectocele

Ease of Use

1. Messy to insert
2. May interfere with sex act
3. May be inserted several hours before anticipated sex act
4. Requires some dexterity
5. Requires storage place
6. Requires fitting by practitioner

Absolute Contraindications

1. Allergy to latex
2. Allergy to spermicide
3. Inability to achieve satisfactory fit
4. Inability of client or partner to learn proper insertion and removal techniques

Danger Signs

1. Severe itching or burning with device and spermicide in place

Side Effects

1. Irritation from cream or jelly
2. Discharge of jelly or cream following diaphragm removal
3. Discomfort (bladder or bowel) if left in place over 6–8 hours
4. Decreased sensation for male or female partner due to reduction of friction

Adapted from Hatcher, 1978; Lieberman, 1978; and Miller, 1976.

IUD

Mechanism of Action

Suggested:
1. Foreign body reaction of endometrium making inhospitable to implantation
2. Immobilization of sperm
3. Increased motility of ovum in tube

Effectiveness

Theoretical — 95–99%
User — 90–94%

Relative Contraindications

1. Recurrent pelvic infection
2. Acute cervicitis
3. History of ectopic pregnancy
4. Abnormal pap smear
5. History of fibroids
6. Recent history of undiagnosed vaginal bleeding
7. Severe dysmenorrhea

Ease of Use

1. Sex independent
2. May stay in indefinitely (Lippes, Saf-T Coil)
3. May stay in place three years (Cu7, Copper T)
4. May stay in place 1–2 years (Progestasert)

Absolute Contraindications

1. Active pelvic infection
2. Pregnancy
3. Distortion of pelvic cavity due to tumor
4. Uterus under 4.5 cm with sounding

Danger Signs

1. Inability to find string in vagina
2. Feeling device partially expelled
3. Suspected pregnancy
4. Pelvic pain
5. Severe cramping
6. Irregular vaginal bleeding

Side Effects

1. Uterine perforation
2. Expulsion
3. Severe pain
4. PID
5. Dysmenorrhea
6. Heavy menstrual bleeding
7. Infertility secondary to PID
8. Increased risk of ectopic pregnancy
9. Cervicitis

Adapted from Greenwald, 1977; Hatcher, 1978; Huxall, 1978; and Hyde, 1975.

Natural Family Planning — Symptomothermal Methods, Periodic Abstinence, Cervical Mucus Testing

Mechanism of Action	Relative Contraindications	Absolute Contraindications	Side Effects
1. Use of various methods to determine time of ovulation and abstain from intercourse during periods in which the woman may be ovulating 2. The combination of several methods is thought to increase the chance of success of this periodical abstinence	1. Very irregular cycles 2. History of anovulatory cycles 3. Irregular temperature charts	None	1. Frustration due to long periods of abstinence 2. Anxiety because of highly variable nature of physical signs

Effectiveness	Ease of Use	Danger Signs	
No conclusive data reached in use of all methods combined	1. May require long periods of abstinence 2. No interference with sex act during safe days 3. No need for prescription 4. Requires cooperation of both partners 5. No cost except for basal body thermometer	None	

feelings of frustration with the complicated nature of Susan's history, and was then able to best assist Susan in coming to her own decision. The reality of the situation must be faced—if a client is forced into using a form of contraception that is not acceptable, the chances of her using it correctly and consistently are quite poor.

CONCLUSION

The role of the nurse in dealing with clients who are seeking contraception is threefold: patient education, patient counseling, and patient advocacy. As an educator, the nurse must be certain the client fully understands the potential benefits and risks involved in the use of any contraceptive. For quick reference, the reader is advised to refer to the charts on the following pages, which summarize actions, contraindications, side effects, effectiveness, ease of use, and danger signs for the more effective contraceptive methods.

In fully informing the client about the methods of contraception available, the nurse acts as patient advocate, allowing and encouraging the patient to assume an active role in his or her sexual health care.

Finally, as with all counseling, the client ultimately makes the decision regarding which contraceptive, if any, should be used. Except in cases of medical contraindications, it is inappropriate for the nurse to advise the client to avoid a particular method. Once the patient is fully educated and counseled, the nurse's goals have been achieved. The final decision is the patient's.

References

Bing, Elizabeth, and Colman, Libby: *Making Love During Pregnancy*. New York, Bantam Books, 1977.

Burbach, Cindy A.: "Contraception and Adolescent Pregnancy." *JOEN Nursing*, Vol. 9, No. 5, October, 1980.

Canavan, Patricia Ann, and Lewis, Claudia Ann: "The Cervical Cap: An Alternative Contraceptive." *JOEN Nursing*, Vol. 10, No. 4, July/August, 1981.

Crist, Robert, and Hickenlooper, Gale: "Problems in Adolescent Sexuality." *In* Barnard, Martha, Clancy, Barbara, and Krantz, Kermit (Eds.): *Human Sexuality for Health Professionals*. Philadelphia, W. B. Saunders Co., 1978.

DIGEST: "Large Majority of Americans Favor Legal Abortion, Sex Education, and Contraceptive Services for Teens." *Family Planning Perspectives*. Vol. 10, No. 3, May/June, 1978.

Freidson, Eliot: *A Study of the Sociology of Applied Knowledge*. New York, Harper & Row, 1970.

Gara, Ellen: "Nursing Protocol to Improve the Effectiveness of the Contraceptive Diaphragm." *MCN*, Vol. 6, No. 1, January/February, 1981.

Goldstein, Bernard: *Human Sexuality*. New York, McGraw-Hill, 1976.

Gordon, Linda: *Woman's Body, Woman's Right*. New York, Penguin Books, 1976.

Greenwald, Judith: "Rating the Latest Methods of Birth Control." *Focus: Human Sexuality 77/78*, Connecticut, Dushkin Publishing Group, Inc., 1977.

Greenwood, Sadja Goldsmith: "Warning: Cigarette Smoking is Dangerous to Reproductive Health." *Family Planning Perspectives,* Vol. 11, No. 3, May/June, 1979.

Hatcher, Robert A., Stewart, Gary K., Stewart, Felicia, Guest, Felicia, Schwartz, David W., and Jones, Stephanie: *Contraceptive Technology 1980–1981*. New York, Irvington Publishers, Inc., 1980.

Hyde, Janet Shibley: *Understanding Human Sexuality*. New York, McGraw-Hill, 1975.

Huxall, Linda, and Sawyer, Suzanne: "Counseling Regarding Birth Control Methods." *In* Barnard, Martha, Clancy, Barbara, and Krantz, Kermit (Eds.): *Human Sexuality for Health Professionals*. Philadelphia, W. B. Saunders Co., 1978.

Jones, Elise F., Beninger, James R., and Westoff, Charles F.: "Pill and IUD Discontinuation in the United States, 1970–1975: The Influence of the Media." *Family Planning Perspectives,* Vol. 2, No. 16, November/December, 1980.

Lieberman, E. James: "Teenage Sex and Birth Control." JAMA, Vol. 240, No. 3, July 21, 1978.

Masters, W., and Johnson, Virginia E.: Human Sexual Response. Boston, Little, Brown and Co., 1966.

Miller, Warren B.: "Sexual and Contraceptive Behavior in Young, Unmarried Women. *Primary Care,* Vol. 3, No. 3, September, 1976.

Nadelson, Carol C., and Notman, Malkah T.: "Treatment of the Pregnant Teenager and the Putative Father." *Current Psychiatric Therapies,* Vol. 17, 1977.

Ory, Howard W., Rosenfield, Allan, and Landman, Lynn C.: "The Pill at 20: An Assessment." *Family Planning Perspectives,* Vol. 12, No. 6, November/December, 1980.

Paul, Eve W., and Scofield, Giles: "Informed Consent for Fertility Control Services." *Family Planning Perspectives,* Vol. 11, No. 3, May/June, 1979.

Pickett, Robert S.: "Sanger to the Seventies: An Historical Analysis of American Attitudes Toward Heterosexuality, Human Reproduction, and Birth Control." *AASECT Convention,* St. Louis, April 16, 1971.

Reichelt, Paul A., and Werley, Harriet H.: "Contraception, Abortion, and Venereal Disease: Teenagers' Knowledge and the Effect of Education." *Family Planning Perspectives,* Vol. 7, No. 2, March/April, 1975.

Sandberg, E. C., and Jacobs, R. I.: "Psychology of the Misuse and Rejection of Contraception." *American Journal of Obstetrics and Gynecology,* Vol. 110, pp. 227–242, 1971.

Seaman, Barbara: "The Dangers of Oral Contraception." *In* Dreifus, Claudia (Ed.): *Seizing Our Bodies: The Politics Of Women's Health.* New York, Vintage Books, 1977.

Sharpe, Jean: "The Birth Controllers." *In* Dreifus, Claudia (Ed.): *Seizing Our Bodies: The Politics of Women's Health.* New York, Vintage Books, 1977.

Zelnick, Melvin, and Kantner, John F.: "Sexual and Contraceptive Experience of Young, Unmarried Women in the United States, 1976 and 1971." *Family Planning Perspectives,* Vol. 9, No. 2, March/April, 1977.

ABORTION

FACTUAL OVERVIEW

Historical Status of Abortion — Through Nineteenth Century

Abortion is an emotionally compelling issue in our society. Rarely do people report neutral feelings about abortion. For some, the issue is clearly one of rights and political import, while for others an area of intense emotional involvement surrounds the issue of when life begins. Still others are most involved with the medical aspects and long term effects of the procedures themselves.

Regardless of an individual's views on abortion, one fact becomes clear in investigations of the history of abortion — induced abortion has probably occurred throughout the history of humanity (Green, 1977). Records of induced abortion can be found in ancient Chinese writings, which recorded abortions by use of mercury-based materials in the years 2736–2696 B.C. (Himes, 1936).

It has been postulated that birth control was not necessary in preliterate societies, since abortion and infanticide filled the need to limit unwanted children. In those times, fetuses and infants were probably killed without guilt, since the fetus/infant usually was not considered to be sacred until after passing through a ceremony of tribal initiation or recognition. In some tribes, this recognition may not have come until the individual married.

In our present culture, all people have inherent biases for or against abortion. For example, the view that life is not sacred until puberty is foreign to our way of thinking. However, the differing views that people have historically had about abortion must be identified and discussed so that we may better understand both the historical aspects of abortion and our own biases about the subject.

In ancient Greece, Aristotle and Plato openly advocated abortion to limit family size. Both philosophers suggested that the government should deter-

---

Note: In this chapter, the feminine pronoun "she" has been used almost exclusively in referring to the nurse. This is not intended to be a sexist comment. Instead, it is recognized that most nurses who choose to work with abortion patients are women. The use of female pronouns reflects only current practice, not necessarily what is desired or the best practice.

mine the optimum family size and provide abortion for those who exceeded that number. Abortion for women who conceived after the age of 40 was also considered necessary. Today, the possibility of governmental limitation and regulation of family size is an issue that is often raised in arguments against the legalization of abortion. The objections have been based largely on the notion that government has neither the obligation nor the right to interfere to this extent in the reproductive lives of individuals.

Not all ancient Greeks supported the notion of abortion. Physicians were notably opposed to it. Their objection may have risen from the fact that they sometimes witnessed severe complications following harsh abortion techniques. Perhaps the primitive techniques and the pressures placed on the physician to "fix" the problems caused by abortion contributed to this opposition. Certainly, physicians of the time had their own private reasons for trying to reduce the incidence of abortion.

We find in the Hippocratic oath a statement condemning the practice of abortion. Hippocrates opposed abortion, especially when it was performed by people who were not physicians, although there were rare instances in which he supported the procedure. The Hippocratic oath requires that the physician promise ". . . nor will I give a woman a pessary to procure an abortion" (Green, 1977).

The ancient Romans seem to have practiced abortion often. The procedures followed were often dangerous, leading to severe complications. Curettage, scraping the lining of the uterus with a sharp instrument, was often complicated by uterine perforation and sepsis, causing death. The antibiotics that we use today were not available to reduce the likelihood of infection. The two popular abortion methods used by the Romans were strong purgatives and caustic douches, which also caused high death rates. Despite the extreme risks faced by women undergoing such dangerous procedures, abortions were common and women seem to have been willing to accept the inherent risks, as they accepted the risks of childbearing. The need to prevent the birth of unwanted children was as strong then as it is now.

Abortion seems to have been generally accepted in most preindustrial societies. The fetus was usually seen as a part of the mother until it was born, much as a piece of fruit is seen as part of a tree until the fruit ripens and falls. Since the fetus was not seen as separate from the mother until after it "fell down" or delivered, the dilemma of taking human life did not enter into the abortion issue (Gordon, 1976).

The idea that abortion is a crime probably came into being with the advent of Christianity, when abortion at any point of gestation was considered an act of murder. By deciding that "the fetus possesses a soul from the moment the ovum is pierced by the sperm," theologians clearly and irrevocably changed the nature of the abortion problem. When the fetus is no longer seen as an extension of the mother, its rights as a separate individual become an important part of the issue.

Prior to the nineteenth century, in the United States, abortion during the first few months of pregnancy was largely ignored in the legal literature. Generally, abortion was allowed until the time of "quickening," the time when the woman "felt life." Abortion beyond this time was regulated or generally forbidden (Gordon, 1976).

The incidence of abortion appears to have increased following the Industrial Revolution, as general health and infant survival began to improve. At this time, the large agricultural family was beginning to lose its importance, and more women began to seek out ways to limit family size. Most early abortion laws dealt separately with the different methods of abortion used at that time. As the number of abortions increased, so did the laws governing abortion. During the years since the Industrial Revolution, the legal aspects of the abortion issue have become more and more tangled.

As in ancient Rome, the primary methods of abortion during the Industrial Revolution involved the use of abortifacients and curettage. The abortifacients did not specifically affect the fetus to produce abortion. Rather, the materials ingested or used in douching preparations irritated or poisoned the body of the woman. This led to rejection of the embryo as a side effect. Such drastic measures often resulted in the death of the woman. Other methods, which were less dangerous, had no real effect other than to cause digestive upsets or minor irritation; they did not have the desired effect of producing abortion. Curettage was widely used (and is still used today), with some success. The primary complications of this method are uterine perforation, sepsis, and the potential for death due to hemorrhage or infection (Gordon, 1976).

Abortion in Contemporary America

Legal Aspects.   As a result of one of the most tragic events of modern times, abortion became an issue of great public sentiment during the 1960's. During this time thalidomide, a tranquilizer, was in wide use by pregnant women. The results of this usage were devastating. The offspring of women who had been given this drug during pregnancy were born with severe malformations that included, among others, absence of limbs and severe retardation. The results of this drug usage were widely reported, and many women who had taken the drug demanded the right to termination of their pregnancies. Also during this time period there occurred a nationwide epidemic of German measles (rubella). Women who had the disease, especially during the first trimester of pregnancy, learned of the potentially awesome results of the infection on the unborn fetus and demanded elective abortions. The children born to these women were often congenitally blind, deaf, and severely retarded.

Largely as a result of these two conditions, the American Law Institute in 1962 proposed a model law concerning abortion. The law allowed abortion when the pregnancy might impair the physical and mental health of the mother, when the child might be born with severe mental or physical damage, or when the pregnancy resulted from rape or incest (Green, 1977). Most states ultimately adopted this law, with some modifications. In 1966, the first reform laws to expand the indications for therapeutic abortion were passed.

In March of 1970, the state of New York repealed the old abortion statute and passed a law that permitted physicians to perform abortions on any consenting woman, provided that the fetus was not older than 24 weeks of gestation (Pakter, 1975). The enactment of the new law brought about a dramatic increase in the number of abortions performed in New York, as women from all over the nation flocked to New York to obtain safe, legal abortions.

On January 22, 1973, all restrictive state laws regarding abortion were invalidated by the Supreme Court, when two landmark cases (Roe v. Wade, Texas, and Doe v. Bolton, Georgia) were declared unconstitutional. The decision was supported mostly on the grounds that a woman's decision to either terminate or continue her pregnancy was part of her right to privacy.

Under the new law, the state was forbidden to interfere with a woman's decision to terminate her pregnancy during the first trimester of the pregnancy. During the second trimester, the state could regulate only the procedures of the abortion, which would serve to protect the health of the mother. Finally, the state could intervene to prohibit abortion only at fetal viability on the grounds of protecting the rights of a potential citizen, and then only in cases in which the mother's life would not be endangered by having the child.

Following the 1973 rulings, most first trimester abortions were performed in nonhospital clinics. These clinics offered less costly pregnancy terminations and were generally more convenient for the outpatient procedures utilized in first trimester abortions. Second trimester abortions usually required a hospital setting because of the increased risk to the mother that is inherent in these procedures (Pakter, 1975).

The controversy surrounding the abortion issue did not end with the Supreme Court decision. Strong political opponents of abortion continued to push for repeal of the permissive abortion rulings of 1973.

In June of 1977, the Hyde Amendment was passed. According to this ruling, states were no longer required to furnish Medicaid funds for abortions of Medicaid-eligible women. Despite protests that limiting abortion funding for poor women was discriminatory, the Hyde Amendment was passed and put into effect. Proponents of more restrictive abortion laws pushed for this amendment on the basis that the state should not have to support a practice that is unacceptable to so many of the taxpayers.

In the Supreme Court rulings, several interesting points were discussed. The court ruled that the state does have a "valid and important interest in encouraging childbirth" and that there is nothing in Medicaid legislation or in the Constitution that bans the state from furthering this interest by refusing to pay for "nontherapeutic" abortions. Further, the decision by the state not to pay for abortions that the state deemed unncessary was not seen as discriminatory, since financial need alone was not a basis for involving the Fourteenth Amendment's guarantee of equal protection. The court held that the state was not creating an obstacle by refusing to pay for abortions in the first trimester. The state was merely not removing an already present obstacle, that of poverty, and was exercising its legislative power in not removing this obstacle in order to encourage childbirth (Digest, 1977).

In August of 1977, the Department of Health, Education, and Welfare restricted abortion funds to cover only those abortion procedures that were considered to be necessary to save the woman's life. In February of 1978, the indications for Medicaid-covered abortion were expanded to include the following (Gold, 1979):

1. Cases where "severe and long-lasting physical health damage" to the woman would result if the pregnancy were carried to term. This damage or potential damage was to be certified by two physicians.
2. Cases in which the pregnancy resulted from statutory or forcible rape or incest, provided the incident was reported to a law enforcement agency or government health service within 60 days of occurrence.

Following these decisions, which essentially eliminated Medicaid funding for abortion, a great deal of research was conducted by both Pro Choice and Pro Life groups, in order to determine the effects of reduction of federal support for abortion. Most studies indicate that predicted increases in mortality and morbidity due to sharp increases of self-induced and illegally obtained abortion did not occur (Cates, 1979; Gold, 1979). The research indicates that most women who were eligible for Medicaid funds prior to the rulings were able to fund their abortions by utilizing private funds. In addition, some large public hospitals and private family planning agencies responded to the decrease in Medicaid funding by reducing the charges for abortion for low income women. A significant finding in the studies evaluating the effect of eliminating Medicaid funding for abortions was the fact that Medicaid-eligible women were delaying their abortions for one to two weeks because of the lack of public funds. That is, the abortions were being obtained at a later date, reportedly because of the additional time necessary to secure the private funding for the procedures. In terms of potential complications from abortion, this delay certainly can be seen as a significant time of risk for these women that could be shortened if funds for abortion were readily available. Any policy that delays the abortion procedure increases the risks of complications and death to the woman (Gold, 1979).

In early 1980, the Hyde Amendment was declared unconstitutional by a U.S. District Court judge in New York. In the McRae v. Harris ruling, the court held that to deny Medicaid funds to poor women for abortion was unconstitutional under the First Amendment as well as the Fifth Amendment. In this case, the court ruled that the government's argument that inability to pay for an abortion does not deny the right to one was rejected. It was decided that the possible state interest in preserving a fetus was not sufficient when "weighed in the balance with the woman's threatened health" (Thom, 1980). The life endangerment standard was found unconstitutional on the basis that it may be impossible to detect a condition that might become life-threatening early enough to terminate the pregnancy. Further agreement by two doctors before an abortion could be performed was ruled to be meaningless, since the required delay could potentially threaten the woman's health.

In terms of the religious freedoms guaranteed in the First Amendment, the court stated: "The irreconcilable conflict of deeply and widely held views on this issue of individual conscience excludes any legislative intervention except that which protects each individual's freedom on conscientious decision and conscientious nonparticipation." A woman's decision to have an abortion was felt to warrant protection as a conscientious decision to the same degree that religiously mandated decisions are given First Amendment protection.

The McRae case has been appealed to the Supreme Court, and will doubtlessly be argued at great length. Because of the depth of documentation of this case, it is felt by some that the issue of deciding the fate of abortion by other means than a new constitutional amendment will be impossible. It is impossible at the time of this writing to determine or even speculate on the outcome of this case. Clearly, the Pro Choice and the Right to Life organizations are strong and are firmly committed to their views. Public opinion seems to favor abortions for women who wish to have them. However, as can be seen by the 1977 ruling, public sentiment is not always taken into consideration in highly charged issues such as this. The fight to produce a final statement on the legal aspects of abortion in this country is not likely to end in the foreseeable future.

Moral Aspects.   In categorizing the moral issues involved in the highly emotional question of abortion, three main interest groups emerge: women's groups and religious factions, legal experts, and physicians. Obviously, the members of these groups may fall into more than one of the above categories.

For ease of discussion, however, we will discuss the moral aspects of abortion in the light of these three groups as if they were distinct.

The major concern of the women's and religious groups is the issue of the rights of the fetus versus the rights of the woman. From this distinction evolves the discussion of when sacred human life begins. Callahan (1970) has presented three major theories of the beginning of sacred life that clearly identify the distinct views of the women's and religious groups.

1. *The genetic school.* According to the genetic school, sacred human life begins at the time of conception. At conception "the individual is whoever he is going to become." This is the view held by the Roman Catholic Church.
2. *The developmental school.* In addition to the genetic requirements for sacred human life, proponents of the developmental school usually believe that some development of form and function is necessary in order to define life as "human." The amount of time and the degree of development are not generally agreed upon by members of this group.
3. *The social consequences school.* This school includes both the genetic and developmental schools. In addition, social values are considered to be of great importance. For example, the social consequences of an unwanted pregnancy are considered a major influencing factor in the decision of the woman to terminate her pregnancy if she wishes in order to maintain or enhance her quality of Life. The Pro Choice groups generally fall into the social consequences school.

Currently, the genetic school proponents, notably the Right to Life and Pro Life groups, continue to press for new restrictive legislation regarding abortion, and are pushing for a constitutional amendment that would allow for the rights of the fetus and deny abortion for any reason (Green, 1977). As of this writing, no constitutional convention has been planned.

Legal experts have had the task of determining a legal definition of fetal viability. Technically, fetal viability refers to the point at which a fetus can survive outside of the mother's uterus. With the recent strides in technology in the field of neonatology, the age at which the fetus can survive outside of the mother has decreased significantly. It has become apparent that to try to finally define the point of viability may be an impossible task. It is possible that in the future fertilization and gestation could be technically accomplished completely outside of the uterus. With the advent of such technology, all attempts to define viability would fail. The legal question of when the fetus becomes "human," then, is nearly impossible to answer.

Finally, the interest of the medical profession concerning abortion must be considered. Regardless of personal feelings about abortion, physicians are generally concerned with the effects, both immediate and long term, of abortion on future conception, prematurity, and perinatal mortality and morbidity.

Research investigation of the long-term effects of a single abortion have generally concluded that a small percentage of women who have had one abortion, primarily those who have had an abortion by dilatation and curettage (D and C) procedures, may be more likely to have a spontaneous abortion in the second trimester of a later pregnancy (Maine, 1979). The risk of later miscarriages following one abortion seems to be linked more with the method of abortion than with the abortion itself. Vacuum aspiration abortions do not seem to carry the long-term risks the D and C procedures do.

The long-term effects of repeated abortion procedures on the future fertility of the woman are not clear at this time (Leach, 1977; Maine, 1979; WHO, 1979). Some studies cite higher rates of miscarriage, premature infants, and low-birth-weight infants, while others show rates for these complications that are comparable with those of control groups.

Regardless of the long-term effects that may follow repeat abortion, the fact remains that women are obtaining repeat abortions. In 1974, 13 per cent of the women in the United States who had an abortion had had a previous abortion (Leach, 1977). The repeat rate should not be misunderstood. The rates do not suggest a decline in the contraceptive efficacy among American women as a result of the legalization of abortion. The rates reflect and are consistent with the contraceptive failure rates of the currently available forms of contraception.

The moral aspects of the abortion controversy are varied and complex. Given our history and our current beliefs in the sanctity of human life, it is unlikely that this issue will be decided in the foreseeable future.

NURSING INTERVENTIONS AND ABORTION

Client Feelings About Abortion

Women's attitudes toward abortion change from time to time and from situation to situation. Attitudinal and situational factors must be considered in dealing with clients with unplanned pregnancies (Green, 1967).

Cultural and social experiences of individuals have profound effects on their attitudes toward abortion. Religion has a definite effect on some women's attitudes toward termination of pregnancy. The nurse should be careful, however, to avoid jumping to conclusions based on the client's reported religion. According to most studies, it is the degree of religiosity perceived by the client that is important in determining her views.

Educational background is another social experience that will affect a woman's views on abortion. In many cases, the woman who becomes pregnant has not yet completed her education. Incomplete education may itself be a rationale favoring abortion. On the other hand, the pregnant adolescent may see continuing a pregnancy as a means out of an educational system that she feels does not meet her needs.

Race is a cultural factor that must be considered in counseling women about abortion. In some racial cultures, abortion is seen quite differently than in the predominantly white, middle class background shared by the majority of nurses.

Situational factors vary with time and tend to assume different degrees of importance with each pregnancy. The age of the mother at the time of the pregnancy is obviously a factor. The very young woman and the woman over 40 will necessarily examine pregnancy differently than will the 25 year old. Gravidity, the number of previous pregnancies experienced by the woman, including their outcome, is a second situational factor to be considered by the woman and the nurse counseling her. Finally, marital status may be an important factor. The nurse must keep in mind that it is the effects of these factors *on the woman* that are significant. The nurse's own perceptions of the factors are not relevant to the decision to terminate or to continue the pregnancy.

The woman most likely to choose an abortion when confronted with an unplanned pregnancy is the young, unmarried woman who is not yet ready to begin a family *or* the older woman who has completed her family (Green, 1977). Feelings of ambivalence about having an abortion have been found to be normal and do not constitute a contradication to counseling for an abortion (Freeman, 1978).

The short- and long-term psychological effects of abortion have received a great deal of research interest in recent years. Overall, the most common post-abortion attitudes reported by women soon after the procedure were relief and happiness. Most women reported that they were happy with the decision to have the abortion, and that they felt that abortion was the right decision for them (Freeman, 1978; Green, 1977; Leach, 1977). This is not to imply that there are no feelings of loss and depression following abortion. The initial response, though, is one of relief.

Some women do report at least transient depressive symptoms following abortion. The woman may also feel guilty. These feelings are usually mild and tend to decrease over time. It seems that the more advanced the gestation, the greater is the likelihood that the woman will experience guilt and depression over terminating the pregnancy.

A significant finding about clients' feelings of guilt and depression was that it was related to the perceived attitudes of the medical and nursing staff toward the abortion and the patient. Nurses in particular were seen as having a great effect on transmitting the message that depression or guilt was or was not expected of the client. Such messages are often nonverbal in nature, and may even be on a subconscious level. They represent the biases of the nurse (in both directions) and must be recognized and dealt with.

In more long-term followup studies of post-abortion patients, it was found that many women need emotional support after the abortion as well as prior to the procedure (Freeman, 1978). According to the self-report measures, women especially felt the need for support from their male partners following the abortion procedures.

Surprisingly, emotional distress experienced before abortions was not an adequate indicator of successful resolution of the abortion experience. The woman's ability to cope with ambivalence and negative feelings was the best indicator of successful resolution. Of the women sampled, the majority of those who felt that they had successfully resolved the experience also reported changes in their behavior or attitudes that were suggestive of increased self-management (Gould, 1980).

For many health care professionals who deal with abortion patients, the repeat abortion patient is the most difficult. Despite the fact that the health care worker can be very nonjudgmental about one accidental pregnancy, two or more "failures" may be more difficult to accept. The tendency toward irresponsibility and the use of abortion as a method of contraception are suspected. The victim is blamed before the nurse actually finds out the specifics. Undoubtedly, some women do utilize abortion as a form of contraception. Contraceptive counselors may even encourage this when they counsel women to consider abortion as a backup should their form of contraception fail. In fact, the increase in the rate of repeat abortions does not indicate a relaxation of contraceptive use on the part of women. The repeat rate is consistent with the use of the most effective methods of contraception available (Parker, 1975). That is, even if women utilize the most effective methods of contraception following an abortion (the birth control pills and IUD) there is still the possibility of a repeat pregnancy due to a method failure. This failure rate corresponds to the repeat abortion rate found in most studies.

Women who have more than one abortion do tend to see themselves differently than their counterparts who are having their first abortion. Many feel an inability to control their lives, especially in the areas of sexuality and reproduction. Interestingly, a full 25 per cent of the repeat abortion clients in one study had received no counseling at all following their first abortion (Leach, 1977). This finding tends to confirm the conclusion that post-abortion counseling is at least as important as the preabortion counseling that most women receive.

The Adolescent Seeking an Abortion

Because of her developmental status, the pregnant adolescent presents a very different picture from that of her more mature pregnant sister. The decision to carry the pregnancy to term or to terminate the pregnancy may be the first decision with lifelong implications that the adolescent has ever had to make. To further complicate the situation, this decision must often be made very quickly. For a variety of reasons, pregnancy may be discovered much later in adolescents than in older women. The adolescent is more likely to have irregular menstrual cycles. Because of this, she may not become alarmed about the possibility of pregnancy until she is well into the pregnancy. In addition, denial, fear, and ignorance play an important part in the delay of recognition of pregnancy. For example, many adolescents do not know that a woman can become pregnant if she has intercourse only once. Others may have incorrectly determined that they had intercourse when they were in a "safe period" and may therefore deny the early signs of pregnancy. Regardless of the reasons for the delay, the reality of the situation is that many pregnant adolescents have to decide under very rushed circumstances whether or not to continue the pregnancy, in order to be able to have the less dangerous and complicated first trimester abortion if they choose to terminate the pregnancy.

The pregnant adolescent may have very unrealistic expectations of what life will be like for her if she continues the pregnancy and keeps the child (Nadelson, 1977). The adolescent woman who feels that her life is empty and deprived may see this as an opportunity to fill the emptiness with love for, and of, this other person. In this sense, the baby may be viewed as a gift. Closely related to this is the expectation that having the baby will be like having a live doll. The child may be seen as a possession of the young mother. Having a child of her own may be considered a way to get herself out of a home situation that she finds intolerable. Once she has a child, she will be eligible for federal assistance and will therefore, she reasons, be able to live on her own. The reality of living at the poverty level of federal assistance and the "trapped" feelings reported by many in this situation are not understood by the pregnant adolescent. To her, the money she will receive seems like a large amount, which she could surely live on with the new child.

If the adolescent, given guidance, still decides that she wants to continue the pregnancy, realistic planning is essential. The pregnant adolescent is at greater risk than the more mature woman during her pregnancy. She is more likely to experience toxemia, premature birth, infection, and complications in labor and delivery. These risks, which can be decreased if she is provided proper and consistent prenatal care, must be discussed in a nonthreatening manner with the client. Exposure to other adolescents who have made the choice to keep their babies should be planned, if possible, so the adolescent can hear from her own peers the impact that having a baby can have, both positive and negative. In all counseling with adolescents, the use of peers who have been in the same situation is very helpful. Providing peer counseling demonstrates an understanding of the importance of the peer group to the adolescent.

The adolescent who decides to have an abortion will also need a great deal of teaching, counseling, and support. The nurse must educate the client, to prevent another unplanned pregnancy due to ignorance. Incorrect ideas must be corrected in a supportive nonjudgmental fashion. Again, realistic planning is essential. It is not unusual to hear an adolescent declare that she will not be having intercourse ever again, and refuse any contraception or contraceptive counseling. The alert nurse will realize that even if the client feels strongly that she will not have intercourse again, the possibility still exists that, in time, she will change her mind. Ultimately, of course, the decision is the adolescent's. She should leave the abortion procedure and follow-up visits with the understanding that contraception is available to her, even if she refuses it at this time. She should be educated in all methods of contraception as a form of anticipatory guidance. The nurse must keep in mind that only after the young woman can see herself as a sexual person will she be likely to be a conscientious contraceptor.

First Trimester Abortion

Despite the Hyde Amendment in 1977, public opinion continues to favor the legalization of abortion (Digest [A], 1979). In a 1979 Gallup Poll, 80 per cent of the sample reported that they felt abortion should be legal in all or some circumstances. This is a 3 per cent increase in this area since the last poll in 1977. Of these 80 per cent in 1979, 70 per cent felt Medicaid should pay for at least some of the abortion for Medicaid-eligible women.

In a 1979 Harris Survey, 60 per cent of the respondents reported that they supported the 1973 Supreme Court decision that made abortion legal. In 1977, only 53 per cent of the sample had indicated this support.

Overall, then, there seems to be greater public acceptance of abortion as a legal alternative to pregnancy than the complex legislation would indicate. For most individuals, it is the safe, first trimester abortions that are the most acceptable.

The suction method of abortion utilizes minimal cervical dilation and a mild suction to withdraw the contents of the uterus. This procedure can generally be performed between eight and 12 to 14 weeks of gestation. Determining gestational size is an important component of this procedure. If, for example, the fetus is less than six weeks by size, it is very possible that the suction will not remove all of the contents of the uterus, and the fetus may remain. Similarly, if the fetus is too large, the gentle suction used will not be sufficient to dislodge the products of conception from the wall of the uterus.

Two less commonly utilized methods of early abortion are menstrual extraction and dilation and evacuation (D and E). Menstrual extraction is performed before the woman misses a menstrual period when the endometrial lining is removed. It is felt that if there is a pregnancy in the uterus, it too will be removed during the procedure. Many women report that they find this method very acceptable, since it frees them from actually having to make a decision as to whether or not to have an abortion. If the woman merely suspects a pregnancy, she can have the procedure done prior to the time at which pregnancy could be detected by the conventional pregnancy tests. One of the negative effects of menstrual extraction, however, is the relatively high failure rate caused by missed abortion. What this means is that when the products of conception are so small that they are missed during the procedure, the pregnancy can continue without the woman's knowledge.

In dilation and evacuation, the cervix is dilated and a sharp curette is used to remove the contents of the uterus. This procedure carries the risk of uterine perforation and bleeding because of the use of the sharp curette. This may be the method of choice for the woman who is approaching the end of the time in which she can obtain a first trimester abortion (Hatcher, 1979). This procedure is implicated in higher risks for future pregnancies.

Potential complications of any of these three methods of early abortion include infection and Rh sensitization. During the preabortion counseling, women are instructed to report any post-abortion temperature elevation immediately. In addition, they are instructed to contact a physician if they notice that the vaginal discharge which follows the procedure becomes foul smelling, or if they begin to experience abdominal pain. Intercourse is usually restricted for at least two weeks or until the vaginal flow stops. Some facilities that specialize in early abortions may choose to give their clients antibiotics for prophylactic purposes. The rationale for this treatment is that the risk of antibiotic therapy is considered less than that of the complications that occur with pelvic infection. In any case, the woman must be instructed and understand under what conditions she should contact her physician.

Increasingly, women who are found to have Rh negative blood are given immune globulin at the time of the abortion. Rh sensitization can occur during abortion. This sensitization has potentially significant negative effects on future pregnancies.

Second Trimester Abortions

A woman undergoing a second trimester abortion is at much greater risk than the woman undergoing a first trimester abortion. The risk of maternal death from the second trimester procedure is nine times greater than that from the first trimester procedure.

The most commonly utilized method for second trimester abortions is saline abortion. This procedure is generally performed between 16 and 20 weeks of gestation, although it may be performed up to 24 weeks, according to the accepted guidelines for legal abortion. During this type of abortion, hypertonic saline is injected into the amniotic fluid through the mother's abdomen. The fetus usually dies as a result of this procedure, probably from electrolyte disturbances brought about by the saline. Within a few hours, most women who have had the saline instillation will begin labor and will deliver the fetus, usually within the next 24 hours. About 3 to 5 per cent of patients do not spontaneously go into labor as a result of this procedure. Some will go into labor following a second instillation of saline.

The major and most serious complication of saline induction abortion occurs with accidental intravascular injection of the saline. Even in small doses, injection of saline into the woman's vascular system may lead to hypotension, loss of consciousness, and cardiac arrest.

Hypernatremia is a second potential complication of saline induction abortion. Thirst, nausea, and abdominal burning or pain reported immediately following the procedure indicate a significant degree of hypernatremia. The condition is characterized by lethargy and drowsiness, and may be accompanied by seizures. If these symptoms appear, the prognosis is generally poor. It is normal for almost all saline induction abortion patients to experience thirst one to two hours following the injection. This is considered to be within normal limits and is not to be confused with hypernatremia.

Finally, disseminated intravascular coagulation (DIC) may occur as a result of saline induction second trimester abortion. The woman experiences a change in her blood coagulation parameters, which may lead to an increased risk of severe hemorrhage. This condition generally responds well to evacuation of the uterus and the administration of fresh whole blood.

Because of the seriousness of the complications of the saline method of abortion, some practitioners have begun to use injections of prostaglandins rather than saline to stimulate the abortion. The prostaglandins are usually injected intra-amniotically, as is the saline. Occasionally, though, they are introduced intravaginally. Prostaglandins cause abortion through direct oxytocin-like myometrial stimulation. That is, the drugs cause uterine contractions.

The use of prostaglandins for second trimester abortions has raised an important moral issue. Following prostaglandin injection abortion the fetus may be born live. In the earlier gestational periods of 16 to 20 weeks, the chances of survival of the fetus are quite small. By the twenty-fourth week of gestation, however, the fetus may be successfully supported until it can mature sufficiently to live outside the mother. The staff of the facility performing the second trimester abortion can be in a very precarious moral and legal position. Many feel that they are trained to save lives and that they are being party to murder if they do not make every attempt possible to save any fetus born live following a second trimester abortion. The question of whether such a child should become a ward of the state, be put up for adoption, or be considered to be the child of the mother that had undergone the abortion still requires a definitive answer. In one case in Boston, a physician was charged with manslaughter when he did not attempt to save a fetus that was born live following a hysterotomy procedure performed to abort the fetus. Because of the potential of a live birth, and because of the current difficulties in defining viability, many facilities have formed a policy under which no abortion past 20 weeks of gestation will be performed. While this usually is sufficient, a more final decision will have to be made. As expertise in the field of neonatology increases, it is logical to assume that even 20-week fetuses may be saved.

The primary physical side effects of prostaglandins are GI disturbances and occasional bronchospasms. It is estimated that between 55 and 85 per cent of women experience vomiting and/or diarrhea (Green, 1977). The rates for hemorrhage, retained placenta, and infection following prostaglandin abortions are comparable to those following saline abortions. The failure rate, that is, the percentage of women who do not abort following one instillation of the prostaglandins, is between 15 and 20 per cent. These women will require a repeat injection. As stated, the failure rate for saline abortions is usually between 3 and 5 per cent.

Post-abortion teaching following a second trimester abortion is essentially the same as that following a first trimester abortion. The client should be informed that she can begin to have intercourse in several weeks, when the vaginal flow has stopped. Even though the second trimester abortion causes the woman actually to experience delivery, she will not have an episiotomy or the attendant discomforts of perineal stitches.

The client must be taught to be aware of and to report danger signs in the post-abortion period, such as foul smelling lochia, abdominal pain, fever, and/or abnormal bleeding. Post-abortion contraception should also be discussed. The nurse should fully inform the client of all the options that are available to her so that she can avoid future unwanted pregnancies. The client must understand the mechanism of conception prior to being taught how to prevent pregnancy. This is well within the province of the nurse.

The Nurse and Abortion

Joan was a 16-year-old student at the local high school. Her parents were prominent members of the community. Joan was seen in the Planned Parenthood abortion clinic for the first time for pregnancy testing. It was determined that she was in her eighth week of pregnancy. In discussing her options in dealing with this unplanned pregnancy, Steve, the nurse, asked Joan some routine questions. He determined that Joan had been sexually active for the past four to five months with her boyfriend, Larry, who was a senior in high school. Larry was not aware that Joan might be pregnant. She had decided not to discuss this with him until she received the test results.

When asked about contraception used, Joan reported that she and Larry were using the rhythm method. They did not have intercourse during the times they thought were her fertile periods. In discussing Joan's menstrual cycle with her, Steve learned that her cycle was irregular, with periods from 23 to 45 days. The couple abstained from intercourse on days 12 through 18 of each cycle.

As the nurse and Joan established a rapport, the nurse asked Joan if she knew about the various types of contraceptives available to the couple. Joan was aware of the clinics in her neighborhood that specialize in birth control for teenagers, but her knowledge of the actual methods was poor.

Joan's reluctance to utilize the birth control clinics was not, as the nurse had assumed, based on fear that she would be recognized. In fact, Joan stated that this had not occurred to her. Joan and Larry had agreed that the most "beautiful" love was a spontaneous love. Not wishing to become pregnant, Joan had limited their lovemaking to her perceived "safe" periods.

As the counseling session continued, the nurse found that he was having difficulty in dealing with Joan. It appeared that she was going to elect to terminate the pregnancy. Although Steve had no negative feeling about this, he found it difficult to accept the fact that Joan had decided not to tell Larry about the pregnancy prior to termination. He also found himself angry that a young woman who was obviously intelligent had failed to prevent the unwanted pregnancy in the first place. The teen clinic was easily accessible to her and was obviously well known to her from her own report.

Steve, the nurse, confronted Joan with his feelings that she should at least consider allowing Larry to take part in the decision. After some discussion, Joan continued to feel that she did not want Larry to know, fearing that he would be angry with her for not being sure about her fertile periods. She agreed to think about it, however, in light of the possibility that Larry could be a support person for her during the procedure.

Steve did not discuss his anger with Joan about her lack of use of available resources. She clearly stated that she knew that even though she did not want to think about sex now, she probably would want to be sexually active again, but this time she did not want to have to worry about another unwanted pregnancy. After some discussion before the procedure and in the post-abortion counseling, Joan decided to have an intrauterine device inserted several weeks after the abortion. Larry did come to the clinic with Joan, and was present during the procedure and the post-abortion counseling. He had wanted her to have the baby but was supportive when it became clear that Joan did not want this responsibility or the marriage that Larry proposed. Although the couple split up two weeks after the procedure, Joan still kept her appointment to have the post-abortion intrauterine device inserted.

One of the questions most commonly asked of women who become accidentally pregnant is what type of contraception was used prior to the pregnancy. Studies indicate that approximately 45 per cent of women seeking a first abortion report that they were not using any form of contraception in the four to five months prior to the unplanned pregnancy (Freeman, 1978; Fylling, 1979). Of those who reported use of contraception, more than 70 per cent used the less effective contraceptive methods, that is, creams, jellies, or douching. In one study, 78 per cent of the total sample stated that they had tried to prevent pregnancy mostly by limiting intercourse during the times they perceived to be not "safe" (Freeman, 1978).

Teenagers tended to use contraception prior to pregnancy less than the older primigravidas. Sporadic use or nonuse of contraception resulting in unwanted pregnancy is sometimes judged by nurses involved in the counseling of these women to be more negative than pregnancy resulting from contraceptive failure. The woman who becomes pregnant because of contraceptive failure may be viewed as an unfortunate victim of the currently unacceptable forms of contraceptives available, whereas the nonuser of contraception may be viewed as an irresponsible woman, who more or less "deserves" to be "caught" and "punished" for her carelessness and lack of responsibility. Rarely are these feelings clear-cut in the mind of the nurse. If they were, nurses would not report such difficulty in dealing with abortion patients who were not using contraceptives at the time of conception. Punitive attitudes toward sexual activity and responsibility must be evaluated by the nurse and dealt with before she can adequately counsel women with unplanned pregnancies, regardless of the cause of the pregnancy.

Post-abortion use of contraception is utilized by the vast majority of these women. Most choose the more effective methods of birth control available (birth control pills, IUDs, diaphragms, sterilization) and report a high continuation rate following their abortion procedures (Freeman, 1978; Fylling, 1979; Leach, 1977). At one year post-abortion, the overall continuation rate for use of birth control pills was about 79 per cent, while the rate for IUD continuation was 93.1 per cent. Part of the rationale for the higher rate for IUD's was explained by the fact that many of the women who chose to discontinue the pill during the first year changed to the use of an IUD (Fylling, 1979).

The increase in effective practice of contraception following abortion procedures confirms the usefulness of instruction and the provision of contraceptive information at the time of the abortion. The post-abortion counseling period is of great importance in helping the client to resolve her feelings about the procedure and is also an excellent time, in terms of learning readiness, for contraceptive teaching.

An interesting finding in one study concerns the nonuse of contraception among teenagers, despite the current availability of family planning services. Fylling (1970) concluded that nonuse among adolescents reflects impaired motivation to utilize contraception, rather than a lack of available services. The fact that these women are highly motivated contraceptors following abortion tends to support this notion (Burr, 1980).

Attitudes of the Nurse

Many nurses and nursing students avoid confronting their own feelings about abortion until they find themselves in the situation of having to deal with abortion directly — that is, by experiencing an unwanted pregnancy themselves, by helping a close friend through an abortion, or by being assigned a patient who is to have an abortion. Ideally, each nurse will thoroughly assess her feelings and attitudes about abortion before the issue becomes pressing. One of the first steps the nurse must take is to assess her own ability to separate her private views on abortion from her professional views. For example, a nurse who does not find abortion to be an acceptable alternative for herself can be highly effective in counseling a client who is deciding whether or not to have an abortion. The separation of the nurse as a professional from the nurse as a friend or confidant is essential in all counseling — abortion counseling is no exception.

Assessing Nurses' Attitudes — Self-Assessment. All nurses who will potentially be counseling women with unplanned pregnancies should ask themselves if they feel that abortion is a valid solution to unwanted pregnancy. If they find that they cannot consider abortion an acceptable solution for others, they probably should not counsel women with unwanted pregnancies, since they will be unable to present these women with a view of all the alternatives that are currently available to them. Still, since they encounter women in all areas of health and sickness, it is probable that they will be approached at times by women with unwanted pregnancies. If these nurses are able to state their views on abortion to clients without sounding judgmental or punitive, they may choose to do so. It is their responsibility, however, to refer these clients to someone who can counsel them regarding *all* of their options in dealing with the unplanned pregnancy. If the nurse is unable to state her feelings without projecting a negative attitude, she should not express these feelings but, rather, should refer the client to another individual for counseling.

Regardless of the role of the nurse as counselor or caretaker during and/or following the abortion procedure, she must have adequate knowledge of the resources available for women who are terminating pregnancies and for those who choose to continue their pregnancies. The nurse not only must know the resources that are available but also should have a working knowledge of the quality and policies of the referral agencies. For example, in some areas of the country an organization called Birthright advertises that they counsel women with unplanned pregnancies. Not included in their advertising but included as part of their policy is the fact that they will not refer women who decide on abortion to any abortion facility. The woman who chooses this agency, then, may have to delay her abortion in order to find, on her own, an agency that will perform the procedure. The nurse who refers a client to such an agency should inform her of these policies and let her know of the alternatives she could choose should she decide to terminate the pregnancy.

A second question nurses should ask themselves before dealing with women with unplanned pregnancies is whether they feel that women should be punished for sexual behavior. The notion that pregnancy is a kind of punishment for sexual activity is common among both clients and health professionals. The nurse who feels that pregnancy is the "just" punishment for sexual activity (whether within or outside marriage) can have a potentially destructive psychological impact on a woman with an unplanned pregnancy. A nurse with this attitude who is caring for a second trimester abortion client experiencing labor can be very punitive toward the patient, even to the point of telling her that the pain of labor is her punishment for her sexual activities. The nurse must understand that her actions and words will have a profound effect on whether the client can successfully reconcile the abortion experience without undue stress. Most health care professionals are aware of the dangers to future mothering skills of women who view pregnancy as a punishment for sexual activity. It is not a big step to imagine the impact that a nurse transmitting this negative information to a client could have on the woman's future self-concept as a mother caring for her child. Clients tend to listen to and remember comments and attitudes of nurses far more than they remember those of nonprofessionals.

A third issue the nurse must confront is that of who should make the decision about abortion in the case of a minor. Some nurses feel that the parents of the minor have the right to be informed of their daughter's pregnancy, while others feel that informing the parents against the wishes of the pregnant woman constitutes an infringement of her confidentiality rights. Although a nurse who feels the parents have a right to be informed can still work with the client effectively, it is not appropriate for the nurse to inform the parents. It must be recognized that a significant number of young women seeking counseling may be pregnant as a result of incest and/ or rape by a family member. To disclose a pregnancy in this situation could have devastating long-term effects on the pregnant adolescent.

Finally, the nurse should examine her own feelings about the role of the father of the baby in the decision-making process. Currently, no approval from the father of the baby is required, although termination of pregnancy without the consent of a husband has been utilized as grounds for divorce in some states. In some cases, the woman's partner may be included in the counseling procedures and may, in fact, be present during the abortion, if that is the method chosen.

The aforementioned questions and the answers that each nurse finds lead to the question of whether all nurses should be required to work with abortion patients. This becomes especially salient in terms of second trimester abortions, since they are usually performed in hospitals on an inpatient basis.

Should All Nurses Work with Abortion Patients?   Nurses who wish to avoid working with first trimester abortion patients can usually do so by choosing not to work in the clinic settings that are the primary sites of first trimester abortions. For the office nurse in a private OB/Gyn office the choice may be a matter of informing the physician of her decision not to work with abortion patients. In rare cases, though, the office nurse may not have the option of refusing to work with such patients.

Second trimester abortions may be more problematic. According to federal regulations, second trimester abortions must be performed in settings in which the woman could receive prompt, round the clock medical attention should an emergency occur. Because of this, the bulk of all second trimester abortions are performed in inpatient departments of hospitals. Frequently, the setting is an obstetrical or gynecological unit. The laboring woman may be placed in a private labor room to deliver the fetus, and may then recover on the regular postpartum unit. It is in these inpatient units that difficulties may arise. Some nurses may wish to avoid working with abortion patients and may ask not to be given such patient assignments. The result of this may be animosity from other nurses, who may eventually feel that they have become the "abortion nurses" because the others are unwilling to take their share of abortion patients. This situation is especially likely to occur in obstetrical units when second trimester abortion patients are placed with normal postpartum patients. The happy postpartum patient is more pleasant for most nurses to deal with than is the woman undergoing a second trimester abortion.

The problem is difficult. Second trimester abortion patients may suffer if all nurses are required to work with them, since the patients have to be exposed to nurses who cannot give them the encouragement and support that is so important to them. The important post-abortion counseling may also be neglected by the nurse who wishes to avoid contact with the patient as much as possible. (Avoidance of patients who are seen as undesirable is not uncommon in nursing, although it is far from therapeutic for either nurse or patient. For example, the demanding patient is undesirable and is the one who is most likely to be ignored by the nursing staff. Avoidance of these patients by the unwilling nurse can be a conscious or subconscious act.)

If it is determined that only those nurses who feel comfortable caring for abortion patients will care for these patients, then these nurses will eventually become less enthusiastic, since the experience may take more and more time away from the care of the types of patients that the nurse originally chose to work with.

As a compromise, some hospitals have worked out a system of care for abortion patients that more adequately divides the time spent with them. Careful assessment of the nurse's feelings usually uncovers specific areas of discomfort for the nurse. For example, some nurses may feel that they do not wish to be present for the procedure itself but may find that they can work with the patient following the procedure. Other nurses may feel that they can work with the patient after the abortion, providing post-abortion counseling and contraception teaching, but are unable to work with the patient during the actual delivery or immediately following the procedure. In order for the staff to devise compromises in such situations, much time, effort, and willingness to be open to alternatives is required. Staff must specifically define their own level of comfort in caring for abortion patients in terms of what will ultimately result in the best care for the patient and the most pleasant conditions for the nurses. Not working with any stage of the abortion experience is an option usually kept by a few nurses.

ABORTION TEACHING

Counseling women with unwanted and/or unplanned pregnancies can take place in a variety of settings. Regardless of the area, the role of the counselor should be the same. The counselor should be an individual who can help the client to understand her motivations, explore her ambivalences, consider her alternatives, and help her to work through any family problems that may be related to the current pregnancy (Nadelson, 1977). The decision of whether to carry or terminate a pregnancy must ultimately be the client's. In order to function as the patient's advocate, the nurse must possess a great deal of technical information as well as the skill to simplify the options according to the patient's level of understanding. Listening skills are essential.

All procedures must be thoroughly explained with both verbal and written illustrations. The client must be informed of all options available to her, including termination of the pregnancy, delivering the child and then putting it up for adoption, the possibility of short term foster care, and keeping the child. Regardless of the woman's choice, she should be informed what to expect in each of her options. For example, should the woman choose to have an abortion, complete instructions as to what will actually be experienced should be provided. If, instead, the woman elects to carry the child to term, utilizing a clinic for her prenatal care, the general policies to be followed at the given clinic should be explained thoroughly to the client.

In dealing with clients with unplanned pregnancies, the nurse should always regard the situation as an emergency and should utilize the techniques of crisis intervention (Gray, 1979). The time limitation necessarily imposes an even greater sense of crisis if the woman decides to have an abortion. Counseling must be thorough, fast, and nonjudgmental. Not all nurses feel prepared to perform the type of crisis intervention needed in such situations. If this is the case, they should remain well informed of organizations and individuals to whom the client who needs such treatment can be referred.

In helping the client to reach a decision as to the best alternative for her, the nurse should assess the patient's current sexual and contraceptive knowledge. This evaluation includes a determination as to whether the client is aware of how she became pregnant. Unfortunately, many nurses overlook this essential issue, assuming that all women know how they become pregnant. Often, the nurse who avoids this discussion does so to avoid embarrassing the client. Many women do not know the exact mechanism of conception. The vast majority, even those who do know that intercourse is usually needed for conception to occur, cannot accurately predict their "safe periods."

Contraceptive knowledge may be inadequate or incorrect. The nurse is the appropriate individual to correct misinterpretations about contraception and to fill in the empty areas of the client's knowledge. In terms of the pre-decision counseling, the nurse is primarily interested in an assessment of knowledge. The bulk of the teaching will usually take place following the procedure (if the client decides on an abortion) or at the end of the pregnancy, when contraception again becomes an issue.

Since current research indicates that the support of a significant other, especially the father of the baby, following the abortion procedure is important in later resolution of the termination procedure, some researchers advocate that the counselor spend time with the client investigating the role of the father of the baby in the current pregnancy (Villanueva, 1978). Discussions of whether the father has been informed and how he feels about the situation will help the counselor to assess the support systems of the client. Under no circumstances, however, is it appropriate for the nurse to inform the father of the baby about either the pregnancy or the client's decision regarding the outcome of the current pregnancy. This must be the patient's decision. For the nurse to take any action in this area would be to infringe upon the client's right to confidentiality. In most cases, if the patient wishes, she may have a significant other present with her during the abortion. If this is the case in the facility that the patient will utilize for the pregnancy termination, she should be informed of this so that she can plan for her significant other to be present to give her support before, during, and following the procedure.

If the client decides upon abortion, the nurse is the appropriate person to initiate teaching about the procedure and what to expect after the abortion. Potential danger signs should be discussed and reviewed until the client is able to repeat, in her own words, those things that she will be expected to report should they occur. These signs include 1) persistent bleeding; 2) foul smelling discharge; 3) persistent uterine cramping; 4) elevated temperature; 5) pain, frequency, or burning on urination; and 6) continued depressed state.

Following the abortion, most patients will be able to resume their normal activities within a few days, provided there are no complications arising from the abortion. They are usually instructed to avoid the use of tampons or douches for at least two weeks, in order to protect them from infection. This may be an appropriate time to instruct women that douching is not really recommended in any event, because the vagina is a self-cleaning organ and because douching places the woman at greater risk of infections that arise from upsetting the pH levels of the vagina.

Intercourse can usually be resumed within two to three weeks, if the vaginal flow has stopped. Most women will resume their menstrual periods in about four weeks. They may notice that the flow during the first period is somewhat heavier, and they should not be alarmed by this. Excessive bleeding, saturating more than one pad or tampon per hour, is not normal and should be reported immediately.

All abortion patients should be seen two to four weeks after the procedure to determine that normal healing is taking place. It should be stressed that this post-abortion check is essential to determine if normal involution is taking place. Counseling on contraception should take place prior to this visit, since some of the clients may resume intercourse before their recheck, and could become pregnant again. *All clients should be informed that they can indeed become pregnant before the period following an abortion.*

As in most patient situations, the nurse is the individual who spends the most time with the client. The quality of this time, especially in terms of resolution of the abortion experience, is crucial for the patient. The nurse must be aware of her own feelings and biases in dealing with abortion patients in order to effectively provide the most positive experience possible for the client. Nurses must attend to their own needs as well as those of the patient in order to be effective. Only the individual nurse can assess comfort levels on the issue of abortion, and only she can decide ultimately whether her skills and counseling will be beneficial to both the client and herself. This decision is one that cannot be made passively. The nurse must work to examine and understand her feelings about abortion, and must then act upon her conclusions to the best end for her and for her clients.

References

Burr, W. A.: "Delayed Abortion in an Area of Easy Accessibility." *JAMA*, Vol. 244, No. 1, July 4, 1980.

Callahan, D.: *Abortion, Law, Choice and Morality.* London, MacMillan Co., 1970.

Cates, Willard, Jr., Kimball, Ann Marie, Gold, Julian, Rubin, George, Smith, Jack, Rochat, Roger, and Tyler, Carl, Jr.: "The Health Impact of Restricting Public Funds for Abortion October 10, 1977–June 10, 1978." *American Journal of Public Health,* Vol. 69, No. 9, September, 1979.

Digest (a): "80% of Americans Believe Abortion Should Be Legal, 70% Approve Medicaid Funding." *Family Planning Perspectives,* Vol. 11, No. 3, May/June, 1979.

Digest (b): "Supreme Court: States Need Not Pay for 'Nontherapeutic' Abortions via Medicaid." *Family Planning Perspectives,* Vol. 9, No. 4, July/August, 1977.

Freeman, Ellen W.: "Abortion: Subjective Attitudes and Feelings." *Family Planning Perspectives,* Vol. 10, No. 3, May/June, 1978.

Fylling, Petter, Svendsby, Torunn: "Contraceptive Practice Before and After Therapeutic Abortion." *Fertility and Sterility,* Vol. 32, No. 1, July 1977.

Gerrard, Meg: "Sex Guilt in Abortion Patients." *Journal of Consulting and Clinical Psychology,* Vol. 45, No. 4, p. 708, 1977.

Gold, Julian, Cates Willard: "Restriction of Federal Funds for Abortion: 18 months Later." *American Journal of Public Health,* Vol. 69, No. 9, September, 1979.

Gordon, Linda: *Woman's Body, Woman's Right: A Social History of Birth Control in America.* New York, Penguin Books, 1976.

Gould, N. B.: "Post Abortion Depressive Reactions in College Women." *Journal of the American College Health Association,* Vol. 28, No. 6, June 1980.

Gray, Mary Jane: "The Role of the Sex Counselor." *AASECT Convention — Presentation,* Washington, D.C., 1979.

Green, Karen, Resnik, Robert: "The Abortion Issue: Past, Present and Future." *Current Problems in Pediatrics,* Vol. VII, No. 10, August, 1977.

Hatcher, R. A., Stewart, G. K., Stewart, F., Guest, F., Schwartz, D. W., and Jones, S. A.: *Contraceptive Technology 1980–1981:* 10th ed., New York, Irvington Publishers, Inc., 1980.

Himes, N. E.: *Medical History of Contraception.* Baltimore, Williams & Wilkins Co., 1936.

Leach, Judith: "The Repeat Abortion Patient." *Family Planning Perspectives,* Vol. 9, No. 1, January/February, 1977.

Maine, Deborah: "Does Abortion Affect Later Pregnancies?" *Family Planning Perspectives,* Vol. 11, No. 2, March/April, 1979.

Nadelson, Carol C., Notman, Malkah T.: "Treatment of the Pregnant Teenager and the Putative Father." *Current Psychiatric Therapies,* Vol. 17, 1977.

Pakter, Jean, Nelson, Frieda, and Svigir, Martin: "Legal Abortion: A Half Decade of Experience." *Family Planning Perspectives,* Vol. 7, No. 6, November/December, 1975.

Thom, Mary: "The McRae Decision on Abortion: Seizing the Moral Imperative." *Ms. Magazine,* April, 1980.

Villanueva, Cesar, and Clancy, Barbara: "Counseling and Abortion." *In* Barnard, Martha, Clancy, Barbara, and Krantz, Kermit (Eds.): *Human Sexuality for Health Professionals.* Philadelphia, W. B. Saunders Co., 1978.

WHO: "Induced Abortion and the Risk of Spontaneous Abortion." *Family Planning Perspectives,* Vol. 11, No. 39, 1979.

10

HOMOSEXUALITY

INTRODUCTION

"Imagine that you are a heterosexual in a homosexual society. One out of ten are heterosexual, but they are not clearly identified. Do not assume that all masculine males and feminine females will be heterosexual. All of you will be expected to date and marry the same sex. There will be jokes about you in most social circles. . . . If your heterosexuality is discovered, you face possible job loss, rejection by family and friends, being labeled a criminal, etc. . . ." (Smith, 1979.)

After reading this quote, think about and try to understand the way a homosexual person may feel in our society. Take several minutes to consider the implications of being homosexual in a heterosexual world — the effect on your self-image and on your happiness. Experiencing discrimination on any basis is a blow to the self-concept that is difficult to overcome; experiencing discrimination and stigma on the basis of sexual orientation can be a particular burden because the expectation of heterosexual orientation is fundamental to all of our social and legal institutions.

Sexual expression in our culture takes many forms. Some alternative life styles are accepted by society — celibacy, for example, is time-honored among religious groups. Other alternative life styles are being gradually accepted by society — in 1980, census forms for the first time provided a separate category to identify "persons of the opposite sex sharing living quarters," in recognition of the great number of unmarried couples living together. In this text, homosexuality is being discussed in a separate chapter because it is a life style that involves a large number of people, whose behavior ranges from fantasizing about homosexuality to openly expressing a complete homosexual orientation, including a choice of permanent same-sex partner for sex and lifelong companionship. Attitudes of society toward this life style range from those who consider homosexuality abnormal and in need of change to those who consider it a legitimate form of sexual expression.

In the past two decades it has become recognized that the number of homosexual people in the United States is significantly greater than was previously thought. It is likely that at some time, almost all nurses will care for or work with individuals who are homosexual. In order to give care consistent with the standards of professional nursing, the nurse must understand homosexuality from the perspective of society, the perspective of the homosexual person, and finally from the perspective of the health care delivery system.

INCIDENCE ESTIMATES

Approximately 3 to 5 per cent of the populations in several studies (Bell, 1975; Money, 1976; Money, 1977) reported that they were exclusively homosexual in terms of their erotic partner. In addition to this exclusively homosexual group, one third of the population who described themselves as primarily heterosexual admitted to some homosexual experience at some time in their lives after the age of puberty. A continuum for sexuality and sexual expression has been proposed to explain commonly encountered sexual orientations and behaviors. In this proposal, all individuals are placed on a continuum according to the relative frequencies of their homosexual/heterosexual ideation, affect, and behavior (Davison, 1976). If one utilizes this scale approach, it becomes clear that the significant portion of people fall somewhere between the extremes of the scale, and that people who are exclusively homosexual or heterosexual are actually quite rare. Placement of individuals on such a scale includes factors such as orientation as well as behavior. Based on orientation, an individual may be somewhere in the middle of the scale, although he or she participates only in heterosexual acts.

Most research and self-reports by homosexuals support the idea that most homosexuals are aware of their sexual orientation from very early childhood (Gochros, 1978; Hunt, 1978). In some cases, the child of five or six may be aware of the preference for members of the same sex, according to the level appropriate for a child of that age group. A common misconception is that it is not until adolescence that sexual orientation is determined. Many believe that the spontaneous homosexual investigations common during adolescence form the basis for the decision to become homosexual or heterosexual. In fact, most people, especially males, report some homosexual play during adolescence despite the fact that most of these people later become exclusively heterosexual in behavior. A commonly accepted rationale for the same-sex play so prevalent in adolescence is the comfort level of adolescents with members of their own sex. In many cases, the adolescent may not feel secure enough to engage in sex play with a member of the opposite sex. Consequently, behaviors may be "tried out" on members of the same sex. The social interactions are essentially the same, regardless of the sex of the participants. The behaviors do not indicate homosexual orientations.

Not all people are certain of their sexual orientation from an early age, however. Some individuals may feel confused about their sexuality and may feel pressured to "decide" one way or the other as to their sexual orientation. These people are especially vulnerable to the social pressures that result from rigid social expectations. On the one hand, they hear quite clearly that homosexuality is bad, sinful, pathological, and perverse. On the other hand, they may be subjected to pressures from those in the homosexual community who say that if people experience any homosexual feelings, they are homosexuals and should admit that fact. Some politically active homosexuals may try to convince individuals who are trying to sort out their feelings that their heterosexual feelings and aspirations are products of the social pressures of a heterosexual society to conform and, as such, should be ignored (Bancroft, 1975). There is no reason to consider either of these views as "right." Utilizing the continuum for sexuality and sexual expression, the individual with uncertain sexual preferences may be one of the group of people who feel that they are happy with both homosexual and heterosexual life styles. The pressure to decide one way or the other is one imposed by society, and it can be detrimental, forcing a decision that will necessarily involve giving up some pleasurable aspects of sexual expression.

Lesbians are generally less likely to be subjected to violence and other overtly negative sanctions than are homosexual men. This has many possible reasons. Perhaps the most obvious one is society's concept of acceptable behavior from men and women. It is not uncommon to see women embrace in public or for women to live together for many years. Women roommates are often viewed as living together for mutual protection and for financial reasons. This greater tolerance does not apply to men. Public embracing by men in the United States is likely to be met, at best, with stares and feelings of discomfort from observers. Adult men who become roommates are quickly suspected of being gay, regardless of their orientation. If men deviate at all from the accepted "masculine" role in our society, they may be ridiculed and harassed.

Weinberg (1972) has postulated that homosexuality in men is seen as more negative and threatening than that in women because of the special benefits afforded men in our society. It is precisely because of the greater status and power given to men that it is considered worse for a man to "act like a woman" than for a woman to "act like a man." It is beyond the comprehension of many why a man would "choose" to give up status and power to follow a homosexual life style. People tend to take a broader view when a woman wishes to act more like a man, since she is then seen as striving for power and status, an issue separate from her sexual orientation. In general, sexual orientation and sexual behavior have little or nothing to do with wanting to be one sex or the other. Although there are differences in the social attitudes toward men and women, homosexuals of both sexes are susceptible to the whims of a hostile society in terms of jobs, housing, physical safety, and legal rights.

The homosexual person is the victim of blatant discrimination in our society. In some cases, discriminatory treatment is performed unconsciously, by uninformed individuals without malicious intent. In other situations, homosexual persons or persons suspected of homosexuality may be harassed purposely in order to force them to quit a job or may be fired, solely on the basis of sexual orientation.

There is no definitive answer to the questions that arise when homosexuality is the topic. Clearly, homosexuality and homosexual behavior are much misunderstood. Among the topics discussed in this chapter are misunderstandings in terminology, differences in theories of the origins of homosexuality, misunderstandings that lead to homophobia, and misconceptions that prevail about the psychological adjustment of homosexuals and their ways of expressing sexuality. In each of these discussions, contemporary theories and research are presented to dispel the misunderstandings of both homosexual and heterosexual readers. In the final section of the chapter, two case studies are presented to show the kinds of problems homosexual people may encounter in the health care system. The feelings of the nurses involved are discussed, and positive nursing actions that can be taken are explored.

BACKGROUND

Brief History

In our culture, society's view and evaluation of homosexuality has become entangled with the medical professional's approach to the treatment of homosexuality. This medical view has, in turn, become enmeshed with earlier religious views on homosexuality.

Early in the eighteenth century, a "medicalization" of the church's sexual morality began (Bancroft, 1975). What had been the Church's condemnation of any form of nonprocreative sex came to be viewed as a medical prohibition of nonprocreative sex, particularly masturbation and homosexuality. Both came to be seen as exceedingly harmful to health. The medical view of these behaviors, unlike the church's, placed great emphasis on their harmful effects.

By the mid nineteenth century, the medical profession seemed to be split on the issue of homosexuality. Some physicians condemned homosexuality and all forms of homosexual behavior as fundamentally sinful, while others sought to tolerate such variances of human behavior (Bancroft, 1975). In efforts to view homosexuality as a variant rather than deviant behavior, sympathetic physicians sought to reduce the pressure on homosexuals by removing the responsibility for their homosexuality from them. It was hypothesized that homosexuality was caused by a congenital anomaly or a "congenital reversal of sexual feeling." Later, the Neo-Freudians would carry this idea further by hypothesizing that homosexuality represented arrested development at an early age. In both explanations, the homosexual was not responsible for the condition and therefore could not be punished for it.

The twentieth century has brought many theories on the origins, need for treatment, and treatment of homosexuality. Some of these are discussed in this chapter. For the greater part of the twentieth century, homosexuality was viewed as an illness. In fact, prior to a 1974 vote, the American Psychiatric Association defined homosexuality as a psychiatric disorder. Since that time, it has been removed from the list of psychiatric disorders (APA, 1974), although the social stigma has not been removed.

Definitions

At the root of much of the discomfort about homosexuality is the fact that most people either poorly understand or completely misunderstand much of the terminology used in discussing homosexuality. For example, the term homosexual is often incorrectly defined to identify a man or woman who engages in sexual relations with a member of the same sex. This cannot be assumed.

When a person states to a nurse that he or she is homosexual, the nurse or anyone, for that matter, should conclude nothing more than that the particular person becomes erotically aroused by people of the same sex and/

or that the person engages in sexual behaviors with people of the same sex (Bell, 1975). Stated somewhat differently, a homosexual is a person whose primary erotic, physiological, emotional, and social interests are in members of his or her own sex (O'Leary, 1979). Note that in both of these definitions it is the *interest in* and the *arousal by* members of the same sex that is used to define the orientation. The individual need not act on these feelings to be considered homosexual. Sexual feelings and desires may be the most important indicators of sexual orientation. It is entirely possible for a person to be exclusively homosexual in feeling but exclusively heterosexual in behavior (Bell, 1975). Indeed, many homosexuals marry and have families, despite their erotic preference for members of the same sex (Gochros, 1978). In discussing homosexuality in the remainder of this chapter, behavior and orientation will be specifically stated in order to avoid confusion.

Homosexuals are sometimes incorrectly described as bisexuals. *Bisexuals are individuals who respond sexually, although in different ways and on different bases, to a variety of people, regardless of their sex.* These individuals define themselves as unwilling to deny themselves the opportunities for sexual exchange out of regard for the highly restrictive cultural expectations forced on them by our society (Bell, 1975). Bisexuals choose to engage in sexual behaviors with members of both sexes, if they wish. Again, some individuals may feel an attraction to members of both sexes but may, in fact, actually have sexual relations with members of only one sex. The concept of bisexuality is not new. Freud hypothesized that all people have an innate capacity for bisexuality that could be released in a less restrictive society than ours.

Many political "gay" (homosexual) people consider bisexuality to be a "cop-out" by other gay people who are unwilling or unable to admit that they are attracted solely to members of their own sex. The bisexual is seen by these active gays as having given in to the societal pressures of a "straight" world.

Other, less political, groups may view the bisexual as one who is on the way to an exclusive homosexual orientation but who may not yet be ready to totally give up heterosexual encounters. If the premise of inherent bisexuality of all human beings is accepted, it can be seen that individuals who have been exclusively homosexual in both desires and contacts could potentially be educated to such a point that they could learn to release their own innate heterosexual capabilities. It is from this belief that many therapists have sought to "cure" homosexuals and guide them into a heterosexual life. Remembering the definition of sexual orientation, though, it can be seen that even in such cases the individual's sexual *orientation* may remain intact. What happens is that the sexual *behaviors* may change. Some people deeply desire a change in their sexual behaviors. If this is the case, such re-education with a therapist can be useful. It is important that neither the therapist nor the client think of the client's homosexuality as being "cured," but, rather, that they understand the nature of the re-education.

Transsexuals are often labeled as homosexual. As a rule, the transsexual is not an individual with a same-sex preference. *Transsexuals are people who are genetically of one sex but psychologically and emotionally of another* (Hutchinson, 1979). It is the transsexual who may seek out sex change operations so that his or her external appearance can "match" the felt emotional and psychological makeup.

Transvestites are often thought to be homosexual, although they are usually heterosexual men. *Individuals who take pleasure in dressing in the clothes associated with the opposite sex are termed transvestites.*

Homophobia is a fairly new term in the vocabulary of homosexuality. By definition, *homophobia is an irrational fear of homosexuality that manifests itself in a broad spectrum of hateful and angry behaviors toward homosexual persons — from subtle discrimination to murderous assault.* Homophobia may occur in homosexuals as well as in heterosexuals. When it appears in homosexuals, it is manifested as self-loathing (Weinberg, 1972). Homophobia is discussed later in this chapter.

PUBLIC ATTITUDES TOWARD HOMOSEXUALITY

Introduction

In a 1976 study on attitudes toward homosexuality, more than 72 per cent of the surveyed sample believed that homosexual relations were "always wrong" (Nyberg, 1976-77). Of those who felt this way, Catholics and Protestants were more negative about homosexuality than were Jews or people who defined themselves as having no religion.

Because of the widely held negative views of homosexuality and homosexuals, some startling legal precedents have been established and enforced. For example, it is not illegal nor is it considered in any way unconstitutional to deny housing or refuse a job to a known homosexual. Despite some well publicized cases challenging military regulations, the armed forces can still discharge any service person on the basis of homosexuality. In case of severe illness in a homosexual, his or her lover is not allowed to sign for any treatments, as a husband or wife could sign for a spouse. Instead, the next of kin, who may be estranged from the individual, has the legal power to make potentially life and death decisions. If the individual should die and no valid will exist, his or her property would not automatically go to the remaining partner, as in a heterosexual marriage, but would be divided among the homosexual's family (Weinberg, 1972). In various cities, efforts have been made to pass referendums to overturn these rulings, particularly regarding housing and jobs. Most of these attempts have failed.

On the basis of sodomy laws 42 states prohibit sexual acts between persons of the same sex (Messer, 1975). Of course, most states also ban some acts between willing participants of opposite sexes (such as fellatio and cunnilingus) under the same laws. Although these laws are rarely enforced, they remain on the books and could potentially be used against an individual. Most often, homosexuals are jailed for so-called "crimes against nature." In such cases, the sodomy laws may be utilized against them.

Myths and stereotypes about homosexuals abound in our society. For example, many people believe that male homosexuals are universally effeminate, whereas female homosexuals are seen as cigar smoking, "butch" dressing women who wish they could be men (Bell, 1975). More damaging than these stereotypes are the beliefs that homosexuals seduce young children. This mistaken belief has led to prejudice against the employment of homosexuals as teachers or in any occupation in which they could contact children. In most cases, homosexuals in such positions must hide their homosexuality or lose their jobs. In fact, according to statistics (Weinberg, 1972), homosexuals are less likely to seduce young children than are heterosexuals.

Some people see homosexuals as generally untrustworthy and may believe that all homosexual women hate men and that all homosexual men hate women. This belief is based on the idea that unless an individual hates members of the opposite sex, he or she will develop "normal" sexual attractions for them. In fact, many homosexuals have long-term friendships with members of the opposite sex, much as heterosexuals have same-sex friendships.

Another common misconception is that all homosexuals invariably regret their sexual orientation and would jump at the chance to be "cured" (Bell, 1975). This is not true, but the fallacy has not been recognized because society prefers not to recognize the existence of happy, well-adjusted persons who are homosexual. Today, there is an increasingly vocal group of homosexuals who openly assert their satisfactions with their sexual preferences and their life styles and whose acknowledged goals are to be allowed to share affection publicly, as heterosexual couples are allowed to do.

It is also true, however, that some homosexuals are not happy to be homosexual. Many marry in the hope that marriage and regular heterosexual practice will cure them of their "illness" (Gochros, 1978). The expected "cure" rarely exists, even in cases where the homosexual completely gives up homosexual behavior. The person's orientation, fantasies, and desires are generally still directed toward members of the same sex. Other homosexuals may marry to conform with family and social expectations, while still others may marry to achieve the intimacy and special exclusive, committed relationship with another person that is enjoyed and sought after by persons who marry. Some homosexuals have married each other in ceremonies not unlike heterosexual marriage procedures. These marriages are not legally binding and are performed more as a display of commitment.

Homophobia

In practically all social attitudes toward homosexuality there is a marked degree of homophobia. The five reasons that have most often been cited by way of explanation for this are (Weinberg, 1972): 1) religious objections; 2) secret fear of becoming a homosexual; 3) repressed envy; 4) threat to values; and 5) existence without vicarious immortality.

Two of the most commonly quoted religious objections to homosexuality are the story of Onan, from the Torah, and the story of Sodom. According to the story of Onan (Genesis 38:4–10), Onan spilled his seed on the ground rather than lie with the wife of his dead brother. According to the customs of the times, Onan was guilty and punished not for spilling his seed but for disobedience of the command to "raise up issue." By spilling his seed, though, Onan precluded procreation. As Christianity developed, sexual intercourse became codified as having procreation as the only goal, according to St. Augustine. Onanism has variously been cited as a Biblical injunction against masturbation as well as against homosexuality, since both are seen as not leading to procreation. In fact, however, it was for his disobedience that Onan was punished. According to the Christian view, however, homosexuality is seen as seeking sexual pleasure without the excuse of procreation and is therefore a sin (Weinberg, 1972).

The story of Sodom (Genesis 18:20) is another often cited reference against the "sin" of homosexuality. In fact, there is no evidence that Sodom's sin was homosexuality. In every other passage in the Bible referring to Sodom, the sins are vain sacrifices, pride, and inhospitality (Isaiah 1:10, Ezekiel 16:48–49, Jeremiah 23:14, Matthew 10:14–15, Luke 10:10–12) (Weber, 1979). According to Weber, even if the men of Sodom had intended homosexual acts against the angels, the passage could only be seen as a condemnation of homosexual rape.

It is far beyond the scope of this chapter to discuss and debate the religious objections to homosexuality. It seems that virtually every passage that is in any way related to sex has been used at various times to support views of homosexuality and its place in religion. For the reader who is interested, many scholarly works have been written on this topic alone and should be consulted.

The second reason for our society's homophobia is the secret fear experienced by many that they themselves will become homosexuals if they are not careful to guard against it. This defense mechanism, called reaction formation, consists of defending against an impulse in oneself by taking a stand against its expression in others (Weinberg, 1972). In short, individuals who experience homosexual feelings that are normal and not an indication that the individual wishes to become a homosexual may fight against homosexuality vehemently in order to protect their own sexuality. Obviously, this can cause a great deal of paranoia among those who oppose homosexuality. Indeed, it has been utilized as an effective tool to quiet individuals who had been speaking out against homosexuality. Intimating that an individual is strongly against homosexuality because of fear of homosexual feelings in himself or herself, however, feeds and supports the negative attitudes held about homosexuals.

Repressed envy is a third reason given for our society's homophobia. Because of our rigid sex role requirements, many people find that they must struggle to achieve even a precarious sex role identity. This is considered especially prevalent among men who are striving to maintain the "masculine" image revered by our society. To such men, homosexuals who apparently are disdainful of the basic requirements of manhood in our society may be seen as highly threatening. The heterosexual man may wish that he too could escape from the rigid "macho" image required. Being unable to do so, he may feel great anger toward the homosexual who is "free" from this striving.

Closely related to repressed envy is the notion that homosexuality is a threat to the values of our society. Many believe that the family forms the cornerstone and the very basis of our society, and homosexuals are seen as undermining that base. The anger focused on homosexuals may be rage against nonconformity in homosexuals in particular and against nonconformists in general.

The objection that homosexual behavior leads to a lack of immortality in the form of offspring is not exactly the same as the religious objections to homosexuality, which are based on the notion that sex is acceptable for procreation only. The accepted roles for adults in our society are to better the world for future children and to invest in the future of our world by having children and instilling in them the proper socially acceptable behaviors and beliefs. By not having children, the homosexual is viewed as not meeting societal expectations and responsibilities. Homosexuals are seen as free from the financial responsibilities of a family. They are viewed as having increased free time and a lack of ties, which enables them to have a freer life style than the heterosexual who is married and rearing children. Envy has a part here as well.

Although therapists are generally not considered a part of the general "public," their attitudes and treatment of homosexuals have definite effects on the public's attitudes toward homosexuality. Treatment techniques utilized will be discussed later in the chapter. The very existence of programs designed to treat and/or "cure" homosexuals is seen by many as a direct form of discrimination against homosexuals, in that they reinforce the notion that homosexuality is an illness in need of cure. Begelman (1975) has stated the opinions of many others in the field regarding the treatment of homosexuals (Bancroft, 1975; Davison, 1976; Sturgis, 1978):

"The efforts of behavior therapists to reorient homosexuals to heterosexuality by their very existence constitute a significant causal element in reinforcing the social doctrine that homosexuality is bad."

Therapists who agree to a treatment goal with homosexual clients convey ethical and philosophical approval of the change of orientation. The power of the approval is significant in shaping the homosexual's view of homosexuality, as well as in shaping the views of the population in general. By implying that homosexual orientations can be modified (as opposed to modification of behavior) pressure is brought to bear on all homosexuals to seek such modification. This pressure is seen as yet another threat to homosexual freedom (Bancroft, 1975).

The issue of free choice in seeking a change of orientation must also be addressed. Given that our society has a strong cultural bias against homosexuality, it has been expressed that free choice in the decision to seek change of orientation is impossible (Davison, 1978). By the time therapy is sought, the homosexual has spent years in an environment that has repeatedly urged the change. Homosexuals who seek change of orientation therapy may enter the therapy because of the feelings of guilt, shame, and loneliness that they have endured as a result of keeping their sexuality a secret. There are individuals who do wish, for whatever reason, to change their orientation, or who wish to determine what their orientation actually is. The right to counseling to deal with these feelings must exist for those who wish to undertake such therapy, and for those who are unsure of their sexual orientation.

THEORIES ON THE ORIGINS OF HOMOSEXUALITY

Introduction

To date, there are still no definitive studies that prove the origin of homosexuality. For years a battle has been fought between those who feel that homosexuality is an inborn trait acquired in the prenatal period, those who feel that it is environmentally induced, and those who feel that a mixture of the two is responsible.

Homosexuality exists. Whether its origins are determined or not, it will probably continue to exist. We must hope that this alternative life style will be viewed as the variation it represents rather than as a deviation, as it has in the past.

Freud on Homosexuality

It comes as a surprise to those not familiar with Freud's original works that Freud did not define homosexuality as illness or deviation from "normal sexuality" (O'Leary, 1979). Freud did speak to homosexuality as a variation of sexual functioning. Because of the health orientation to homosexuality, Freud did little to determine its origins.

Neo-Freudians and Homosexuality

Freud's work on psychosexual development did, however, form the basis of the Neo-Freudian view of homosexuality, which sees homosexuality as a manifestation of psychological immaturity stemming from fixation during the individual's psychosexual development. Normally, individuals are seen as progressing through a number of psychosexual stages (oral, anal, genital, etc.). Following the successful progression through a given stage, the individual leaves some psychic energy in this phase and continues to the next phase of development. According to Neo-Freudian theory, a person may become homosexual in several ways (Weinberg, 1972): 1) through fixation; 2) as a result of exaggerated castration fear; 3) through narcissism; or 4) through overidentification.

Fixation occurs when the individual overinvests psychic energy in some particular phase of development. It is seen as the primary mode through which an individual becomes a homosexual.

Fear of castration as a factor causing homosexuality explains the male homosexual's preference for men only. According to this theory, the man withdraws his penis from the vagina to avoid the castration of intercourse. By withdrawing his penis from women, the homosexual man turns his affections (and his penis) toward members of the same sex, who are not seen as threatening.

Narcissism, or falling in love with one's own contour, has also been postulated as an explanation for homosexuality. Instead of finding the form of the opposite sex sexually attractive, the homosexual is perceived as not being able to let go of the self-love of childhood to advance to the mature sexual love of a member of the opposite sex.

Overidentification with the parent or with members of the opposite sex is the final source of homosexuality cited by Neo-Freudians. This overidentification is thought to occur especially in cases of men who have strong, domineering mothers and weak, submissive fathers. The man is viewed as wishing to emulate the mother for her strength. In overidentifying with the strong mother, the son takes on the mother's sexual preference for men. Interestingly, in the cultural group known most for having domineering mothers, Jews have been found to have a lower than expected incidence of homosexuality (Weinberg, 1972).

The parents are often found to be at the root of the homosexuality of their children. That is, homosexuality is seen as the result of a "botch job" by the parents. Male homosexuality has consistently been attributed to a seriously disturbed father-son relationship. It has been hypothesized that if a loving, constructively related father were present, homosexuality would not occur in men, even if a neurotic mother-son relationship existed (Bieber, 1976). In cases of divorce in which the mother retains custody of male children, the importance of male role models for the child is stressed, with the underlying notion that the boy will need male role models in order to escape homosexuality (Hunt, 1978).

Feeling guilt for what society tells them are unnatural sexual preferences in their child, parents are often very upset when their son or daughter tells them that he or she is homosexual. Even in cases where the child is happy with the homosexual orientation, the parents tend to ask themselves, "Where have we gone wrong?" An organization of parents of gays has been formed and will be discussed later in the chapter. It is a support group for the parents of gays and for the gays themselves, to help them deal with the familial explanation for the origin of homosexuality.

According to Neo-Freudian thought, there is no way an individual can become a homosexual except by some kind of failure. Each of the four causes discussed above requires some type of failure by the individual. This failure is seen as the root of the homosexuality. Of course, given such an orientation, homosexuality will be viewed negatively.

Sex Typing of the Brain

In the chapter on sexual development, sex typing of the brain was discussed and will be reviewed here in terms of its relevance to homosexuality. John Money (1972) proposed that during fetal growth, the fetus develops sexually in several stages. First, chromosomal sex determines whether the individual will be genetically male or female. This sex determination occurs at the moment of conception. Next, the fetal gonads will either secrete or fail to secrete fetal androgens. If the male testes secrete fetal androgens, male structures will develop. Even in a chromosomally male fetus, if the androgens are not secreted, the fetus will develop female reproductive structures. In addition to the formation of the male structures, the androgens cause the secretion of an inhibiting substance that prevents further development of the female duct system. The third step in determining biological sex is the sex typing of the brain, in which the pattern for the release of pituitary gonadotropins is established. For males, the release is noncyclic, while for females the pattern is the typical cyclic one.

During the sex typing of the brain, prenatal hormones that facilitate or hinder the masculine or feminine dimorphism of psychosexual development are activated. It is hypothesized that this is the point at which homosexuality may be determined, depending on the prenatal hormones. Closely related to this is the theory that homosexuality is due to a severe androgen deficiency after birth in early infancy (Weinberg, 1972). In attempting to check this theory, however, James (1977) found that the androgen levels had no etiological significance in the treatment-seeking homosexuals, and had no relevance as indicators of the treatment outcome. Further, there were no significant differences between androgen levels in homosexuals and members of the control groups.

These biological theories of the origins of homosexuality have for many years served as the basis of thought about sexuality and have led to treatments aimed at altering androgen levels to "cure" the problem. These approaches have all been unsuccessful. Most theorists now combine the biological explanation with a social learning one.

Exposure to Homosexuals

Another hypothesized cause of homosexuality is exposure in early life to homosexuals. This exposure includes both active seduction in childhood by an individual of the same sex and the common adolescent homosexual experimentation (Harris, 1977). This fear of contamination forms the basis for many of the objections to homosexual teachers in schools. On examination, this fear has no basis in fact. First, sexual behavior of any type, homosexual or heterosexual, is not usually discussed by teachers in any school setting, particularly where small children are involved. The topic of sexuality is still sufficiently emotional to prevent most teachers, regardless of sexual orientation, from risking such discussion. Secondly, studies have shown that sexual encounters between adults and children of the same sex are far more frequent between heterosexual males and young males than between homosexuals and young children. If the reader can put aside fears of contamination, the situation becomes more clear. Like heterosexuals, homosexuals are seeking relationships that will fulfill emotional as well as physical needs. This type of emotional fulfillment cannot be found with a young child. The individual who seeks sexual fulfillment with a child is not considered normal in either the homosexual or the heterosexual world.

Homosexual behavior in adolescence is very common, particularly among boys. As discussed earlier, it is felt that this type of behavior is the early experimentation in the roles of sexual behavior performed in the relative safety of the peer group that serves as a practice run for future heterosexual behavior. Indeed, some adolescents do prefer homosexual behavior to heterosexual behavior, but this preference is established far earlier than at the sexual experimentation stage. The adolescent homosexual is rarely going to try to seduce a friend to homosexuality if the friend is not already homosexual. As a rule, the homosexual is rarely attracted to the heterosexual who makes it clear that his sexual behavior is heterosexual. Of course, the same is true for heterosexuals.

Feminist View of Lesbianism

An interesting addition to the literature about homosexuality has been inclusion of the feminist view of lesbianism. It has been proposed that women may turn to lesbian relationships as one strategy for coping with the fundamental dilemma of being born female in our society (O'Leary, 1979). According to this notion, girls are all aware of their inferior status from a very early age. They learn that their mother values her husband and sons more than her daughters. The daughter can secure her mother's love by being ingratiating to her and becoming more like her (and thus developing a heterosexual identity), or she may instead identify with the male, thereby attaining independence from the need for security from the male. This view is dangerously close to an interpretation of homosexuality as an illness rather than as a viable alternative for women who find themselves in a bad position as a result of our society's restrictive role definitions. The emphasis is on the limitations placed on women by society's definition of the female role. Apart from the decidedly Neo-Freudian view presented above, feminists propose that women who feel compelled to constantly reject the traditional female role may find that an intimate relationship with a woman is more rewarding than one with a man, since the woman will be able to maintain an egalitarian relationship based on mutual respect and the potential for individual growth. A fundamental weakness of this theory is that this application does not speak to the basic difference between sexual orientation and behavior. Another flaw is the idea that only through a relationship with a woman can egalitarian relationships exist.

The Healthy Homosexual

Not all theories about homosexuality rely on the theme that homosexuality is an illness or deviation. The healthy homosexual is defined as an individual who has discovered that the heterosexual ideal believed in since childhood is inapplicable in his or her own life (Weinberg, 1972). This person is not guilty about or ashamed of his or her homosexuality. Rather, he or she regards homosexuality for himself or herself as healthy. Healthy homosexuals have freed themselves from misgivings and have accepted the homosexual life style.

In determining the "cause" of homosexuality from this healthy view, social learning theorists propose that homosexuality is a result of positive associations with homosexual stimuli (O'Leary, 1979). This learned preference is not necessarily accomplished by psychological disturbance.

A term used to describe the revealing by a person of his or her homosexual orientation is "coming out." Many persons who choose to stop hiding their preferences report an increased sense of freedom and self-esteem, and increased opportunities to meet, identify with, and perhaps make sexual and social contacts with others who have similar orientations (Gochros, 1978). The "coming out" can be a very positive step toward healthy homosexuality. The homosexual subculture can be remarkably useful in helping the newly "out" homosexual (Hart, 1978). It can serve to solidify the homosexual identity and the commitment to develop successful ways of managing a homosexual life style. This support function is a positive one that should not be overlooked. The homosexual "subculture" will be discussed at greater length later in this chapter. One recently organized support group reveals much about society's attitudes about homosexuals. This group, called Parents of Gays, has the following four goals (Smith, 1979):

1. To eliminate prejudice and discrimination and to change attitudes and legislation to ensure gay people's individual freedom and civil rights.
2. To help parents through the "coming out" period.
3. To offer support to other gay women or men who have not yet told their parents or who have been rejected by their parents.
4. To provide a consciousness raising group.

Perhaps the best explanation of the Parents of Gays comes from their own literature:

"We will not contribute by bigotry or by silence to the ongoing persecution of our Gay daughters and sons. We have a commitment to 1) actively help ourselves through increasing our understanding, and 2) actively help our Gay daughters and sons by working for the same basic human rights, liberties, and opportunities for them enjoyed by others. As proud parents of Gay persons, new windows of understanding have been opened to us which have enriched our lives.

We recognize that this new-found pride did not come easily and some parents may still have doubts. We had to do a lot of thinking and talking together. That is why we founded Parents of Gays. If you are a parent of a Gay, please join us."

Viewing homosexuality as a healthy alternative is extremely difficult for some people. For many, homosexuality is synonymous with illness or deviation. The existence of such a large number of individuals who consider themselves happy and well-adjusted forces society to re-evaluate homosexuality from the health perspective.

TREATMENT OF HOMOSEXUALITY

In order to fully cover the topic of homosexuality, some of the more popular treatment methods concerned with reorientation of homosexuals will be briefly discussed. As discussed earlier, the very existence of such treatment does lend credence to the view that homosexuality is an illness. In no way is this discussion meant to be an endorsement of these methods. The methods do exist, however, and the health care professional should be informed of all the alternatives available for dealing with homosexuals.

Systematic Desensitization

Joseph Wolpe is generally credited with the development of systematic desensitization (Weinberg, 1972). The basic idea in such desensitization programs is that the homosexual's desires are attributed to anxiety surrounding encounters with members of the opposite sex. Rather than deal with these anxieties, the individual chooses to avoid them, following, instead, a homosexual pattern of sexual expression.

In treating homosexuals with systematic desensitization, small steps are taken to deal with successively more anxiety-producing situations. For example, the first step in the program may involve just talking with a member of the opposite sex. When the client is able to do this with a minimal amount of anxiety, he or she proceeds to the next step, which involves kissing. Using this step-by-step method, the client is helped to progress through embracing, being physically in the bedroom, being in bed, kissing goodnight, preliminary sex play, and finally to intercourse with a person of the opposite sex. This type of therapy has the aim of altering sexual behavior, and does not attempt to deal with sexual orientation. The person is defined as "cured" when homosexual behavior is stopped, even if he or she continues to fantasize about and yearn for homosexual relationships.

Aversive Techniques

Aversive techniques utilize reinforcement of one kind or another to condition the homosexual to respond sexually to members of the opposite sex. In the masturbation method (used primarily with males), the client is instructed to masturbate in a darkened room. When the client is close to orgasm, pictures of scantily dressed women (or men for female clients) are flashed in the room. The reason for this type of conditioning is to help the individual to associate erotic feelings with the form of a member of the opposite sex.

Emetic persuasion is a more severe technique. In this method of conditioning, the individual is shown nude pictures of members of the same sex. While the homosexual is shown these sexually arousing pictures, he or she is rendered acutely ill by being given medications that cause severe nausea and vomiting. It is thought that this "persuasion" will lead to a conditioning in which the client will no longer associate sexual feelings with members of the same sex. This does not ensure that the homosexual will later feel sexually aroused by members of the opposite sex.

Closely related to emetic persuasion are aversive techniques that utilize electric shocks as a form of negative reinforcement. Again the intent is to form a negative feeling toward members of the same sex as erotic partners.

It is questionable whether these aversive techniques actually help the homosexual. Politically active homosexuals who define homosexuality as a normal variation of sexual expression are strongly against such methods, stating that they are brutal and may be far more damaging to the homosexual's psychological health than the homosexuality itself, assuming homosexuality is damaging at all.

Despite the severity of some of the approaches to "curing" homosexuality, individuals do seek out treatment. It is probably impossible to determine if they seek such treatment completely of their own free will, given societal homophobia, but the fact remains that some self-described homosexuals wish to change their sexual orientation and are willing to undergo treatment in the hope of being "cured."

Homosexuals Anonymous

This organization functions very much like Alcoholics Anonymous. Groups of "cured" homosexuals form a type of club with mutual support mechanisms. If one of the members feels unexpectedly overwrought with homosexual urges, he is urged to call another "cured" person to come to his home and be with him until the feeling passes. An important basis for the formation of such a group is the notion, as with alcoholism, that there is no cure for homosexuality. Only through complete avoidance of the behavior can the individual expect to lead a "normal" life. It is assumed that the individual will always be a homosexual and will always have to fight off the sexual urges felt toward members of the same sex.

PSYCHOLOGICAL ADJUSTMENTS OF HOMOSEXUALS

Early studies of homosexuals and their psychological adjustment led to the commonly held misconception that homosexuals were universally in psychological turmoil. They were viewed as poorly adjusted, unhappy people.

Bell (1975) stated that "it is impossible to predict the nature of any patient's personality, social adjustment, or sexual functioning on the basis of sexual orientation." His assertion has been validated through much research of the adjustment of homosexual samples versus heterosexual samples (Davison, 1976; Hart, 1978; O'Leary, 1979; Siegelman, 1979). In some older research, differences in the adjustment between homosexual and heterosexual samples were indeed found. The controlling factor seems to be in the sampling techniques utilized rather than in the samples themselves. In many studies, the samples of homosexuals included prison inmates, institutionalized patients, and other nonrepresentative groups. This inherent bias in the research negates its value.

When nonclinical samples of homosexuals are compared with matched nonclinical samples of heterosexuals, however, very few, if any, differences in psychological function are found (Bell, 1975). These findings are significant in attempting to deal with society's homophobia. The picture of the unhappy, maladjusted homosexual is simply not a true one.

SEXUAL EXPRESSION IN HOMOSEXUALS

Despite the homophobia that is common in our society, there is great curiosity about the sexual activity of homosexuals. People who have always been exclusively heterosexual in behavior often want to ask the homosexual what he or she actually "does" during sexual encounters. Contrary to popular myth, anal intercourse among homosexual males is not the primary mode of sexual expression (Bell, 1975; Masters, 1979; O'Leary, 1979). Expecting this to occur is an essentially heterosexual view of homosexuality. It is hypothesized that the homosexual man will seek sexual fulfillment by placing his penis inside of a receptacle. As the heterosexual male is seen as enjoying penis-vagina intercourse, it is assumed that the homosexual male will wish to have penis-anus intercourse. While this is one type of sexual expression reported by homosexual males, it is by far not the most commonly reported method. Mutual masturbation and oral-genital sex are far more commonly practiced. As with heterosexuals, kissing, holding, and caressing are very important.

Similarly, the use of penis substitutes (dildoes) is reported by lesbians less frequently than is generally accepted. Again, the notion is that the woman receives sexual gratification primarily through penile-vaginal contact. It has been shown that for both homosexual and heterosexual women the primary site of sexual stimulation is the clitoris. For most women, then, intercourse alone will rarely provide full sexual satisfaction.

In their research on homosexuals and their sexual behavior, Masters and Johnson (1979) found no real differences between homosexual men and women and heterosexual men and women in the physiologic capacity to respond to similar sexual stimuli. Like heterosexuals, homosexuals differ in the amount of attention they give to the sexual aspects of their lives (Bell, 1975). For both men and women in the Masters and Johnson research, the response to masturbation was the same.

Oral-genital sex among homosexuals was found to be deliberately slowed in the entire stimulative process. The goal orientation (toward orgasm) found in heterosexual couples was noted much less often among homosexual couples. Particularly with homosexual women, oral sex was found to be significantly more effective in satisfying partners than in heterosexual couples. It has been postulated that this is due to "gender empathy" (Masters, 1979). Another possible explanation for this is that in our society many men view oral sex as a necessary preliminary to be finished with, so that the couple can then proceed to genital intercourse.

Masters and Johnson found no significant quantitative differences in response at orgasmic levels to the techniques of masturbation, partner manipulation, and fellatio/cunnilingus, regardless of the gender of sexual preference of the subjects. In both homosexual and heterosexual samples, however, women were more likely than men to emphasize the importance of the emotional context in which their sexuality is expressed (O'Leary, 1979).

THE GAY SUBCULTURE

Geographic areas in which homosexuals tend to congregate exist in most large cities. There may be areas of homes or apartments occupied almost exclusively by homosexuals. Certain neighborhoods may be well known as "gay sections," just as other areas may be known for concentrations of certain ethnic groups. Gay areas may be recognized by both heterosexuals and homosexuals. Often businesses such as restaurants, clothing stores, bookstores, and bars will cater specifically to homosexuals and the public homosexual life style.

The attraction of living in an area where homosexuals can feel freer to be openly affectionate with a same-sex companion can be readily seen. A further benefit, one enjoyed by many who choose to live in ethnic neighborhoods, is the familiarity of living among a group of people who share some important aspect of their lives.

Such congregation or "ghettoization" has negative effects as well. The chief negative effect is that it creates an area primarily identified with sexual activity. Whereas people who choose to live among members of their ethnic group are assumed to do so because they have common ties of religion, language, culture, and political opinions, homosexuals are identified by their sexual activities. No one would describe a neighborhood as "heterosexual" or "incest-oriented." Yet homosexuals are labeled by this one aspect of their lives. This sexual identification and constant reminder of sexual activity contributes to a life style in which sexual activity is tremendously accentuated. If society sees all homosexuals as promiscuous, homosexuals themselves may begin to believe in the myth. The level of sexual activity varies among homosexuals, as it does among heterosexuals.

Some homosexuals who choose to live in "gay neighborhoods" may do so in part out of an interest in the increased sexual activity. Others may find that the emphasis on sexuality in the neighborhood leads to more sexual activity than they had experienced before living there. Still others may pass up the benefits of the gay subculture to avoid the emphasis on sexual activity. Many of the myths about homosexuals, particularly those concerning high levels of indiscriminate sexual activity, are based on heterosexual fascination with the behavior of a small minority of homosexuals.

A disadvantage to living in a gay "ghetto" is the reality of being openly identified as a homosexual. Outsiders with intense homophobia may find a gay neighborhood an inviting place in which to express their violent anger toward homosexuals. Violence directed toward homosexuals occurs at times in gay bars.

Although the life style of the open gay subculture is one nurses should be aware of, by no means do all homosexuals live in gay areas or participate in the subculture. Homosexuals live in wealthy enclaves, in middle-class suburbs, in working-class neighborhoods, and in small towns. Some homosexuals live quietly together as couples in the same neighborhoods for decades; others prefer a big-city "singles" atmosphere. Some homosexuals are open about their sexual preference, participating in the political process to eliminate legal discrimination. Other homosexuals live "closeted," denying even to close family members their sexual behavior.

The variations in life style and sexual behavior among homosexuals are great. As a professional, a nurse cannot make generalizations about people based on their sexual preference any more than he or she can make generalizations based on race, religion, ethnic background, or any single aspect of an individual's life.

HOMOSEXUALITY AND THE HEALTH CARE DELIVERY SYSTEM

The Nurse and the Homosexual Patient

Many homosexuals tend to delay seeking medical help, especially in situations that would necessitate disclosure of their homosexuality to the nurse or the physician (Maurer, 1979). The reluctance to disclose a homosexual orientation should not be taken lightly. Patients who admit their sexual orientation leave themselves open to some severe consequences, such as loss of job and loss of housing should the health care professional choose to disclose this information to others. Of course, such disclosure is not ethical and does violate the clients' rights to confidential treatment. However, homosexuals who do disclose this preference place themselves in a precarious position. Rather than risk this disclosure, many will avoid or greatly delay seeking care. Some will find physicians and nurses who are known throughout the gay community to be sympathetic to gays. This is not always posssible.

Once the homosexual client has sought care from the nurse or physician, the risk of judgmental treatment exists. Although passing judgments is not a nursing function, and although such judgments can have a negative effect on care, judgments may be made (Lawrence, 1975). A commonly encountered error is the conclusion that sexual difficulties reported by a homosexual patient reflect a general dissatisfaction with the homosexual life style. The same health care professional would not necessarily assume that the heterosexual client who reported a sexual problem was really reporting a dissatisfaction with heterosexuality (Bell, 1975)!

Regardless of the problems that the homosexual patient presents to the health care worker, an air of acceptance is a necessary prerequisite to the establishment of a trusting relationship in which both participants feel comfortable. The nurse gives verbal and nonverbal cues to homosexual patients as well as to heterosexual patients. Homosexual patients may be more sensitive to the cues, especially if they fear rejection from the nurse. One negative nonverbal cue is generalized body tenseness in the practitioner. This body posture conveys general anxiety. This, coupled with crossed arms, may be interpreted by the client as an expression of resistance to the information being presented. Raising the eyebrows, particularly as the client tells the practitioner of his or her sexual orientation, gives the client a message of rejection (Maurer, 1979). These nonverbal cues and their effects are found in dealing with heterosexual patients as well, but are repeated here in the context of the homosexual patient to stress their importance.

Verbal cues also convey an air of acceptance or rejection. Extensive use of highly clinical language with any patient can increase the patient's anxiety. In the case of a patient who is trying to disclose a homosexual orientation, the increased use of technical language by the practitioner may signal the client that the topic being approached is not "O.K.," and may act as a signal to stop discussing homosexuality. On the other hand, awkward use of commonly known "street" language can have just as negative an effect. The practitioner who tries to use language that is not comfortable merely tends to sound condescending. Condescension is a subtle but effective form of rejection.

As with any sexual concern, there will be nurses who feel that they cannot adequately deal with homosexual patients. Professional ethics require the health care professional to refer any patient he or she cannot respect (Maurer, 1979). The referral should be explained honestly to the client, and the nurse should be sure that the client will receive nonbiased care at the place to which the nurse has referred him or her. Some nurses may not even be aware of the biases they feel until faced with an unusual situation. To illustrate some of our biases more clearly, several situations will be discussed.

Situation #1: The lesbian patient and the outpatient women's clinic.

The setting for this example is a women's clinic in a large university. The clinic is a nurse practitioner clinic which offers yearly pelvic exams and Pap smears, contraception, VD treatment and screening, and treatment of vaginal infections. Five full time RN nurse practitioners make up the staff.

In response to an active gay community on campus, the coordinator of the clinic arranges a continuing education meeting for the clinic personnel to coincide with Gay Awareness Week on campus. As part of their commitment to continuing education, the nurses are to attend a group discussion on "Women's Health Care Needs for Lesbians." The speaker is an attractive, well-spoken woman who has been known at the women's clinic, and has been seen by several of the practitioners. At the end of her presentation on the needs of gays, she discloses that she is a lesbian, and has, in fact, come to the discussion with her lover (another woman who has been writing important points on the blackboard).

The general reaction to the woman's disclosure is surprise, quickly covered. In speaking of the care she received at the clinic, she points out several areas in which her rights as a homosexual were blurred:
1. At each visit, she was asked if she was

sexually active. When she answered yes, she was asked if she used birth control. When she stated that she did not, at each occasion she was advised about the risks of unprotected intercourse.
2. When being treated for a vaginal infection, she was repeatedly advised either to abstain from intercourse or to have her partner wear a condom.

Clearly, her points were well taken. Since the clinic was primarily utilized by the college population as a birth control clinic, the nurses were all biased in the direction of heterosexual activity. The problem regarding treatment for vaginitis which, in her case, was persistent, was more serious. It was later discovered that she and her lover were passing the infection back and forth, resulting in what appeared to be a recurrent infection. Had the staff been alert to the possibility of homosexual contact, both partners could have been treated, thus eliminating the need for repeated treatment and reinfection.

The reader may ask, as did one of the nurses, why the client had chosen to be silent about her homosexuality until that point in time. The woman reported that she had feared that the information would be recorded on her chart and would become part of her permanent health record. She did not wish to risk the full disclosure that could follow her should she have her medical records sent from the university to her own physician.

Following the presentation, lively discussion followed, and it seemed that the situation was one of easy acceptance. How- ever, several weeks later, the lover of the woman who had presented the talk called the clinic to make an appointment. Four of the nurses refused to see her. After much discussion, it was determined that all four of the nurses felt uncomfortable performing a pelvic exam on the young woman who they all now knew was a lesbian. The nurses feared that the lesbian patient would "enjoy" a pelvic exam performed by a woman. Pointing out to the nurses that heterosexual women do not "enjoy" pelvic exams performed by men did cause the nurses to think about this but did not dispel their anxiety about the possibility of sexually stimulating this lesbian during the routine pelvic examination. When asked if they thought that heterosexual male practitioners became aroused from performing pelvic exams on women, all of the nurses answered that they did not, but there was some hesitation.

For many months, only the one nurse who did not share the fears of the others saw the clients known to be homosexual. The word spread among the gay community that this nurse could be trusted and that she would not state the sexual preference on the client's record. As a result, she saw a great number of lesbians seeking gynecologic health care. Gradually, the other nurses began to face their own fears about homosexuality and the relations of the fears to their own anxiety. A full year later, two of the nurses who had refused to care for homosexual patients were able to begin to see these patients. The other two did not feel that they could adequately treat these patients, and therefore did not do so.

The Homosexual Patient in the Hospital

In society at large, the homosexual generally lacks societal affirmation, recognition, or support. In the hospital, the limitations placed on the homosexual can be more severe. The most obvious loss that the hospitalized homosexual patient may have to endure is separation from the loved one at the stressful time of hospitalization. In cases in which permission for procedures cannot be obtained from the patient, the patient's lover is not legally permitted to grant permission. Instead, the family, with whom the client may not have been in contact at all, must give such permission. If the family was unaware or unaccepting of the patient's relationship with the lover, the decisions may be made without the input of the patient's most significant other.

The exclusion of one's significant other can slow the patient's progress. The additional stresses encountered as a result of such separations may even cause problems for the ill homosexual's recovery. Lawrence (1975) has stated the following rights of homosexuals in hospitals:

"Every homosexual patient has every right to know if his potential care givers are willing to accept and respect his life style and relationships as at least potentially healthy alternatives to heterosexuality. He also has the right to expect that his same sex mate or close friends will be regarded as significant others, and that, as such, they will be permitted to be involved in his treatment."

These rights do not seem to be outlandish, but they are simply not given to most homosexuals in most hospitals. Since no differences aside from choice of love object have been found between homosexuals and heterosexuals, one would think that these rights would be freely granted (Maurer, 1979; O'Leary, 1979).

The homosexual patient who discloses his or her homosexuality on admission is likely to receive different treatment from that of the heterosexual patient or the homosexual patient who has not discussed his or her homosexuality. The following situation illustrates some fairly commonly encountered aspects of care that the homosexual patient may experience.

Situation #2: The homosexual male patient in the hospital.

Steve is admitted to a surgical floor on the night before his scheduled surgery. His lover, Mike, accompanies him. Steve and Mike inform the nurses that they have been living together for some time, and that Steve would like to have Mike listed as his significant other. The two men are openly affectionate toward each other. During the admission procedures, Steve's roommate has been out of the semiprivate room that they are to share for the next few days. Following the initial admission procedures, the nurse contacts the supervisor, requesting that Steve be given a private room and that the physicians be notified to limit Steve's visitors.

Later that evening, Steve is moved into a private room. This is somewhat upsetting to him, since his insurance will pay only the cost of a semiprivate room. When Steve asks why he has been changed, the nurse tells him that it is their policy to separate homosexuals to avoid any unnecessary contact with other same-sex patients. Steve attempts to protest, but by that time, the entire floor, including his old roommate,

seems to have been informed that Steve is a homosexual. His old roommate refuses to have Steve move back into the room, saying, "I'm not going to be able to get any rest wondering if that guy is going to be lurking around in the same room with me. That queer stuff isn't natural, you know."

Steve and Mike decide that they will bear the burden of the extra cost of the private room to avoid further conflict. At the end of visiting hours, Mike is asked to leave, despite the fact that on this unit, significant others are usually granted unlimited visiting rights. Again, Steve questions this change and is informed that, for his own good, limiting Mike's visiting will decrease the discomfort that Steve will feel as a result of the general negative feeling about homosexuals. The couple is told this by a sympathetic nurse, who assures them that it is in their best interest to comply. Not wishing to further upset Steve, Mike leaves. Steve then sits in his private room, alone, thinking about his impending surgery. He feels that the nurses are avoiding him but is unsure if this is real or if he is imagining it. He passes a sleepless night and is depressed on the morning of his surgery.

The possible repercussions of this treatment are clear. The patient, solely because of his sexual orientation, is separated by the staff from his lover and, indeed, from contact with most of the other staff members in the hospital. At the time when Steve can most benefit from the support and teaching of the medical staff, this support is denied to him because of prejudice toward his life style. The fact that Steve's illness is in no way related to his homosexuality does not seem to have an effect on this prejudice. Depression prior to surgery has been shown to have negative effects on the recovery of the patient, regardless of the reason for the depression.

Counseling Homosexuals About Homosexuality

Thus far, the discussion regarding homosexuals and the health care delivery system has focused on the homosexual seeking care for conditions not related to homosexuality. This is usually the case. Some homosexuals, however, do seek treatment for sexual problems, as do heterosexuals. The counselor must not jump to the conclusion that the patient is actually presenting a sexual problem as a way to approach discussion of dissatisfaction with homosexuality as a life style. All individuals may experience sexual difficulties, regardless of their sexual orientation. For the same reason that a heterosexual is not questioned about his or her satisfaction with heterosexual life when presenting a sexual problem, it is inappropriate to ask this of a homosexual patient.

In cases where the homosexual wishes to discuss homosexuality, either in terms of changing orientation or in terms of more successfully adapting to the chosen life style, the counselor must first determine that the patient has sought treatment of his or her own free will, as much as possible given societal attitudes toward homosexuality (Bancroft, 1975).

Homosexuals have many decisions to make about themselves, about homosexuality, and about the effect of their homosexuality on others. These decisions can be roughly broken down into three main areas (Weinberg, 1972): 1) decisions about attitudes toward oneself; 2) decisions about other individuals in one's life; and 3) decisions about homosexuals as a group. These decisions are difficult ones that the counselor can assist the client with but that must ultimately be decided by the client. Clients must decide whether they will try to change to adopt a heterosexual life style. They must also decide whether to lament their homosexuality. Finally, they must decide whether they wish to pursue homosexual life with the full commitment to the relationship and to the attendant homosexuality.

Once the client has determined how to deal with his or her own homosexuality, the decisions that surround others in their lives become more significant. Disclosure or nondisclosure of homosexuality is a tremendous issue for most homosexuals. If the homosexual decides to share knowledge of his or her homosexuality with parents, friends, or others, the decision must be made about how the presentation will be made. For example, the homosexual who has determined to lament and generally feel guilty about homosexuality may inform close associates about his or her homosexuality much differently than will the homosexual who has decided that homosexuality is an appropriate choice. When clients decide to tell others of their homosexuality, the decision must be made about being seen with other same-sex partners, about disclosing the orientation at work, and about other problems of this type. This issue is more complex. Things taken for granted by heterosexual couples, such as walking arm in arm in public, must be carefully weighed by homosexuals in terms of the potential effects of such public displays.

Finally, the homosexual person must decide where, if at all, he or she fits in with other homosexual people. For some, the homosexual subculture can be invaluable as an entry into the homosexual world. For others, though, this subculture is entirely unacceptable. Indeed, some homosexuals, perhaps in an attempt to remain undiscovered, are the strongest opponents of gay rights. Regardless of the decision made, the homosexual must at some time or another make the decision.

The role of the counselor working with homosexual clients will depend on the stage of decision-making the client is in when he or she approaches the therapist. If, for example, the client reports confusion about sexual orientation, the role of the counselor is to help the client explore different types of relationships, and to help the client achieve a balanced perspective regarding what is bad and what is good for the client about sex. The counselor should attempt to offer help and encouragement in establishing rewarding sexual relationships, whether they are homosexual or heterosexual. As with any sexual counseling or teaching, the health care professional is interested in assisting the client to utilize sex as a method of communication that can serve as a binding force in interpersonal relationships.

If the client has decided to pursue a homosexual life style, the health care professional may be consulted to assist him or her to more easily adapt to the homosexual role. This may be particularly important for the homosexual who has decided to "come out." The counselor, through acceptance and nonjudgmental support, can help the homosexual client to deal with some of the stigmatizing consequences of the homosexual role in our culture. In doing this, the guilt experienced by many homosexuals can be reduced. Finally, the counselor can help the homosexual deal with interpersonal or sexual problems that may arise in the particular homosexual relationship, much as the counselor would help in a similar situation with a heterosexual client (Bancroft, 1975).

CONCLUSION

Regardless of the origin of homosexuality, it is becoming a more visible alternative life style in our society. Attitudes toward homosexuality and homosexuals are changing very slowly. The nurse may be the initial contact that the homosexual patient has with the health care delivery system. The treatment the client receives from the nurse can set the tone for all other encounters with the medical system, and can therefore have a significant effect on the health care activities of the client. As with most situations in which the nurse deals with the sexuality of clients, the nurse must spend time analyzing how he or she feels about homosexuality. If the nurse finds that homosexuality can be seen as a viable alternative to heterosexual expression, and that she or he can care for homosexual clients in the same nonjudgmental fashion as for other clients, the nurse can be a great asset to the gay community, as an educator, advocate, and counselor. As discussed and illustrated with the patient situations, biases and negative feelings are often hidden from the nurse until a specific situation surfaces. At that time, however, the nurse must analyze his or her feelings, and begin to work in the most appropriate role possible to best give care to the large number of homosexuals.

References

American Psychiatric Association: Position Statement on Homosexuality and Civil Rights. *American Journal of Psychiatry,* Vol. 131, 1974.
Bancroft, John: "Homosexuality and the Medical Profession: A Behaviorist's View," *Journal of Medical Ethics,* Vol. 1, No. 4, December, 1975.

Begelman, D. A.: "Ethical and Legal Issues in Behavior Modification." *In* Hersen, M., Eisler, R., and Miller, P. M. (Eds.): *Progress in Behavior Modification.* New York, Academic Press, 1975.

Bell, Alan P.: "The Homosexual as Patient." *In* Green, Richard (Ed.): *Human Sexuality: A Health Practitioner's Text.* Baltimore, The Williams & Wilkins Company, 1975.

Bieber, Irving: "A Discussion of Homosexuality: The Ethical Challenge." *Journal of Consulting and Clinical Psychology,* Vol. 44, No. 2, April, 1976.

Davison, Gerald C.: "Homosexuality: The Ethical Challenge." *Journal of Consulting and Clinical Psychology,* Vol. 44, No. 2, April, 1976.

Davison, Gerald C.: "Not Can but Ought: The Treatment of Homosexuality." *Journal of Consulting and Clinical Psychology,* Vol. 46, No. 1, 1978.

Earle, Ken: "A Homosexual Teacher's Argument and Plea." *Alive!,* 1978.

Gochros, Harvey: "Counseling Gay Husbands." *Journal of Sex Education and Therapy,* Vol. 4, No. 2, Winter, 1978.

Harris, Barbara S.: "Lesbian Mother Child Custody: Legal and Psychiatric Aspects." *Bulletin of the American Academy of Psychiatry and Law,* Vol. 5, No. 1, 1977.

Hart, Maureen, Roback, Howard, Tittler, Bennett, Weitz, Larry, Walston, Barbara, and McKee, Embry: "Psychological Adjustment of Nonpatient Homosexuals: Critical Review of the Research Literature." *The Journal of Clinical Psychiatry,* Vol. 39, 1978.

Hunt, Samuel P.: "Homosexuality from a Contemporary Perspective." *Connecticut Medicine,* Vol. 42, No. 2, February, 1978.

Hutchinson, Bill: "Now What?" *In: Understanding a Life Style: Institute on Sexism Component on Homosexuality.* Miami, Florida International University, 1979.

James, Sheila, Carter, R. A., and Orwin, A.: "Significance of Androgen Levels in the Aetiology and Treatment of Homosexuality." *Psychological Medicine,* Vol. 7, No. 3, August, 1977.

Lawrence, John C: "Homosexual, Hospitalization and the Nurse." *Nursing Forum,* Vol. 14, No. 3, 1975.

Masters, William H., and Johnson, Virginia E.: *Homosexuality in Perspective.* Boston, Little, Brown and Co., 1979.

Maurer, Tom B.: "Health Care and the Gay Community." *In* Kowalski, Karren (Ed.): *Women's Health Care: Nursing Dimensions.* Vol. VII, No. 1, Spring, 1979.

Messer, Henry D.: "The Homosexual as Physician." *In* Green, Richard (Ed.): *Human Sexuality: A Health Practitioner's Text.* Baltimore, The Williams & Wilkins Co., 1975.

Money, John: "Bisexual, Homosexual and Heterosexual: Society, Law and Medicine." *Journal of Homosexuality,* Vol. 2 (3), Spring, 1977.

Money, John: "Statement on Antidiscrimination Regarding Sexual Orientation." *Journal of Homosexuality,* Vol. 2 (2), Winter, 1976-77.

Nyberg, Kenneth L., and Alston, Jon P.: "Analysis of Public Attitudes Toward Homosexual Behavior." *Journal of Homosexuality,* Vol. 2 (2), Winter, 1976-77.

O'Leary, Virginia: "Lesbianism." *In* Kowalski, Karren (Ed.): *Women's Health Care: Nursing Dimensions.* Vol. VII, No. 1, Spring, 1979.

Siegelman, Marvin: "Adjustment of Homosexual and Heterosexual Women: A Cross-National Replication." *Archives of Sexual Behavior,* Vol. 8, No. 2, 1979.

Smith, Jean: "Homophobia." *In: Understanding a Life Style: Institute on Sexism Component in Homosexuality.* Miami, Florida International University, 1979.

Sturgis, Ellie, T., and Adams, Henry E.: "The Right to Treatment: Issues in the Treatment of Homosexuality." *Journal of Consulting and Clinical Psychology,* Vol. 46, No. 1, 1978.

Weber, Joseph C.: "What the Bible Seems to Say." *Engage/Social Action,* Washington, D.C., June, 1975.

Weinberg, George: *Society and the Healthy Homosexual.* New York, Doubleday Books, 1972.

11

RAPE

INTRODUCTION

The fear of rape is inculcated into girls from an early age, particularly in this culture, in which women are often emphasized as sexual objects in the media. The notion of the "macho man" who takes his pleasure where and with whom he will is not uncommon. Closely linked with the "machismo" belief is the commonly held misconcept that all women secretly wish to be raped. Actually, rape is an act of violence in which sex is used as a weapon. It is not a sexual crime. The application of force to induce an individual to perform any act against her or his will cannot rationally be seen as anything but a potentially severely damaging situation.

Records of rape and other assaults on women are almost without number in our history. Unfortunately, they are not just a part of our history. According to the Federal Bureau of Investigation (FBI), rape is the fastest growing crime in the United States today, even though it has been estimated that more than 90 per cent of rapes are never reported (Sredl, 1979). It has been suggested that more women are now coming forward to speak out about their rapes, and that this has artificially inflated the claim that rape has increased. The facts do not bear this out. Most women are still very reluctant to come forward after they have been sexually assaulted (Brownmiller, 1975). If a woman who has been raped does decide to press charges, the judicial process is usually painful and difficult — and one in which she will need continued support and counseling.

The nurse is usually the first health care professional that the rape victim encounters, generally in the emergency room. The meeting with the nurse and the relationship established at that time can have a profound effect on the later recovery of the woman. It is essential that nurses be aware of the proper treatment, legal ramifications, counseling, and teaching that victims will require. Anticipatory guidance is essential for the nurse. Because most nurses are women, and because most women share the realistic fear of sexual assault, victims of rape who are seen in the hospital may not receive the unbiased care that they so desperately need. The nurse may unconsciously not wish to face the fact that she too could be the victim of such an attack. In her own denial, she may seek a "reason" for the rape, such as that the victim was foolish or careless in her behavior. This type of blame-finding can be devastating to the victim, who may already be questioning her own actions. Nurses must be knowledgeable about the realities of assault and its effects on victims. In addition, nurses must evaluate the myths about rape that abound and examine their own values to determine whether they hold biased beliefs. For example, the nurse who believes that "a virtuous woman" cannot be raped will give different care than will the nurse who is free of such a myth.

In this chapter society's attitudes about rape, the motivations for rape, the personality of the rapist, and, most important, nursing care and interventions in dealing with the victim of rape are considered.

Rape is not a simple crime. There are different types of rape, and many definitions of rape exist. For this chapter, however, the following definition has been used ... *"intercourse, cunnilingus, fellatio, anal intercourse or any intrusion of any part of another's body, or any object manipulated by the other into the genital or anal opening of the victim's body, or the intentional touching of the victim's sexual parts by another when this is accomplished by force or threat of force, or against the victim's will"* (NIMH, 1977). This definition, it will be noted, does not discriminate by sex or by age. Rape is not a crime limited to women. Men can and have suffered rape, as have children. However, this chapter will focus primarily on rape and sexual misuse of women and girls.

Regardless of the motivations for rape or the type of rape, the central fact is that rape is a brutal act of subjugation. The trauma of this subjugation accounts for much of the victim's suffering (NIMH, 1977). Feminists assert that rape is a political crime against women, arguing that "... rape is the quintessential act by which a male demonstrates to a female that she is conquered — vanquished — by his superior strength and power" (Brownmiller, 1975).

The anger that people feel toward rapists and their victims is very real and must be dealt with. The nurse is in a position to give desperately needed support and care for the victim.

HISTORICAL VIEW OF RAPE

Rape in War

Perhaps the most blatant examples of the acceptance of rape can be found in history books and other accounts of war. Often the reader reads of the "raping and pillaging" of villages by the conquerors. We see this so often that we seldom pause to consider the effect of these rapes or the meanings behind them. In the context of war, rape can be seen primarily as an act of conquest. The effect of the rape on the brothers and husbands is to demoralize and intimidate them with the enemy's greater show of strength. In fact, the rape is seen as a crime of a man against another man. The woman involved is viewed primarily as the property of the "injured" man (Brownmiller, 1975). Despite the fact that in the United States rape in war is punishable by death or imprisonment (under Article 120 of the American Uniform Code of Military Justice), it persists as a common act of war. The literature documenting this is readily available (Brownmiller, 1975).

The issue of women as property is at the root of this view of rape. Historically, when a man paid for a woman or was paid to take her (as with a dowry), he expected that his property would be delivered intact. That is, he expected that the woman would be a virgin. If a crime was committed against her body, it was viewed legally as a crime against the man's estate.

One can see from current rape laws that the notion of women as property continues. For example, in most states a man cannot be charged with raping his wife. By law, the man in the marriage has the right to sexual relations with his wife, even if obtained against her will.

In terms of rape in war, depersonalization of the victim allows for the crime to be more "acceptable." The woman is seen as a possession of the enemy, to be spoiled much as the land is spoiled by way of retribution exacted by a conquerer. While the attitude is repugnant, it does help explain the near universality of rape in wartime.

Rape is a complex issue that has apparently been a part of humankind throughout time. Our current beliefs about rape and our current rape laws reflect some of the historical biases discussed here.

CONTEMPORARY VIEWS OF RAPE

Myths of Rape

Probably the most easily defended statement about the current views of rape is that the myths surrounding it abound. The notion that women enjoy rape or that they need force to enjoy sexual relationships is only one of the myths surrounding the topic of rape. To gain a better understanding of the biases most people have about rape, some of the more commonly accepted myths are presented here (Brownmiller, 1975; NIMH, 1977):

Myth 1. All women secretly wish to be raped.
Myth 2. A virtuous woman either cannot get raped or does not get into situations that leave her open to assault.
Myth 3. Once a woman has consented to one man, she will thereafter consent to many.
Myth 4. Rapists only assault pretty women. Unattractive women having a weak self-image would be willing to fabricate rape charges to get attention.
Myth 5. If the woman is not hysterical after the rape, it is implied that she is lying or is abnormal. If she is hysterical, her testimony is not to be trusted.

Myth 1. All women secretly wish to be raped. It is common to blame the victim of rape. The basis for this tendency can be found in the psychoanalytic literature, and particularly in the writings of Helene Deutsch and Sigmund Freud. It was largely through their writings that the idea of the "rape fantasy" became accepted. According to this notion, all women are masochistic by nature.

Masochism was perceived by Freud and Deutsch as an essential element of femininity and as a condition of erotic pleasure. Stated more simply, women were considered primarily hysterical creatures who needed pain to enjoy sex. It is only a short step from the view that women are sexually masochistic to the notion that all women secretly wish to be raped. Indeed, many men have been taken in by this myth. The pressure on a man to exercise his "masculinity" by forcing a woman until she submits is great. Pressuring a man to force sexual relationships reinforces the notion that male power and domination are essential to masculinity, much as female submission is a requirement for femininity. These views are harmful to both men and women.

Another argument put forth by those who blame the rape victim is that these women were "asking for it." The claim is made that the women were dressed in a provocative fashion, that they were out alone at night, or that they behaved or looked "sexy," thus making them responsible for the attack. Rape is not a crime committed by a sexually frustrated person, it is a crime of violence; therefore, such arguments should be irrelevant. They are, however, an accepted part of the mythology surrounding rape.

It is not unusual that advice be given women concerning what they should do if they are sexually assaulted. Often the advice includes the innuendo that they relax and enjoy the situation. (Naturally, it is rarely stated quite so bluntly.) In advising women to relax and enjoy themselves, the actual physical violence and violation are made light of. Furthermore, an assumption is made that inevitably the rapist will triumph over the woman. Finally, the notion is reinforced that all women wish to be raped anyway (Brownmiller, 1975).

Myth 2. A virtuous woman cannot be raped.   Believing that a "virtuous woman" cannot be raped is at best a self-deception of women who feel that rape "happens to other people." By denying the possibility that virtuous women will be attacked, these women achieve some degree of security in their own minds. In fact, however, many women are raped in their homes by unknown assailants (Mahan, 1980). A more insidious effect of the belief that only "loose" women get raped is the tendency to blame the rape victim for the attack. In no other type of assault is the victim so routinely blamed for the attack.

Advising women not to place themselves in situations where they could be raped returns the victim again to self-blame. Some women cannot avoid being outside at night. Women who work nights have to come home after work. If they are indeed targets for rapists (who tend to premeditate their attacks), surely they cannot be expected to stop working to avoid the possibility of such an attack. It is the attacker's behavior that is in need of change, not the victim's.

Myth 3. Once a woman has consented to one man, she will consent to others.   Past sexual experience is another basis given for doubting the woman's claim of sexual assault. The issue to be examined in situations of alleged rape revolves around the force or the lack of force used against the victim. If one does not believe that all women wish to be forced against their will to engage in sexual activities, the notion that past sexual relationships that have been consenting have any relationship to a forced encounter is clearly ridiculous.

Myth 4. Rapists only assault pretty women. The belief that rapists attack only attractive women has been disproved in a number of studies. The age of victims varies from those who are only several months old to those who are in their eighties. Because the crime is not one of sexual passion or of sexual frustration, the appearance of the victim, other than the fact that she is someone against whom the anger can be expressed, is irrelevant. Claiming that an unattractive woman would falsely accuse someone of rape again blames her, this time for being too unattractive to attract a man in any other way. It also denies the physical violation and the blow to the self-concept that such a violation includes.

Myth 5. If the woman is not hysterical, she is lying or is abnormal. If she is hysterical, her testimony cannot be trusted. This is a classic double bind. It is believed by some that following a sexual assault the woman will be totally hysterical. Her clothes should be ruined, and her body bloody and beaten (Schwartz, 1978). If a woman who reports that she has been raped does not conform to this stereotypical view, she may very well not be believed. The fact that her attacker may have had a gun or a knife, or that there may have been many attackers, making resistance a life-threatening situation, is generally not considered. It has been well documented that in the time immediately following assault, some women are withdrawn rather than hysterical (Burgess, 1974). Withdrawal is a common reaction, but one that the public is not aware of. Hence, if the woman appears in control of herself the truth of her charge is questioned.

The woman who does conform to the expected picture — hysterical or loudly distraught — may also be doubted. She may be sufficiently upset to become confused in telling her story and may not seem to be a credible source. The result is that no matter how the victim behaves, following the assault, her charge of rape is likely to be doubted.

Reporting of Rapes

With the increase in reported rapes, one would assume that more rapists than ever are being sent to prison. This is not the case. Of the less than 10 per cent of rape cases reported, only 1 per cent actually go to trial. Of this 1 per cent, only 30 per cent are ever convicted. That is, only 0.03 per cent of all accused rapists actually go to jail for their crime (Sredl, 1979). The reason for the incredibly low conviction rate for accused rapists lies in part in the legal system. The American belief that convicting an innocent man is worse than letting a guilty one go free leads to a system that requires the victim to undergo "a virtual ordeal by fire to prove her veracity" (Schwartz, 1978; Sredl, 1979). The mere fact that four out of five rapes are not reported seems to refute the argument that women easily accuse men of rape. In fact, the accusation is often not made because the victim fears she will not be believed.

Two major reasons for reporting rape are the desire and need for medical treatment and the desire to take the rapist off the street (NIMH, 1977). For women who are poor, the only medical treatment, comfort, and support that may be received is from hospitals that are required to report suspected cases of rape. The reporting may be required of the woman, rather than her choice.

More affluent women may be able to seek care privately and therefore avoid reporting, if that is their wish. The desire to take the rapist off the street may have two motivations — to ensure punishment, and to keep the rapist from raping again.

Some reasons for not reporting rapes are fear of retaliation, guilt, fear of what family may say and do, fear of skepticism and suspicion, desire not to cause trouble, and desire for privacy.

Fear of retaliation by the attacker is often thought to be the major reason why women do not report rapes. This is not the case. In at least one major study, fewer than 20 per cent of the subjects who reported that they almost did not report the rape stated that this was the reason (NIMH, 1977).

Guilt is a frequently cited reason for not reporting rape. Women have been subjected to the same mythology about rape that men have. Many of them feel that somehow the attack must have been their fault. This is more evident in some cases (such as cases in which a woman has known her attacker and may have had consenting sexual relations with him in the past) than in others. However, even in cases in which a woman was randomly attacked, guilt and embarrassment about her part in the attack is very common.

Closely allied to embarrassment is fear of what the woman's family might say and do. She may fear that they either will not believe her story or will believe that she somehow provoked the attack. Husbands and boyfriends may react in ways that the woman would not have thought possible. For some men, staying with a woman who has suffered a sexual assault is most difficult and may be nearly impossible, even with counseling. The man may not be able to accept the fact that his partner has been sexually "used" by another man.

The fear of not being believed is based on reality. Women do run a great risk of not being taken seriously when charging rape. Police may doubt her story and may decide not to press charges because of insufficient evidence. More will be said about "unfounded" cases of rape in a later portion of this chapter.

The desire not to cause trouble and the desire for privacy are closely related. The woman who has been raped has undergone a significant life-threatening loss of control and physical violation. She may wish to try to forget the entire event and try to put her life back together. In addition, she will be clearly informed that her past sexual activities and her current living situations will be openly scrutinized should she bring the case to court. For many, this additional lack of privacy may be too stressful to endure.

Demographics of Rape as a Crime

In attempting to understand the crime and its effect on the victim, studies have been conducted to describe the typical victim and the typical rapist. The most common age at which women are raped is between 15 and 20 years of age, although 20 per cent of sexual assaults are reported on girls less than 13 years old. Twice as many black women are raped as white women, far out of proportion to the general population. About 29 per cent of the women victims are raped in their own homes, while 20 per cent are attacked in the rapists' homes. Twenty-nine per cent of the women reported that they knew their attacker well, while 26 per cent knew him superficially.

In terms of the rapists and the rapes themselves, 80 to 90 per cent were reported as premeditated (Mahan, 1980).

Avoiding Rape

Advice given to women on avoiding rape does not guarantee that a woman will be safe, and may have an insidious effect on them, by undermining their own sense of control and confidence (Schwartz, 1978). Look at the typical advice given:

1. Always be suspicious.
2. Never give out any information.
3. Be aware of possible danger at all times.
4. Never tell anyone that you are alone.

In the name of rational caution, women are expected to engage in a tremendous amount of pretense. Essentially, they are told to pretend that they have a male protector even if they do not. They must be constantly on guard not to disclose any facts about their personal identity, life style, or independence. This level of caution can begin to border on paranoia (Brownmiller, 1975):

5. Never go anywhere alone.
6. Keep a large, ferocious dog.
7. Never stop to help strangers.

These cautions clearly tell women that they will not be able to defend themselves, should the situation arise. Despite the fact that it is men who are the rapists, women are taught that their ultimate security lies in being accompanied by men at all times (Brownmiller, 1975). A bind is created as men are identified both as possible protectors and potential rapists.

8. Never daydream while walking.
9. Wear conservative clothing.
10. Don't carry packages.
11. Never drive with less than a half tank of gas in the car.
12. Never have the car windows open.

These last warnings imply that women who value their sexual integrity cannot expect the same amount of freedom and independence that men routinely enjoy. Even small pleasures such as taking the car out with the windows open on the spur of the moment are described as dangerous or even reckless behavior (Brownmiller, 1975).

Obviously, safety is an important matter for all people. However, to impose special burdens on women because of their vulnerability to sexual assault makes them victims who must bear the burden of guilt for the crimes done against them. The crime is not theirs. To force women to accept responsibility for avoiding rape is ineffective, first, because rapes occur regardless of how vigilant a woman is. Secondly, the specially required behavior to avoid attacks may actually cause women to experience the fear, subjugation, and invasion of the self that they are trying to avoid.

THE ACT OF RAPE

Basic Patterns of Rape

The components of rape are power, anger, and sexuality. Sexuality is the means by which the offender expresses the aggressive needs and feelings that operate within him and that underlie the assault (Groth, 1979). The sexual expression is one of power and anger, not one of sexual desire or frustration.

Research has indicated that far more rapes are planned than had previously been thought (Brownmiller, 1975); Mahan, 1980). This is particularly true in cases of gang rape, although planning has been found in a significant number of single attacker rapes as well.

Three basic patterns of rape have been described: anger rape, power rape, and sadistic rape. Each of these patterns will be discussed here (Groth 1979).

Anger Rape.   The anger rape is characterized by physical brutality, usually far more than would be needed to complete the sexual assault. The intent of this type of rape is to hurt and degrade the victim, using sex as a weapon. The motive is often one of revenge. The offender usually feels that he has been wronged in some way, and sees the assault as a reaction to being wronged. The attacker usually is found to view sex as "dirty" and is therefore a significant weapon that can be used to degrade and humiliate his victim. Anger rape is generally impulsive rather than planned, and makes up about 40 per cent of all rapes.

The victims of anger rapes are generally found with considerable physical trauma to all areas of their body. They usually will have sensed the violent anger and experienced the assault as a life-threatening experience. Despite the great physical trauma, there may be some greater psychological recovery from the attack in that victims with these very visible signs of attack may be more likely to be believed than women who are less physically abused. There is generally less suspicion of lying and more supportive care given to the victim of an anger rape.

Survival is the key issue for the victim of anger rape. Her goal, if she found the situation to be life-threatening, was to survive, and she has done that. She may for the first time in her life be aware of life-threatening dangers, and will need guidance to help protect herself better and make her feel less vulnerable. She will also need to understand why the offender behaved as he did. The anger rapist rarely attacks the same woman twice, since women are seen primarily as objects by such men, and therefore are viewed as interchangeable.

Power Rape.   In power rape, the intent of the rapist is to assert his competency and to validate his masculinity. Sexuality becomes an expression of conquest. The aim of the assault is to capture and control the victim. The power rapist usually uses only the amount of force needed to overpower and subdue the victim. Victims are chosen for their availability, accessibility, and vulnerability. In his fantasies, the power rapist feels that the woman will resist initially and then be excited by the rape, as in the "rape wish" fantasy described earlier. Trying to resist in such a case would probably only spur the attacker to greater violence.

The victim is seen by the rapist as a symbol of everything that he dislikes about himself — she is seen as weak, powerless, and effeminate. The rape grows out of the rapist's need to reassure himself of his virility and sexual competency. In fact, most power rapists will report that the woman actually did not resist, but rather enjoyed the situation. The assault may be triggered by what the offender views as a challenge by the woman or by a threat by some man. Power rapes account for about 55 per cent of all rapes.

The victim of the power rape will usually present with little or inconclusive evidence of physical trauma. She may have realized that she should cooperate in order to survive. Having successfully done this, however, her charges may be met with doubt by both police and friends, who may feel that she in some way invited or encouraged the attacker. The victim of the power rape is made to feel helpless by the attacker. She is purposely led to believe that any attempt to escape or any show of power on her part will be useless. In treating the victim of a power rape, the health care worker should help her to realize that the strategy of not resisting the attack was certainly the best, and may have ensured her very survival.

Sadistic Rape. Sadistic rape has as its intent to abuse and torture the victim, using sex as the weapon. The motive for sadistic rape is punishment and destruction. The attacker in this type of rape finds intentional mistreatment of his victim to be intensely gratifying and takes pleasure from her torment, anguish, and suffering. The physical injury and abuse in sadistic rapes usually focuses on the sexual areas — breasts and genitals. Instruments or foreign bodies may be used to penetrate the vagina, anus or mouth of the victim. Often victims of sadistic rape do not survive the attack, which is generally deliberate, calculated, and preplanned. The bodies are often sexually mutilated when they are discovered. The excitement associated with the inflicting of pain on the victim may be a prerequisite for the rapist to achieve an erection. The victim who tries to resist may find that her resistance excites the attacker, allowing him to achieve an erection. Murder may be seen by the rapist as the ultimate satisfaction. For one thing, it eliminates the witness. More importantly to the rapist, killing is viewed as intrinsically pleasurable.

The victim who survives a sadistic rape generally requires intensive therapy. Often the victims fear that they will lose their minds. The terror and horror that they have experienced may even lead them to wish that they had died rather than to have to relive the experience in their minds. Some victims suffer severe depression. If they have sustained permanent injuries (which is not uncommon), they will be continually reminded of the assault.

Sadistic rape accounts for 5 per cent of all rapes. However, they seem to be the cases that receive the most media attention. This is especially true of cases in which the victims were young and attractive. Such biased coverage of this relatively uncommon type of rape reinforces the myths that women cannot successfully defend themselves and that men rape only beautiful women. The myth that "virtuous women" need not fear rape is furthered by the fact that prostitutes are frequently the targets in sadistic rapes.

Rape Described by Age Group

We have defined rape by type in terms of the rapist and his feelings; it must also be defined according to the age of the victims (Brant, 1977; Deni, 1978; NIMH, 1977). In general, children who are sexually misused are most often victimized in their homes by someone they know. Little violence is used. They are usually induced into cooperation by coercion (including threat of physical harm to self or siblings) and tempting, such as by promises of new clothes or of feeling good (NIMH, 1977). Sexual misuse is defined by the child's age, level of psychosexual development, and role in the family (Brant, 1977). In cases of incest, the first sexual experience is usually when the girl is between six and nine years old. Sexual activity may continue over several years (Herman, 1978).

The adolescent rape victim is most often the object of a carefully planned gang rape that takes place over a weekend and is usually related to some social event. More force is generally used in adolescent rape than in child misuse but less than with adult rape.

Gang rape may be planned as an initiation rite or as punishment for failure of the victim to recognize "her place" (Brownmiller, 1975; Groth, 1979; NIMH, 1977). Penile-vaginal intercourse is the most commonly practiced sexual act during the rape. Repeated acts of intercourse by the same offender or group of offenders is common.

Adult women are most often raped indoors after dark by strangers (NIMH, 1977). The adult victim suffers greater physical violence than victims of any other age group during the attack.

THE RAPIST

Rape is never the result of sexual arousal that has no other outlet. It is an expression of power over another person. For the majority of rapists, the act is the result of a specific fear and of feelings of hostility toward women (Bearney, 1978; Goldstein, 1978; Groth, 1979). Most rapists are between 16 and 24 years old. They are evenly split between blacks and whites (Brownmiller, 1975). Black women are raped more often than white women, however (NIMH, 1977).

The danger of accepting the common misconception that the rapist's behavior is primarily motivated by sexual desire and that the rape is directed only toward gratifying this sexual need is in people's tendency to blame the victim for somehow arousing the offender. Most rapists themselves expect that the rape will be sexually rewarding, but find that it is not. They report little if any sexual satisfaction in the act of rape. In fact, the reactions to the sexual aspects of the assault have been found to range from disappointment to disgust (Groth, 1979).

In analyzing the sex offender, the Freudian view is often utilized. In utilizing this idea of the "sexual psychopath," the rapist is the perceived victim of an "uncontrollable urge" that is "infantile" in nature. This urge is in turn perceived to have resulted from the thwarted "natural" impulse of the offender to have intercourse with his mother. The act of rape is viewed as a "neurotic overreaction" that stemmed from his "feelings of inadequacy" (Brownmiller, 1975). The problem with this type of analysis is that it accepts as right and appropriate the theme of supreme rightness of male dominance and aggression.

A less psychoanalytic view of the rapist usually shows him as suffering from either a temporary or a chronic and repetitive psychological dysfunction. He is usually described as feeling desperate and unable to handle the stresses and demands of life. The offender is pictured as emotionally weak and insecure, usually lacking close emotional and intimate relationships with anyone, male or female. He has little capacity for warmth, trust, compassion, or empathy (Groth, 1979). Almost half of the offenders in one study were found to have been victims of sexual assault when they were children (Groth, 1979). Of this group, 68 per cent were sexually assaulted before they were 13 years old. The forms of sexual assaults varied but generally fell into the following groups:

1. Eighteen per cent were pressured into sexual relations by an adult.
2. Eighteen per cent were in a sex stress situation which may have included

severe reaction by others to their early sexual explorations (one example of this can be the severe punishing of a young boy for masturbating).
3. Three per cent reported that they had witnessed upsetting sexual activity between other adults.
4. Two per cent had sexual injuries or some physiological handicap.

In correlating the types of sexual assault suffered by the rapists as children, it was found that men who raped women tended to have been in pressure or sex stress situations. It has been postulated that child molesters tended to have been forcibly sexually assaulted as children.

The misuser of children is often seen as a "dirty old man." In fact, this stereotypical view is inaccurate. Over 75 per cent of offenders against children are less than 35 years old; only 1 per cent are over 55 years old. The offender generally knows his victim at least casually. He is not retarded or sexually frustrated. In fact, the child offender is usually found to be married. He is not insane, and his acts do not become progressively more violent. He is not a homosexual (Groth, 1979). The sexual offender of children generally views himself as inferior. He may feel that he cannot compete with men in an attempt to attract adult women and may therefore turn to little girls for affection and sexual gratification. He is generally better able to control his urges than is the rapist, and he is generally more passive (Peters, 1976).

The use of alcohol has long been linked with sexual abuses in both children and adults. In most studies, about half of the rapists are reported to have been drinking at the time of the rape. Rapists in general have been found to be relatively heavy drinkers, although, according to the criteria of The National Council on Alcoholism, only 35 per cent are actually alcoholics (Rada, 1975).

Alcohol does tend to decrease ego control and judgment and to reduce normal inhibitions. It has been demonstrated that there is a cause-and-effect relationship between drinking and sexual assault. Alcohol may at most serve as a release only when an individual has already reached a frame of mind in which he is prone to rape (Bearney, 1978; Groth, 1979; NIMH, 1977; Rada, 1975).

One effect that alcohol has been found to have on the general male population is that it interferes with sexual performance (Masters, 1970). The effects of alcohol may in part explain the high rate of sexual dysfunction among sex offenders during the sexual assault. More than one in three sex offenders were found to have been sexually dysfunctional during the rape, even when they were not dysfunctional in consenting sexual relationships. Impotence and retarded or absent ejaculation were the most common dysfunctions. Both have implications on testing for presence of sperm. This high rate of dysfunction supports the theory that rape is symptomatic of psychological conflict and anxiety (Groth, 1979).

THE VICTIM

"A world without rapists would be a world in which women moved freely without threat of men. That *some* men rape provides a sufficient threat to keep all women in a constant state of intimidation, forever conscious of the knowledge that the biological tool must be held in awe for it may turn into a weapon with sudden swiftness borne of harmful intent" (Brownmiller, 1975).

The aftereffects of sexual assault are varied. Short- and long-term effects will be discussed here.

Rape Trauma Syndrome

Rape trauma syndrome was first described in detail by Burgess (1974) as the result of a study of 96 adult victims of forcible rape. Rape trauma syndrome is an acute stress reaction to life-threatening situations resulting from rape or attempted rape. The syndrome itself consists of two phases, acute and reorganization.

During the acute phase women tend to react in either an expressed style characterized by fear, anger, sobbing, restlessness, and tenseness or in a controlled style in which feelings are masked or hidden and there is a resultant calm, composed, or subdued effect. In the acute phase, there is great disorganization of the woman's life style. She may experience noticeable physical symptoms and may be very fearful. In the later, reorganization phase she may experience changes in motor activity and nightmares. Phobias may also develop during this time (Burgess, 1974).

Physical reactions during the acute phase include skeletal muscle tension (headaches, fatigue, disturbances in sleep patterns, and startle reactions), gastrointestinal irritability (nausea, stomach pains, and appetite changes), genitourinary disturbances (vaginal discharges, and itching and burning on urination), and general pain. Rectal bleeding and pain are also found in those who have been forced to have anal intercourse.

Emotionally, women in the acute phase of rape trauma syndrome experience a tremendous fear of violence and death. They may also experience self-blame. Other reactions include feelings of humiliation, embarrassment, anger, and revenge (Burgess, 1974).

During the reorganization phase, which usually starts two to three weeks after the rape, many victims change their place of residence. If the woman is unable to move, there is a strong need to get away on a trip. Telephone numbers are often changed and unlisted for fear that the assailant knows her and will attempt retaliation. In the studies by the Burgess group, turning by these victims for support to family members was not frequently observed. In partnership relationships, disruption following sexual assault was common. Fifty-nine per cent of couples reported total disruption of the relationship, and an additional 14 per cent reported a semi-disruption (Burgess, 1979).

Nightmares were common in the reorganization phase. Toward the end of the phase, most women reported mastery in the dream, such as escaping or successfully fighting off some type of attack.

Nearly all women reported fears of being alone during the reorganization phase. Fears of being in the setting in which the attack occurred were common. Sexual fears were also commonly reported (Burgess, 1974).

In some cases victims had a history of physical, psychiatric, or social problems prior to the assault. These women experienced what is called a compounded reaction to the attack. Their symptoms, in addition to those outlined above, included depression, psychotic behavior, psychosomatic disorders, suicidal behavior, alcoholism, drug use, and sexual acting out (Burgess, 1974).

Some women never tell anyone about the rape. The woman who practices this "silent reaction" tends to carry a tremendous burden that may be uncovered later in therapy undertaken for some other reason (Burgess, 1974).

Recovery from rape is a subjective feeling. In a sample of 81, Burgess (1979) found that 37 per cent felt "back to normal" in several months following the rape. Another 37 per cent reported that it took years to recover, while 26 per cent reported that four to six years was not sufficient time to recover from the attack.

Women who recovered from rape quickly were found to have employed common adaptive responses to the attack (Burgess, 1979). Women who tended to have a generally better sense of self-esteem and who evaluated their part in the attack as appropriate recovered more quickly than those who experienced guilt or doubt about their part in the attack.

The use of defense mechanisms such as explanation, minimization, suppression, and dramatization also tended to aid the woman in her recovery. If the woman was able to find some reason for the rape, whether it was an explanation regarding the rapist's motivation or the taking of responsibility herself, she tended to recover more quickly. Even a victim who explained the attack through her own negligence (e.g., hitchhiking) recovered more quickly after a reason had been identified.

Minimizing the attack served to decrease the terrifying aspects of the assault and allowed the woman to think of it in tolerable amounts. (For women who associate rape with death, merely having survived the attack may help in recovery.) Some women found that they could successfully put the rape out of their thoughts through conscious effort, while others seemed to have the need to repeatedly discuss the assault. This discussion tended to reduce the woman's anxiety about the attack.

Increased action on the part of the victim also tended to aid in her return to normal following the attack. As mentioned previously, many women changed their residence or travelled after the attack. It was common to have telephone numbers changed or unlisted. Many women also became involved in rape crisis centers. Of the women who did this, 70 per cent reported that they had recovered from the rape within months (Burgess, 1977). The act of helping others seems to have had a marked effect on self-help in this group.

Unfortunately, not all responses to attacks are adaptive. In the Burgess groups, reliance on drugs and alcohol following the assault was not uncommon, occurring in 14 per cent of the sample (Burgess, 1979). Suicide attempts were also common. In the group of women who reported that they were still not back to normal four to six years after the attack, 43 per cent reported that they had tried one or more of these coping mechanisms (Burgess, 1979).

Recovery Following Rape — Children and Adolescents

Children have been found to be more likely not to report sexual misuse than members of any other age group (Peters, 1976).

Anxiety over parental response and fear of retaliation by the offender were the most commonly encountered reasons for the reluctance to report. The effects of sexual misuse in children include the following: reports of negative feelings toward men, sleep disturbances, decreased interest in school work, uncharacteristic moodiness, and other symptoms of tension including migraine, stomach ailments, skin disorders, and disabling aches or pains (Deni, 1978; NIMH, 1977). These symptoms can, of course, be attributed to other upsetting situations, but the possibility of sexual misuse should not be ignored in diagnosing.

The reaction of the parents upon learning of the misuse may be far more emotional than the child's (Goldstein, 1978). In some cases, the response of the parents may be more upsetting to the child than was the actual sexual activity. Parents should be advised to respond to the rape as they would to any other assault on their child. The child will need expressions of concern and reassurance, and the knowledge that steps have been or will be taken to ensure that she will not be exposed to the misuse again. Overprotection may tend to confuse and cause the child to feel guilty. Family routines should be continued except for any that leave the girl vulnerable to further attack (NIMH, 1977).

The long-term effects of early sexual misuse often include difficulty in trusting men in adulthood (Herman, 1978; Peters, 1976). Low self-esteem is often encountered in women who have been misused. While they may feel that they are not entitled to love and respect, they may view themselves as powerful and dangerous to men. They may believe that they seduced their father (or relative) and can therefore seduce any man. Guilt at having enjoyed a special relationship with the father may lead to further feelings of low self-esteem (Herman, 1978). Hatred of the mother is a common finding in long-term problems experienced by victims of sexual misuse. The anger revolves around the perceived failure of the mother to protect the child (Peters, 1976).

In addition to suffering from feelings of low self-esteem, victims of sexual misuse tend to be socially withdrawn and regressive, and seem to project a feeling of fear and sadness. Nightmares are common (NIMH, 1977). More study is needed on this topic to determine more precisely the effects of sexual misuse.

In counseling child victims, ventilation of feelings is most important. The child who is encouraged to express in her own words what happened and how she felt about it seems to adjust with fewer traumatic changes than the child who is not allowed to discuss the misuse and who is encouraged, instead, to "forget" it; the latter child may feel unprotected and rejected (Peters, 1976).

Many adolescents are afraid to tell their parents about the assault. Sometimes the attack takes place in a situation that the adolescent has been warned about by her parents. If the attack occurs in a social situation or when the adolescent is disobeying authority, she frequently is doubted by the authorities (NIMH, 1977). In addition to the perceived lack of understanding and communication with the parents and the fear of blame or punishment, the adolescent has to face the fact that her acquaintances might be friends of the offenders who could apply pressure on her to be quiet. Hence, even friends are rarely told of the attack (NIMH, 1977).

The age of the adolescent tends to have an effect on the reactions. The younger adolescent initially tends to regress socially and to turn away from her peers, particularly from more sexually experienced friends who they feel may have betrayed them. A return to the family is not uncommon. The adolescent may lack confidence and spontaneity and may see herself as dirty and contaminated. Fear of sexually transmitted disease and pregnancy may continue long after the danger of these has passed. The reaction of the older adolescent depends largely on her support system and her maturity. As in other cases, physical symptoms include changes in eating and sleeping patterns. Many experience nightmares, and a substantial number of adolescents have reported negative feelings toward men and about being alone. Family relations do not seem to significantly change following the attack. More than half of the adolescents decrease their social activities.

Long-term effects of sexual misuse on adolescents include sustained unrest, which may lead to a desire to escape or run away. Sleep disturbances, including nightmares, continue, as do intense and specific fears and phobias. There tends to be psychological evidence of retreat or regression, including the avoidance of complex activities, difficulties in concentration, and a decrease in creative effort (NIMH, 1977).

In the group studied by Burgess (1979) sexual functioning in women who had been sexually active prior to the assault was found to be significantly affected. The majority of women reported disruptions in their sexual functioning within six months following the rape. Thirty-eight per cent were abstaining from sex, 33 per cent had decreased activity, 19 per cent reported no change, and 10 per cent reported increased activity. Frequently encountered sexual symptoms following sexual assault included sexual aversion, flashbacks, vaginismus (involuntary contractions of the muscles of the vagina preventing penetration), and orgasmic dysfunction.

In addition to their role as patient caregivers and advocates, nurses have a role in the legal aspects of the care given to the rape victims. It is to the legal aspect of rape that the next portion of the chapter is devoted.

LEGAL ASPECTS

Founded and Unfounded Rapes

Rape is a crime of aggression against women. It is a crime of rage (Sredl, 1979). Rape is not a medical diagnosis, it is a legal term only. It is not up to the physician or nurse to determine whether or not a sexual assault has occurred. For charting purposes, the event must be called an "alleged rape" until it is proven in court. Additionally, the assailant is to be referred to as the "accused" (Sredl, 1979). These points are significant, since the written records obtained in the hospital can be judged inadmissible if such conclusions have been drawn by the physicians or nurses caring for the victim.

Generally the police are the first people the victim will encounter following an alleged rape. It is the duty of the police officer to have all women or men who allege that they have been raped medically examined as soon as possible, both for treatment purposes and to collect evidentiary material that will later be used to "found" or "unfound" a case of alleged rape (Peters, 1975). Often, women who inform the police that they have been raped will be taken to the police station initially, rather than to a hospital for treatment, so that they can be "evaluated" for the credibility of the allegation. If the police do not believe the woman, she may be discouraged from pressing charges (NIMH, 1977). These delays often last several hours. In one study, 27 per cent of male policemen did not believe the women. Overall, 15 per cent of alleged rape accusations are labeled unfounded and are dismissed because they are thought to present insufficient cause to pursue a charge of rape (Brownmiller, 1975; Goldstein, 1978; Peters, 1975).

Some of the reasons why charges of alleged rape are termed unfounded are listed here (Goldstein, 1978):

1. Delay in reporting the crime
2. Lack of evidence of physical abuse
3. Refusal of the victim to allow collection of specimens
4. Victims were engaged in what the police define as questionable behavior, such as hitchhiking or walking alone at night

If the victim does not immediately report a rape, she is likely to be doubted. In states where the crime of rape has a statute of limitations, the statute is usually of shorter duration than the statute of limitations for similar crimes, such as assault (Peters, 1975). Another reason why a woman is likely to be doubted is that it is believed that she may be accusing the man because she has some desire to strike back at him and has fabricated the story to accomplish this. Again one is presented with the idea that women lie about rape.

Lack of evidence of physical abuse may occur as a result of the woman being threatened with a knife or gun. The victim may choose to comply with the sexual demands more or less in return for her life. Of course, the rapists do not always follow the same rules as the victim. In some cases, however, the woman will not show signs of resistance and force although she was surely raped. The requirement of signs of force is peculiar to victims of rape. "In no other crime is the victim expected to demonstrate such signs of force and resistance to establish her credibility" (Peters, 1975).

Some women may view the physical examination following the rape to be further insult and trauma and may indeed refuse to have specimens collected. With supportive treatment she may be made to see that the collection of the evidence can assist her later if she should decide to press charges, but this is not always possible.

Finally, women who are raped by strangers in situations in which there was demonstrable violence are more likely to be believed than women raped in cars or women who are believed to have been intoxicated at the time of the rape. The police may believe that the woman initially agreed or was somehow angry or displeased with her partner and decided to falsely accuse him of rape. Again, the bias that women freely charge rape is deeply ingrained (Brownmiller, 1975).

A legally prosecutable rape has been defined as "forceful vaginal penetration with the penis by a male of a female who is not his wife." (Goldstein, 1978.) Although proof that the woman physically resisted has been required in the past, many states have omitted this requirement. If sodomy or fellatio occurs or objects other than the penis are inserted into the vagina of the woman, these charges cannot always be prosecuted under current rape laws (Goldstein, 1978). Most states have no rape laws that include male rape.

The Trial

About 0.03 per cent of accused rapists actually go to prison. The low number of convictions may be due to our criminal justice system, which is openly hostile to the victims of rape (Schwartz, 1978). In the past, laws requiring corroboration of penetration and proof of resistance have made conviction harder.

Rules of evidence that allow the victim's entire private life to be attacked publicly have also contributed to the reluctance of victims to bring a case to court. In addition to these impediments, many of which still exist, is the severity of the punishment for rape. It has been thought that very severe penalties would serve to prevent potential rapists from committing the crime. The actual effect has been the reluctance of juries to convict accused rapists. A verdict of not guilty means only that there was not enough evidence to rule out the possibility that he might not have committed the crime (Goldstein, 1978; Sredl, 1979).

A further detriment to the conviction by a jury of an accused rapist is what is called a "cautionary instruction" from the judge to the jury. In his instructions, the judge has been required in some states and may choose in others to recite this statement before the jury begins its deliberation. "A charge such as that made against the defendant in this case is one which is easily made and, once made, difficult to defend against, even if the person accused is innocent" (Geis, 1978). This instruction singles out the rape victim as being a member of a group whose very credibility is suspect. The instruction was once mandatory in California, but has been repealed in the last few years.

A charge of rape is technically prosecuted by the state. The victim does not charge the rapist. Rather, she is a witness for the prosecution. The district attorney will serve as the victim's legal representative. As a witness, the victim is required to speak to substantiate her charge. She is also subject to cross examination by the lawyer defending the accused rapist. Cross examination may include the details of the attack and of the previous sexual history of the victim (Goldstein, 1978; Herman, 1977; NIMH, 1977; Peters, 1975; Sredl, 1979). Proponents of allowing the victim's past sexual experiences to be admissible argue that if it tends slightly to increase the probability that the woman consented or that she is lying, it must be admitted. The myth that once a woman says yes to one man she will say yes to all men is surely at work here. Opponents to allowing the victim's past sexual activities to be admissible argue that it is insulting and demeaning to the victim, and prejudicial to her case (Geis, 1978). While the past history of the woman can be admitted, the alleged rapist need not testify. If he chooses not to, the jury is instructed not to hold this against him (Sredl, 1979). His past criminal record, including past convictions of rape, are not admissible.

Although no state requires that the victims of robbery or assault provide corroboration, some states still require this for rape cases (Goldstein, 1978). Some example of corroboration include (Burgess, 1977):

1. Medical evidence and testimony
2. Condition of clothing
3. Bruises and scratches
4. Emotional condition of the victim
5. Presence of blood or semen on the clothing of victim and accused
6. Evidence of breaking and entering into the home of the victim
7. Opportunity of the accused
8. Conduct of the accused at the time of arrest
9. Speed of complaints to police

Numbers 1 through 5 relate to the role of the health care workers. Most of these items deal with physical evidence, which includes any fragment, particle, or remnant of any substance that can be examined microscopically or chemically to corroborate a crime (Burgess, 1977).

Collection of physical evidence will be covered in the section on nursing intervention. The legal aspect of this collection involves insurance that the evidence, once collected, has not been opened, tainted, or destroyed between the time of collection and the time it is introduced as evidence. The term "chain of custody" is used to describe the systematic method utilized to insure that all persons responsible for keeping or handling the material can be easily traced (Burgess, 1977; Sredl, 1979). The importance of accurate record keeping cannot be stressed enough. At a trial, any discrepancy between the victim's testimony and the record will lead to the instruction that the record be considered to be correct. Any error in recording is likely to be used to discredit the victim (Burgess, 1977). The records must be legible and precise, omitting value judgments and opinions by the nurse or physician.

Proposed Changes in Rape Laws

Much debate surrounds the issue of changing rape legislation. Extended laws that include male as well as female rape and forced acts such as fellatio, cunnilingus, and acts of vaginal and anal penetration by objects other than a penis have been proposed (Geis, 1978). Michigan did adopt a neuter sexual assault law in 1976 (Schwartz, 1978). The law attempts to distinguish between sexual union and coercive genital contact. It also defines sexual assaults on a "degree matrix," which is based on the danger, the amount of coercion used, the infliction of personal injury, and the age and incapacitation of the victim. The law does not require corroboration, does not admit past sexual behavior of the victim, and shifts the burden of proof regarding the possibility of "consent" to the defense. The Michigan law has been called a "model rape law" (Schwartz, 1978).

Reducing rape penalities has been suggested by many in order that juries will not be so fearful of conviction (Brownmiller, 1975; Schwartz, 1978).

Elimination of sexual assault laws completely has been proposed in an effort to demystify rape. Placing rape under current assault laws is seen as achieving many of the aforementioned goals. Corroboration would no longer be required. The law for assault focuses on the behavior of the defendant rather than on that of the victim. Consent or the victim's resistance would be irrelevant. Threat or use of force would be the most significant factor. The question would focus only on whether the defendant used force. It has been suggested that if the law focuses on the assault rather than on the sexual nature of the crime, the tendency to blame the victim or to look for something in the victim's behavior as the cause would be greatly reduced. For example, asking a stabbing victim if he "enjoyed it" seems foolish. The idea that many people may unconsciously want to be punished is not an accepted defense to the crime of assault.

The behavior of the victim is also not a defense to an assault charge. The appearance of the victim is never a defense to such charges. The "asking for trouble" argument is not valid in such cases (Schwartz, 1978). Assault laws are written particularly to proclaim the right of all citizens to the physical integrity of their bodies. Sexual assault under these laws would be seen as a violation of this right. Stating that assault on any other part of the woman's body is assault whereas assault on the genitals is a different crime relates to the idea of women as property.

Regardless of whether or when rape laws are reformed, nurses must be knowledgeable about these laws in their particular state. Rape crisis centers or legal aid centers are generally most willing to discuss this with interested people. If nurses are to give informed care, they must possess this information.

Sue is brought by the police to the emergency room. The police officer informs the nurse that Sue reported she had been sexually assaulted in her home. The accused attacker was not known to her and has not as yet been apprehended.

Marge, the nurse, escorts Sue to a private waiting area used for persons in cases of alleged sexual assault. Marge offers Sue a chair or a couch to sit on, and asks if she would like some tea or coffee. While getting Sue a cup of tea, Marge explains that she will stay with her for the entire time Sue is in the emergency room.

After Sue seems to be a little more relaxed, Marge asks her about the bruise on her face. Sue touches the area and says that her attacker punched her in the face when she refused to "put my mouth on his penis. It was disgusting!" she continues, saying that she should never have opened the door when he knocked on it. She had ordered a pizza, and assumed that he was the delivery man from the restaurant. The attacker had forced his way into the room, and had begun to pull at her clothing. Although the timing is poor, Marge asks Sue to allow an oral swab before she drinks the tea to determine the presence of sperm prostatic fluid in the mouth or throat. Sue agrees and this is done.

With little encouragement other than supportive statements, Sue haltingly tells Marge the story of her attack. The progression of the story is not precise, and Sue frequently begins to cry. When she seems to have stopped, Marge asks her if she would like to call anyone to be with her. Sue becomes very upset, fearing the reaction of her boyfriend to the event. She states that although she wants him with her, she is afraid that he will be furious at her for allowing anyone into the apartment when she was there alone. The nurse offers to call Bob, and Sue asks her to tell him that she is all right, in the hospital, and will call him later. She asks that Bob not be told that she was assaulted. Sue decides to call her sister. Marge suggests that the sister bring along a clean set of clothing for Sue. It is only then that Sue realizes that her clothing is ripped and stained.

After the telephone calls are made, Sue asks the nurse what will happen to her now. Marge explains the procedure for the physical exam, including the collection of evidence, informed consent, medication (if needed), and permission to take photographs. She determines that Sue has just finished her period, and that she has been taking birth control pills for the past two years.

Using the form developed at the hospital for victims of alleged sexual assaults, Marge begins to note Sue's physical condition, including bruises, scratches, etc. Photographs are taken of all injured areas. Sue's clothing is collected in the appropriate bags and labeled by Marge. She is given a hospital gown to wear.

Next, Marge explains that the physician will be in to examine her. She assures her that she will stay with her at all times. The physician on duty is a woman. Sue seems greatly relieved by this information. She had had pelvic examinations in the past and has not had any pain or anxiety about them. She repeatedly states that she feels so dirty and wonders if she will ever be clean again.

As Marge is explaining the procedure for the physical exam and the possible treatment for venereal disease, Sue suddenly remarks that the knife must still be in her apartment. She had not previously mentioned the use of a weapon. Marge notes this on the record. Further gentle questioning revealed that in addition to the forced fellatio, her attacker forced intercourse. He did not insert any objects or his penis into the anus. Sue did not lose consciousness at any time. She states that she wishes she had. "I was so sure that he was going to kill me. It was all I could think of. I'm too young to die. Now, I will always have the memory of what that animal did to me. Perhaps I should have died." Following this statement, Marge tells Sue that survival was her goal and that she had achieved it. She points out that the attack was the act of a sick and terrible person who wanted to disgrace and humiliate her, not because of who she was or what she did, but because she represented something else to him. She assures Sue that her behavior was appropriate and successful. She has survived, and she will get over the attack.

Sue's sister arrives around this time. Marge gives them some privacy but does not leave the room. Sue's sister has brought clothes for her. She doesn't ask questions, but hugs Sue and assures her that she will help her. She asks Sue if she will stay with her and her family for at least a few days. Sue states that she hadn't thought about where she would go, but she is sure that she doesn't want to go back to the apartment alone.

After a brief time, the physician arrives. As Marge had informed Sue, the physician is a woman. She introduces herself as Dr. Joan Smith. Instead of asking Sue to repeat her story, she asks Sue if she may ask Marge to tell her the story as she understands it. Sue agrees, and fills in gaps in the story as Marge tells it to the physician. The physician then asks Sue if she is ready for the pelvic exam. She asks Sue's sister to leave, but Sue begins to become very agitated, wanting her sister to stay with her. The sister is allowed to stay.

Following the exam and treatment of Sue's cuts and bruises, she is given tetanus toxoid and a prophylactic dose of penicillin, since being on oral contraceptives makes her far more susceptible to gonorrhea. She is instructed verbally and in writing to return for further treatment. Sue is allowed to shower before going home with her sister. She still seems shaken, but the relationship between the sisters is noted by both the nurse and the physician to be a strong and supportive one.

As policy, Marge will call Sue the next day, in one week, and monthly for several months. Sue is informed of this, and thanks Marge. Marge assures her that she can call her at any time if she needs to talk or if she needs information.

Following Sue's discharge, Marge gives the carefully labeled and sealed contents of the examination to the police, who have been waiting. The knife was not found in the apartment.

The Nurse as Counselor/Caregiver in the Hospital

In the preceding case study, the essential goals of care for rape victims have been met. The nurse was appropriately and effectively the major contact the patient had with the hospital and hospital staff. The goals she met or helped to meet were (Virginia State Crime Commission, 1978):

1. To provide a relaxing atmosphere and a sympathetic attitude toward all patients while assessing the needs and support required to prevent additional trauma
2. To administer treatment and emergency medical care for physical injury
3. To conduct the medical exam and collect evidentiary material and documentation in a professional and sympathetic manner
4. To prevent unwanted pregnancy and venereal disease
5. To make provisions for the follow-up care for the patient

An additional goal, not covered in the case study but one that will be discussed in this section, is:

6. To recognize the special diagnostic and therapeutic needs of child victims of sexual misuse.

The Atmosphere and Attitude Toward Patients.   In order to give patients support while assessing their needs, it is essential to have a private area in the emergency room for victims of alleged rapes. Often, unfortunately, victims of sexual assault are forced to wait in a common waiting room as other more "serious" cases are treated before them. It is essential to avoid leaving the patient alone during this time (Welch, 1977). She probably views her attack as a situation in which she was totally under the control of another. The loss of control can be devastating. Giving her choices is essential in helping her to regain her sense of self-esteem and control (Goldstein, 1978; NIMH, 1977).

The nurse gave Sue choices on several points — coffee or tea, where she would like to sit down, if she wanted to notify anyone, if she was ready for physical exam, etc.

In addition to allowing Sue to make choices, the nurse allowed her to tell her story in her own way. Forcing the patient to do anything, including telling her story in a systematic way, often contributes to the patient's feelings that she is being assaulted again (Clark, 1976). There are other advantages to letting the patient tell her story in her own way, without a structured interview. People tend to remember better and discuss more points more easily if they talk as the thoughts occur to them. In addition, some new ideas and topics may be uncovered in an unstructured interview that may not have occurred to the interviewer. It also allows the interviewer to note the links that are spontaneously made between topics (Holmstrom, 1975).

Patients should be reassured that forgetting details in a crisis is normal. They may fear that they are losing their minds, and will need this reassurance. The patient must feel that the nurse understands how hard it is for her to talk about the assault. Silence must be utilized effectively to enable the patient to feel comfortable.

In the course of the discussion, the nurse will need to find out some essential data (Goldstein, 1979):

1. When and where did the alleged rape take place?
2. Was there a threat of violence?

3. Did the patient see a weapon or was it referred to?
4. What physical abuse was utilized?
5. Was any foreign object inserted into the rectum or vagina?
6. Were any restraints used?
7. Did the patient lose consciousness at any time?

The immediate support and kindness of the nurse may be the single most important aspect of all the nursing care given to a woman following an alleged rape (NAACOG, 1979). Even when the patient recounts the events of the assault to the nurse, careful, on-the-spot documentation is essential. The information must be noted without judgment of the veracity of the patient's statements. Judgments of emotional trauma should report actual descriptions of the patient's behavior, such as sobbing, tears, trembling, hyperventilation, or extreme withdrawal (Burgess, 1977).

When Sue was ready to attend to the present, she asked the nurse what would happen next. Marge was then able to inform her about the collection of physical evidence and the fact that she had the right to refuse this; about medical treatment, including the pelvic exam and the prophylactic treatment related to pregnancy and sexually transmitted disease; about the collections of photographs to document her injuries; and about her right to contact the authorities (Welch, 1979). In Sue's case, she had already contacted the police, and did intend to pursue the case.

Providing for external support systems is also of great importance. In the case study, Sue rejected the idea of a rape crisis counselor but did want her sister to be with her. It was established that Sue's sister would provide an excellent support system for her. Sue was informed of the available resources and was again allowed to make a choice.

Importantly, when Sue began to voice feelings of guilt and self-blame, the nurse was able to quickly assure her that her behavior was appropriate. Although the assault was a life-threatening situation, the nurse was able to reinterpret the situation as one in which the victim, although suffering during the attack, had ultimately survived. She was able to stress that survival, not escape, was the key (Groth, 1979; Sredl, 1979).

Treatment for Physical Injury and Emergency Medical Care.   Although in Sue's case, emergency medical treatment was not required, in other cases, this may be the first priority. Certainly, bleeding must be stopped and the patient must be adequately hydrated and oxygenated prior to having her try to talk. Life-threatening situations must be dealt with first.

Medical Exam, Collection of Evidentiary Material, and Documentation.   Ideally, all hospitals will adopt some written policy regarding the care and collection of data on rape cases. Specifically, it should be noted who is responsible for the following (Virginia State Crime Commission, 1978):

1. Collection of specimens and other evidentiary material
2. Retaining evidentiary material
3. Obtaining consent for the release of evidentiary material. (Note: If a patient does not give consent for the release of such material, it should be kept for seven days in case the patient should change her ·mind. The patient should be informed in writing and verbally that this will be done.)
4. Chain of evidence
5. Notification of the police to collect the evidentiary material
6. Turning the evidentiary material over to police

In the case study, the nurse was responsible for all of these steps, even though she did not carry out the physical examination herself.

Evidentiary material has been briefly discussed earlier, but will be covered again here in more detail, especially regarding the collection of the material and the physical exam.

"Physical evidence," defined earlier, includes (Burgess, 1977) "Any fragment, particle, or remnant of any substance that can be examined microscopically or chemically to corroborate a crime." As stated earlier, corroboration of some form is still required in most states. In order to prove that materials collected are intact and have not been tampered with in the time between the collection and the time the materials are used in a legal proceeding, limiting the number of people who handle the material is advised. All material collected is to be placed in envelopes, which are to be labeled as to contents and the name of the person collecting and sealing the envelopes. In addition, the date, time, and name of the person who received or transferred each item is noted on each envelope. When the evidence is turned over to the police, it is again signed by the police officer, and the nurse or other hospital representative who has been collecting and labeling the data receives a receipt for the evidence. This procedure, which is basically a systematic method to insure that all persons responsible for keeping or handling the evidence can be easily traced, is called the "chain of evidence" (Sredl, 1979).

Physical evidence of rape includes the clothing of the victim, fingernail scrapings, pubic hair combings, vaginal tampons, and photographs. In the collection of this physical evidence, the woman is directed to stand on a paper while she is undressing in order to catch any particles that may fall from her clothing or her body during the undressing. The paper is then included in the analysis of the evidence (NAACOG, 1979). Clothing is collected in paper bags. Plastic bags should be avoided, since the plastic tends to promote the molding of seminal stains. Prior to putting the clothes in the bag, tears, blood stains, semen stains, and soil marks should be noted (Burgess, 1977; Sredl, 1979).

Fingernail scrapings are not routinely done but may provide further evidence in the identification of the assailant. If the nails are broken, it should be noted in the patient's record. Broken nails are usually accepted as a sign of struggle.

Pubic hair combings are usually performed to collect any further evidence. If at all possible, the victim should be allowed to do the combing herself. The results of the combing are collected in an envelope and sealed with the comb for further evaluation.

If the woman was wearing a tampon during the alleged attack, the tampon should also be saved as evidentiary material. It will be evaluated for the presence of seminal fluid and sperm.

Recently, the addition of the use of photographs has become more widely accepted in courts across the country. By the time a case reaches trial, the victim has usually healed from the physical signs of the trauma. Photographs serve to demonstrate the condition of the victim immediately following the alleged attack. The photographs should be in black and white, since in some cases, color photographs have been inadmissible because they were ruled as being too "sensational" (Burgess, 1977; Sredl, 1979).

Laboratory tests collected are generally aimed at determining the presence of prostatic fluid and semen. Vaginal, cervical, oral, and rectal swabs are collected to determine the presence of these materials. Lab testing is also done to help identify the location of the attack and the attacker. Blood and dirt samples may be used for this purpose.

Alkaline phosphatase tests are used to detect male prostatic fluid. These are especially valuable, since sperm is not needed to determine that intercourse (or other penetration of an orifice) has taken place. The test would be positive in cases where the assailant has had a vasectomy, as well as in cases where ejaculation did not occur. Acid phosphatase tests are valuable in helping to determine the time that has elapsed since the attack. Usually the specimen collected from the vaginal pool is used for this purpose (Burgess, 1977; Peters, 1975).

The patient will especially need sympathetic, supportive care from the nurse during the actual physical examination. The examination may vividly remind her of the experience. She may even become hysterical (Sredl, 1979). If the victim is forced to cooperate during the exam or if she is made to feel that her claim of assault is in question, her trauma may be significantly increased (Goldstein, 1978). In Sue's case, the nurse explained the procedure before the physician arrived. The physician introduced herself and established rapport with the patient before asking her if she was ready for the exam. She did not have the patient in the lithotomy position with her feet in the stirrups for any discussion (Welch, 1979).

During the physical exam, the patient's entire body is inspected for abrasions, bruises, swelling, lacerations, and teeth marks. Particular attention is paid to the arms, legs, neck, breasts, and the inner aspects of the thighs (Burgess, 1977). Prior to the pelvic exam, the patient should be instructed to empty her bladder and save the urine. It will be checked later as a baseline pregnancy test (NAACOG, 1979). Any trauma to any area should be noted and described, despite the fact that photographs may be taken.

The gynecological exam includes inspection of the vulva, perineum, hymenal ring, vagina, and rectum for tenderness, swelling redness, lacerations, and bruises. The specimens mentioned earlier, vaginal, cervical, and anal swabs, are also collected.

The attitude of the physician is particularly important to the later recovery of the patient and the degree to which her testimony will be believed in later legal proceedings. In Sue's case, the physician was nonjudgmental, collecting the evidence required. She at no time decided that it was her role to determine whether or not Sue's story was true. Her role was to collect and record evidence so that any criminal charge would not fail because of inadequate medical or forensic evidence (Stewart, 1978). Unfortunately, not all victims of sexual assault are seen by physicians who view their role in this light. In one medical journal, the following quote was found: "Using commonsense and clinical experience, the doctor may well be able to make some preliminary estimate as to the truthfulness of her story" (Knight, 1976). It must be stressed again that rape is a legal term and is not a medical diagnosis. The attitude presented here can only be damaging to the woman. In stressing the need for having a chaperone during the physical examination, the author of the same article states, "As many complaints of sexual assaults are fabrications, there is the added danger that a female who will offer such spurious accusations will also be more ready to accuse the doctor of some impropriety, making the presence of a chaperone all the more vital" (Knight, 1976). The attitudes are clear — women lie about rape, and they easily accuse men. These stereotypical and negative views, when held by physicians and some nurses in whose care the woman must place herself, can be tremendously damaging. Re-education of physicians and other health care workers who share these views is essential.

Prevention of Unwanted Pregnancy and Sexually Transmitted Disease.   Following the actual physical exam, the physician or nurse should discuss with the patient any treatment that is recommended. Some hospitals routinely prescribe antibiotics and tetanus injections to all victims of alleged sexual assaults. If there is a chance of pregnancy, the patient may be offered a postcoital contraceptive," a menstrual extraction, an abortion, or postcoital IUD insertion. The last of these is contraindicated if the victim was pregnant at the time of the assault (Goldstein, 1978; Sredl, 1979; Welch, 1979). Protection against sexually transmitted disease is often prescribed prophylactically regardless of the method of contraception utilized. The patient may receive penicillin (or an alternative treatment for those allergic to penicillin). She will then be instructed to return for a follow-up serologic test for syphilis in six weeks.

Provisions for Follow-up Care.   Before Sue left the hospital, Marge, the nurse, told her that she would be in contact with her the next day and at intervals for the next several months. While this is ideal, it is not always possible. If such contact is not possible, the need for a specific person, usually one from a rape crisis center, is of even greater importance (Clark, 1976; Goldstein, 1978).

Sue was given a list of resources in her community to help her regain the control she had lost. The list included the rape crisis center that she had refused earlier. Each of the facilities listed was described according to the care given and its goals.

Sue was able to bathe and had a clean set of clothing waiting so that she could leave the hospital in a more dignified and controlled way. Her living arrangements, at least for the night, were taken care of before she left the emergency room. If her sister had not been available, the nurse should have been aware of some safehouses that were available for women in Sue's situation (Welch, 1979).

Long-term care of rape victims focuses around their feelings of control and self-esteem. They need to learn that they have the right to control their body and not be violated. They must also develop a new sense and understanding of their own sexuality and power in the world (Zehner, 1980). The groundwork for this has been established for Sue, because of the excellent care and treatment she received in the hospital.

The rape and events immediately after its reporting, including the police interrogation and the medical exam, make up the first of two major crisis periods for victims of sexual assault (NIMH, 1977). The second of these occurs if the attacker is caught and identified. If the patient decides to press charges, she must then endure an often grueling and long legal process. It may be months or even years before the case comes to trial.

Sexual Misuse of Children — Special Diagnostic and Therapeutic Needs

Child sexual misuse, particularly incest, often elicits the most negative reactions from health care professionals. Many cases go unnoticed because of the influence of the strong taboo against incest in our culture. The very idea that a relative, particularly a father, would sexually misuse his daughter is seldom even considered by health care workers. The statistics do not support our desire to deny the existence of child sexual misuse. In fact, the greatest increase in numbers of cases is among child victims.

Any time a child is brought to the hospital to be treated for signs of physical trauma, sexual misuse must be ruled out as well. Assessment of adolescents who are pregnant must include determining the circumstances under which the pregnancy occurred. The nurse may find out that the pregnancy is the result of sexual misuse, or it may become apparent that the adolescent has no idea how pregnancy occurred. Some adolescents need information about the very basics of human anatomy and reproduction.

Children who have been physically or sexually misused in the past are at high risk for repeated misuse. In some cases, the child herself may provoke a repeated misuse in an attempt to master the traumatic event (Brant, 1977). For many nurses and physicians, the idea that the child may have actually approached the adult is especially difficult to accept. It is important to keep in mind that the sexual nature of the event is beyond the understanding of many children. They are generally unsure of the "rightness" or "wrongness" of the event. The child's attempt to work it out in her own mind is a natural and healthy one.

Children whose own parents were sexually misused are at greater risk of suffering sexual misuse from their parents. Of course, the fact that the parent has been sexually misused does not necessarily mean that the behavior will be re-enacted with the child.

Children of single parents have also been found to be more likely to have been sexually misused. It is postulated that the lonely, needy, isolated parent may turn to the children for warmth and closeness. This may lead to inappropriate stimulation for the child (Brant, 1977). Again, this is not to be taken as an absolute, but it must be considered as a possibility to rule out.

In most cases of reported sexual misuse of children, the parent feels generally positive feelings toward the child victim such as: sympathy toward the child, anger toward the attacker, or guilt for not protecting the child sufficiently (NIHM, 1977). Not all feelings are positive, however. Some parents feel that the child has somehow brought disgrace and shame on the family. The anger may be expressed toward the child.

The response of the parents, especially the mother, is of primary importance in the recovery of the child (NIMH, 1977). If the child anticipates a negative response, the misuse may be kept a secret. In cases where the mother tries to defend the offender, the child may feel isolated, vulnerable, guilty, and somehow to blame. The worst problem for the child occurs when the attacker is the father or a close family member.

An interdisciplinary approach has been proposed for treating the family and the child victim of sexual misuse (Brant, 1977). The team may consist of a physician (pediatrician and/or child psychiatrist), a nurse, and a social worker. Others, such as lawyer, gynecologist, and specialist in child protection, should be utilized as consultants. The focus of treatment is on understanding the symptoms of the sexual abuse in terms of the impact on the child's later development and its meaning within the context of the family system. The capacity of the family to provide safety and protection for all of its members must be determined. If the family cannot provide this safety, protective agencies should be notified.

An important step in helping to prevent sexual misuse is to teach children that they do not have to comply with the adult's requests for physical contact (Coleman, 1980). This is particularly important in the prevention of incest.

In treating the families involved in incest, the development of a trusting relationship is essential. The child must know she will be believed and will not be blamed for the sexual relationship that developed. The child will be urged to experience and express her full range of feelings about herself and the offender and other family members, within the safety of the structured therapeutic situation (Zehner, 1980).

The therapeutic team must understand the roles, secrets, and power dynamics that exist in the family. In most cases of incest an estrangement between the mother and daughter almost always precedes the overt act of incest (Herman, 1978). In Herman's study many of the mothers were for some reason unable to carry out their usual roles in the household. Often the daughter took over these roles, seeing their mothers as helpless, frail, and downtrodden victims who were unable to take care of themselves. Hence, when the sexual advance was made, often the daughter did not feel able to go to her mother, and instead took over the mother's roles in all areas, including the sexual one. A situation such as this places a tremendous responsibility on the daughter to keep the family together. She often experiences a sense of isolation and shame, coupled with the feeling that she has the power to destroy the family by divulging her secret of incest (Herman, 1978).

The resolution of cases of incest and sexual misuse of children need not be hopeless. From the very start, nurses must support the family in any way possible. The very fact, for example, that the child has been brought for help can be positively reinforced by the nurse. This first step may be tremendously difficult for the parent. Educating the parent, particularly the mother, of the importance of her or his response is essential to the later readjustment of the child. The nurse can serve as teacher, counselor, and advocate for the child and the family throughout the treatment. Before treatment can be instituted, however, diagnosis is essential.

LEGAL ASPECTS AND THE NURSE

Part of the nurse's job of guiding and informing the patient in the emergency room is to inform her of the legal procedures that will follow, should the patient choose to take legal action against her alleged attacker (Sredl, 1979). It is essential that nurses become aware of the legal requirements and precedents in their state so they can accurately inform their patients.

Occasionally, the nurse may be called in to the trial as an expert witness. In many cases this will not be necessary if the records have been accurately kept and if they are legible. Sometimes, though, the nurse and/or the physician may be required to appear. It is the role of the nurse (or physician) to provide the judge and jury with the facts pertinent to the case. Only the facts should be presented. Speculation on the part of the expert witness may be used to decrease the credibility of the entire testimony, and should be avoided.

As expert witnesses, the nurse and the physician are expected to establish their credibility as such. They are generally instructed in terms of dress and behavior.

For example, the witness is generally advised to avoid eye contact with the plaintiff (the patient) or the legal counsel of the plaintiff. Eye contact should be with the questioner only. It may appear to the judge or jury that expert witnesses are not sure of their testimony if they look to the plaintiff or her lawyer for what may be construed as confirmation. Questions are to be answered as briefly as possible, after allowing a few seconds after the question for the plaintiff's lawyer to object. Finally, the expert witness should not volunteer any information, and should report only what was actually observed.

SUCCESSFUL RESISTING OF SEXUAL ASSAULT

Primary prevention of rape is a difficult issue for all people, especially nurses who routinely work with rape victims. As mentioned earlier, active resistance is not always the appropriate action and may indeed lead to greater harm of the victim. Reports of rapists who began to assault women and did not carry through with the assault tend to have several factors in common that can be discussed in educational programs intended to help women and girls realistically deal with the possibility of rape (Groth, 1979).

First, women who managed to keep their self-control and refused to be intimidated by the attacker tended to not be raped. This makes sense in light of the earlier discussion of the power rape, in which the intent is to intimidate and subjugate the woman. If the victim does not behave in the expected way, the rapist does not receive the satisfaction he desires, and may leave that potential victim for one who is more easily intimidated.

Secondly, women who did not counterattack were more often left alone than those who did fight back. The lack of fighting back in some cases failed to excite the attacker. Recall that overpowering and subjugation is an essential element in most rapes. If the woman did not fight back, she was not following the "script" of the rapist, who may have reacted in some way other than in anger. Most rapists advised women against carrying a weapon unless they were capable and intended to use it. In many cases, if the woman hesitated, the rapist had the opportunity to take the weapon away, and later to use it on the victim. The fact remains that most men are stronger than most women, and it makes sense that unless the weapon is used immediately, chances are good that the attacker will overpower the victim.

Thirdly, some victims said or did something that the rapist reported registered with him and communicated to him that she was a real person and not just an object. The victims of rape are always objectified by the attacker. When she is seen more as a person, the rapist may find that he cannot carry through with the attack.

Finally, some victims talked the attacker out of the attack. In some cases, she may have confronted him with the enormity of the rape, by asking how he would like it if his sister or wife were raped. In other cases, she may have talked about the futility of his efforts, telling him that the rape will not solve his problems or be a satisfying sexual experience. The potential victim may encourage the attacker to talk. This may serve to decrease the chances of attack further, since the victim again will be seen as a person rather than an object.

In teaching women some of the strategies that have been successful in avoidance of rape, nurses must be very careful to avoid leading women to think that these techniques always work. They do not. The safety measures mentioned earlier are also not foolproof. Women should be encouraged to take reasonable safety precautions and should then focus on positive experiences.

When a woman has been raped, it is the role of the nurse to provide supportive care, education, counseling, and advocacy, and to collect evidentiary materials. It is a difficult role for some nurses. If, despite efforts to explore biases and to learn to give care effectively despite them, nurses find that they are unable to give the care needed and required by the victims of sexual assault, these nurses should not be required to work with these patients. Forcing unwilling nurses to work with rape patients will bring negative results for both the nurse and the patient. The positive, supportive nurse will have a significant impact on the patient's ultimate recovery.

References

Bearney, C., and Phillips, M.: "Understanding Patients Charged with Rape." *Dimensions in Health Service,* December, 1978.

Brant, R., and Tisza, V. B.: "The Sexually Abused Child." *American Journal of Orthopsychiatry,* Vol 47, No. 1, January, 1977.

Brownmiller, S.: *Against Our Will: Men, Women, and Rape.* New York, Simon and Schuster, 1975.

Burgess, A. W., and Holstrom, L. L.: "Adaptive Strategies and Recovery from Rape." *American Journal of Psychiatry,* Vol 136, No. 10, October, 1979.

Burgess, A. W., and Laszlo, A. T.: "Courtroom use of Hospital Records in Sexual Assault Cases." *American Journal of Nursing,* January, 1977.

Burgess, L. W., and Holstrom, L. L.: "Rape Trauma Syndrome." *American Journal of Psychiatry,* Vol. 131, No. 9, September, 1974.

Clark, T. P.: "Counseling Victims of Rape." *American Journal of Nursing,* December, 1976.

Coleman, P.: "WOAR's Child Sexual Abuse Program." *WOAR Path.* Vol. 6, No. 4, April, 1980.

Geis, G., and Geis, G.: "Rape Reform. An Appreciative — Critical Review." *Bulletin of the American Academy of Psychiatry and Law,* Vol. VI, No. 3, 1978.

Goldstein, F. L., Schaeffer, J., and Sullivan, R. A.: "Practical Caring for the Victims of Rape." *Patient Care,* October 30, 1978.

Groth, N. A., and Birnbaum, H. J.: *Men Who Rape: The Psychology of the Offender.* New York, Plenum Press, 1979.

Herman, J., and Hirschman, L.: "Incest Between Fathers and Daughters." *Nursing Care,* May, 1978.

Herman, L.: "What's Wrong with Rape Reform Laws?" *Victimology,* Vol. 2, Spring 1977.

Holstrom, L. L., and Burgess, A. W.: "Assessing Trauma in the Rape Victim." *American Journal of Nursing,* Vol. 75, No. 8, August, 1975.

Knight, B.: "Forensic Problems in Practice; Sexual Offenses." *Practitioner,* Vol. 21, August, 1976.

Mahan, L. "The Reality of Rape." *WOAR Path.,* Vol. 6, No. 4, April, 1980.

Masters, W. H., Johnson, V., and Reina, E.: *Human Sexual Inadequacy.* Boston, Little, Brown and Company, 1970.

National Institutes of Mental Health, U.S. Dept. of Health, Education and Welfare, 78–485, 1977.

The Nurses' Association of the American College of Obstetrics and Gynecology (NAACOG): Treating the Sexual Assault Victim. 1979.

Peters, J. J.: "Children Who Are Victims of Sexual Assault and the Psychology of Offenders." *American Journal of Psychotherapy,* Vol. 30, No. 3, July, 1976.

Peters, J. J.: Social, Legal, and Psychosocial Effects of Rape on the Victim. *Pennsylvania Medicine,* February, 1975.

Rada, R. T.: "Alcoholism and Forcible Rape." *American Journal of Nursing,* Vol. 132, No. 4, April, 1975.

Scott, M. S.: "Rape and the Trauma of Inadequate Care," *Nursing Digest,* Vol. 5, Spring, 1977.

Schwartz, M. D., and Clear, T. R.: "Feminism and Rape Law Reform." *Bulletin of the American Academy of Psychiatry and Law,* Vol. VI, No. 3, 1978.

Sredl, D. R., Klenke, C., and Rojkind, M.: Offering the Rape Victim Real Help. *Nursing 79,* July, 1979.

Stewart, L. A., and Deller, C.: Step by Step Management of Female Victims of Sexual Assault. *Australian Family Physician,* Vol. 7, November, 1978.

Subcommittee on Treatment of Victims. Study of Criminal Sexual Assault Advisory Committee, Virginia State Crime Commission: "Hospital Protocol for Treatment of Sexual Assault Victims." *Virginia Nurse,* Vol. 46, Winter, 1978.

Zehner, M.: "Treatment Issues for Incest Victims: Freud vs. Feminism." *WOAR Path.,* Vol. 6, No. 4, April, 1980

Diseases and Sexuality

SEXUALITY IN MEDICAL CONDITIONS

MEDICAL CONDITIONS

by SHEILA GROSSMAN

INTRODUCTION

Purpose

The purpose of this chapter is to acquaint the reader with the sexual fears
and changes experienced by patients who suffer from chronic and acute
medical conditions. It is important for nurses to increase their awareness of
how physical illness can affect one's sexuality. Health care workers tend to

think of potential sexual changes only in patients who have experienced pathological changes of the reproductive organs; problems with nerves and/ or blood vessels which supply the genitourinary area; hormonal imbalances, and/or muscle and bone changes leading to joint stiffness or immobility. However, all illnesses will temporarily or permanently affect the patient's sexuality. Often this change will be in the psychosexual area and will be manifested by a decrease in self-esteem, a feeling of dependency causing a sexual role problem, or a change in self-concept and body image. Other problems, such as sensory changes (blindness, loss of hearing), communication difficulties (stroke), and depression (caused by long-term hospitalization), may further influence an individual's sexual self.

Patient Response to Medical Illness with Regard to Sexuality

All patients will respond differently to their hospitalizations and diagnoses. Obviously one's response will depend on a variety of factors, including length of hospitalization, degree of illness, and possibly physical or psychological limitations that the diagnosis may impose on the individual. The nature of the medical illness will also affect one's response. For example:

Mr. Ryan, a 31-year-old man recently diagnosed with myasthenia gravis, was relieved that he had finally been given a tangible reason for his frequent intermittent periods of lethargy, depression, and fatigue. His friends and family had perceived him to be a neurotic hypochondriac and had continuously complained of his behavior. His wife, with whom he had had an excellent marriage for five years, had not supported him since his physician had initially (over a period of two years) found no cause for his symptoms. Their marriage had almost completely disintegrated, he had lost his position at the factory, and their savings had been completely depleted nearly six months ago. He felt physically unattractive, had no desire for sex, and had lost his self-esteem. One can easily see the changes in Mr. and Mrs. Ryan's sexual life style which were directly influenced by Mr. Ryan's undiagnosed disease. In this instance, the diagnosis actually might be what the Ryans needed to return to their previous way of life. Many times people have great difficulty in adjusting to a medical diagnosis that will affect their sexual functioning and/or general sexuality.

Some individuals will not be able to prepare for their diagnosis, for, without any warning, they will have a sudden heart attack or cardiovascular incident, or will be involved in an automobile accident. Any sexual limitations or changes they will experience as a result of their illness will need a slow adaptation. Partners of the patients will in many cases be a most supportive and advantageous external resource whom the nurse should fully utilize. Often the nurse will need to assist the patient's partner in coping with the sexual changes and fears that their loved one may be experiencing. Some problems will be strictly related to the patient, while others will involve both the patient and partner.

Effect of Medical Condition on Patient's Sexuality

Patients who are experiencing problems such as draining wounds, loss of body control or function, inability to mobilize independently, and feeling too ill to participate in sexual activities will need assistance and guidance from the nurse. Some patients will be adversely affected in terms of their gender identity, independence, ability to communicate with their partner, and/or their sexual functioning as a result of their illness.

Many will be taking medications for hypertension, inflammation, infectious processes, vitamin deficiency, or other conditions. Many of these drugs affect sexual desire by depressing libido, by decreasing sexual response, or by causing impotency. It is important for the nurse to be aware of the patient's medication habits, for they may be a cause for the sexual changes experienced. As a result of their medical problem(s), some patients will need long-term assistance such as oxygen or humidification, urinary catheterization, or hyperalimentation therapy, or they will need supportive devices such as canes, crutches, or walkers. All of these will have some effect on the individual's sexuality. For example: Ms. Smite, a 24-year-old recently divorced woman, is diagnosed with Crohn's disease, which requires her to have a permanent hyperalimentation line inserted. She will no longer be able to eat through her mouth. Even though her medical condition does not involve her reproductive system, the sexual implications in this case are vast. It may be more difficult for Ms. Smite to cope with these sexual ramifications, since she does not have a steady partner.

Stewart (1976, p. 48) identified several problems chronically ill individuals often experience as a result of their disease: "1) decreased sexual potency and capability; 2) stiffness of joints or muscles, tremors and spasms; 3) breathlessness, palpitations, brittleness of bones, and convulsions; 4) paralysis, paresis, and weakness; and 5) mental and emotional changes." Any of these problems can detract from one's sexuality. Individuals may have difficulty expressing their sexual needs but may easily verbalize the other aforementioned problems. Nurses can assist patients by asking them, for example, how their breathlessness affects their sexual performance and/or sexual desire. Nurses can also share experiences reported by previous patients with similar diagnoses with the new patient. Each patient needs clear and appropriate information concerning sexual functioning. Sexual health care needs should be dealt with as all other health care needs.

Nursing Interventions: The Nurse as a Patient Advocate, Educator, and Counselor with Patients Experiencing Medical Problems

Nurses can assume many roles in sexual health care of patients. As an advocate, the nurse must possess sufficient knowledge to answer the patient or partner's sexual questions accurately. Nurses should be aware of their own sexuality but should not impose their values and opinions on their patients. An atmosphere that will allow free patient verbalization should be encouraged by the nurse.

Information concerning drugs, disease-involved anatomy and pathology, and alternative methods of sexual activity should be explained to the patient and partner when appropriate. The nurse can educate the couple to the available community resources that may aid them in adjusting to the patient's illness.

Many individuals diagnosed with a medical disease will recover quickly and without complications. They do, however, need advice and sometimes counseling as to when they should resume their sexual activities. For example, chronic obstructive lung disease patients should have their respiratory treatments prior to sexual activity and arthritics could limber their joints by taking a shower prior to engaging in sex. Some people will not need hospitalization but will be followed on an outpatient basis by their private physician or nurse practitioner. These individuals will also need some guidelines as to when they may resume sexual activities (for example, after they finish their prescribed medications, before or after their x-ray treatments, or only after the splint is removed). Usually people assume that they should not practice their regular sexual activities until they are recovered. In reality, their sexual actions may have no bearing whatsoever on their physical state. Nurses may need to give these individuals permission to engage in sexual relations. The nurse can be a very supportive and significant person for the client with a medical problem that leads to chronic illness. Often these patients and their partners benefit from a close, one-to-one contact with the nurse. If appropriate, the nurse may refer the patient or partner, or both, to a certified sex therapist or psychologist.

COMMON EXAMPLES OF MEDICAL CONDITIONS THAT CAN AFFECT SEXUALITY

The remainder of this chapter concentrates on three medical conditions that can influence sexuality. The first is cardiovascular disease, with specific focus on the myocardial infarction (MI) patient and his or her partner. The MI is an example of a life-threatening disease. The second condition chosen that affects one's sexuality is a chronic disease, diabetes mellitus. The third condition, renal disease, can be an acute or chronic problem. The focus will be on the patient with irreversible kidney disease receiving a kidney transplant or adjusting to hemodialysis. Each condition will be discussed in relation to 1) patient-partner knowledge of the disease in terms of sexual effect and functioning; 2) changes and fears regarding sexual functioning experienced by patients and partners with the condition; and 3) the role of the nurse as patient advocate, educator, and counselor in working with those experiencing these illnesses.

Cardiovascular Disease

Cardiovascular disease is very prominent in the United States. Most Americans will experience some form of hypertension and arteriosclerosis in their lifetime. The majority of people will go undetected and will not knowingly suffer from their disease. Others will experience dyspnea, chest discomfort, headaches, irritability, and the symptoms due to arterial or venous insufficiency.

This section focuses primarily on the sexual aspects of patients who have experienced a myocardial infarction and/or who suffer from coronary artery disease. There are references to patients who use cardiac pacemakers, who have hypertension, who have experienced a cardiovascular incident, and who have undergone open heart surgery for various degrees of occlusive coronary artery disease.

Patient/Partner Knowledge of Coronary Disease

People with diagnoses of hypertension, arterial insufficiency, venous stasis, and mild congestive heart failure usually do not have limitations on their sexual activity. The effect these conditions may have on an individual's sexual functioning would be in the areas of fatigue and possibly restricted activity. A person who is suffering any of these conditions is unlikely to experience sexual changes. Potential sexual changes should be discussed if the disease should progress and cause the person to be at risk of a cerebral vascular incident, myocardial infarction, or more severe cardiac disease. Many individuals with these conditions are treated with antihypertensive agents and diuretics, which are believed to cause a decrease in libido and in some instances may induce impotency. The patient should be periodically asked if he or she is experiencing any changes in sexual desire or performance.

Littleton has stated that males with occlusive artery disease may have difficulty in maintaining an erection because of inadequate arterial flow to the penis (Littleton, 1977, p. 655). This is usually a result of partial obstruction of the hypogastric artery. Surgical intervention is frequently very successful.

Patients who have extremely high, uncontrolled blood pressure should be cautioned to avoid stressful, anxiety-provoking situations. This would include sex-related activities that the client is unfamiliar or uncomfortable with. These clients should be told not to avoid sexual intercourse or any other sexual functions they are comfortable with. However, they should know their activity limitations and should avoid any exercise, including sex, if their cardiac symptoms occur. The physician and nurse should discuss sexual functioning immediately with the individual who has experienced an uncomplicated myocardial infarction. This not only will answer any questions and relieve any doubts the client may have about sexual functioning but will also serve to reinforce the fact that the individual is getting well and is expected to return to regular activities. A discussion of sexual functioning with patients who have complications from MI can begin either when the person requests information or when his or her condition stabilizes. For patients who have experienced a myocardial infarction, a general policy is that "sexual activity is allowed when the individual can climb two flights of stairs without difficulty" (Littleton, 1977). AASECT (1979) equates this stair-climbing activity with the activity level of sexual intercourse. Vemireddi (1978) agrees with this equivalency of oxygen expenditure during stair-climbing and coitus. He further suggests a time frame of 8 to 12 weeks postinfarction for resumption of sexual activity for a person who has an uncomplicated MI. This is confirmed throughout the literature. Historically, it was felt that the person experiencing a heart attack needed from three to six months for convalescence without sexual activity (Kolodny, 1979).

Vemireddi (1978) further recommended that post-myocardial infarction patients with longstanding, severe hypertension avoid excessive exertion and indicated a more conservative method of resuming sexual intercourse. Labitz

(1975) stated that a person with a heart attack who experiences complications should not begin resumption of sexual activities until 16 weeks postinfarction.

Many researchers have noted the higher incidence of sudden death during extramarital sexual activity. This is probably due more to the anxiety of a new sex partner than to performing the act itself; however, more research in this area is needed. Ueno (1963), the Japanese pathologist, found that intercourse accounts for less than 1 per cent of all sudden deaths. It has been suggested that patients discuss their needs and past sexual habits with health care professionals in order to allow the individual to participate in devising a plan for resumption of sexual functioning. Patients who are more physically fit can usually participate in sexual activities earlier than those who are unfit.

Changes and Fears Regarding Sexual Functioning Experienced by Patient or Partner Following Myocardial Infarction

AASECT (1979) estimated that "eighty per cent of acute myocardial infarction patients under the age of 65 return to a normal schedule of activity within a period of two to four months." Several studies have indicated that the majority of individuals do not receive very extensive guidelines regarding resumption of normal sexual activities following myocardial infarction or any cardiac event. Many studies involving post-myocardial infarction patients indicate that there is a change in many people's sexual functioning. These changes may be due to physiological factors such as decreased oxygen to the myocardium and/or to psychological conditions such as anxiety, fear, or anger.

The literature indicates there is a significant chance that males will develop impotence and a decreased sexual response after myocardial infarction. Although studies do not reflect women's sexual response following myocardial infarction, one would tend to suspect this to be true for them also. Severe vascular diseases can physiologically affect potency, but usually the impotence experienced following myocardial infarction is of a psychological nature. For example, Littleton (1977) states that fear of a heart attack by either the involved person or the partner may cause performance difficulty or may impinge on the enjoyment of the sexual activity.

Males especially may have difficulty dealing with the role changes that usually result from decreased activity and independence limitations during the convalescent period. This whole phenomenon of role change may cause males to fear a loss of gender identity, causing a decrease in self-esteem, which, in turn, can affect their sexual functioning. One's premyocardial infarction sexual relations or sexual desires will greatly influence one's post-myocardial infarction sexual activities.

If patients or partners are extremely fearful, or if the health care provider is skeptical regarding the patient's ability to tolerate the different levels of exercise required in sexual activities, it is advisable to perform stress testing in a supervised cardiac rehabilitation laboratory. Information on the response of the heart to sexual activity can also be collected if the patient wears a Holter electrocardiograph monitoring device in the home during the actual sexual activity. This device will provide tangible proof to the patient and partner that the heart is capable of withstanding the strain imposed by the couple's sexual activities.

There has been some controversy concerning positioning for sexual relations regarding which position assumed by the post-coronary person will allow less energy expenditure (Green, 1979). AASECT (1979) found blood pressure and pulse measurements of post-myocardial infarction patients collected in both the top and bottom positions during sexual intercourse to be within similar ranges. It is currently felt that there is no reason for the post-coronary person to change his or her usual position unless fatigue becomes an interrupting factor. The new, unfamiliar position may cause more stress than assistance to the patient or partner.

Patients with cardiac pacemakers should have no problem with sexual functioning as a result of the pacemaker if the patient and partner understand the purpose and function of the pacemaker. Often this couple needs reassurance regarding the effectiveness of the pacer. There have been people who have, in their words, completely ignored their sexual desires and needs in order "not to tax the pacemaker." After discussion with some of these individuals, it was found that they were more concerned with the thought "we are living on borrowed time and I do not want to waste any of it" than with the assumed thought that they did not trust the efficiency of the machine. It is imperative that the physician or the nurse educate the patient and partner regarding any misconceptions they may have so they can make an educated decision as to the resumption of their sexual activities. The functioning and method of testing for functioning of the pacemaker should be completely explained to the individual and partner to promote better understanding and acceptance of the pacer as part of the individual.

Nursing Interventions with the Patient and Partner Following Myocardial Infarction

Usually the patient who is experiencing his or her initial myocardial infarction has not had the opportunity to prepare for it, since in most cases it happens without warning. The nurse needs to assess the patient thoroughly and to collect data regarding sexual activities and physical exercise habits preceding the myocardial infarction. It is common for most nurses in the Coronary Care Unit to utilize standing orders regarding the major portion of a post-myocardial infarction patient's care. However, the patient's and his or her partner's sexual aspects of care need to be individualized. The information collected can be utilized to help them plan alternative methods of sexual gratification to be utilized until the patient is capable of resuming sexual intercourse. Once a workable plan has been discussed and understood by both patient and partner, the nurse must focus on the patient's present psycho-sexual needs. For example, all coronary patients in an intensive care unit need to be oriented to the equipment they are surrounded by and, for some, dependent on. The nurse must realize that the majority of patients will feel very dependent on these machines and on the nurses and doctors who have been providing 24 hour care to them. This dependency can greatly influence their self-esteem and can damage their self-image.

Nurses should be cognizant of 1) the physiological impact of a myocardial infarction on one's sexuality; 2) the effects of various drugs (antihypertensive agents, antidepressants, tranquilizers, and sedatives) on one's sexual response; and 3) the psychosexual impact a cardiac crisis can inflict on a person and his or her sexual partner. The University of New Mexico College of Medicine and Nursing initiated a sex counseling/education program that provided sessions for both the patient and the partner. They also developed guidelines of precautions for post-coronary patients, which they taught the patients to follow. The guidelines include 1) *awareness of signs of heart strain* (rapid heart rate and respiratory rate persisting 20 to 30 minutes post-intercourse, palpitations that persist 15 minutes post-intercourse, chest discomfort during or post-intercourse, and/or extreme fatigue on the day following intercourse) and 2) *suggestions for avoidance of sexual activities* (immediately after a large meal or alcohol ingestion, during extreme cold or hot temperatures, close to an anxiety-provoking setting or a stressful situation, and before or after strenuous activity) (Puksta, 1977).

Nurses need to review these guidelines with their patients so the patients will be able to notify their health care providers of the presence or absence of heart strain. Most of the time medications can relieve these symptoms. It is of utmost importance for patients to recognize their limitations and problems so appropriate therapy can be instituted to attempt to correct them. At the same time, patients should be made to feel comfortable about and not fear resuming their sexual activities.

There are many resources available to coronary patients. The American Heart Association sponsors screening clinics and many other activities, and also offers educational pamphlets and films. There are support groups such as the Heart-to-Heart group and the Mended Hearts. Most large medical centers have cardiac rehabilitation units. Nurses need to be aware of their patients' needs and, together with patients' physicians, make appropriate referrals to these resources.

Nurses must assist their patients in regaining confidence and wholeness after a cardiac crisis. As already discussed, the psychosexual impact of a heart attack can be very stressful to some individuals. Kolodny (1979) lists the following common sexual concerns that a post-myocardial infarction patient experiences: "1) fear that the excitement and exertion of sexual activity will lead to sudden death; 2) fear that medical advice will preclude sexual activity or will greatly change the nature of participation in a sexual relationship; 3) fear that a heart attack will create physical difficulty in sexual functioning; 4) concern that a heart attack is a warning of the aging process and, therefore, signals an impending deterioration of sexual activity; and 5) concern that excitement and orgasm may precipitate another infarction." Nurses and physicians must take the time to offer support to their patients regarding such fears and worries. Some patients and/or partners will need follow-up counseling on a long-term basis.

Sometimes people will not disclose their concerns or fears regarding changes in their roles and resumption of their sexual activities. The nurse, given his or her close contact with the patient, is in a good position to discuss with either the patient or the partner or both some of the concerns other patients may have expressed. This technique affords an opportunity for the patient and partner to voice their own fears and thoughts.

Diabetes Mellitus

There are approximately ten million people in the United States alone who suffer from diabetes mellitus (AASECT, 1979). Countless others experience symptoms of hypoglycemia and hyperglycemia but do not connect them with this disease and, thus, go undetected. Still others do not manifest any symptoms although their body is undergoing pathological changes. The next section focuses on aspects of sexual functioning with regard to this disease.

Patient and Partner Knowledge of Diabetes Mellitus

There is an abundance of literature on the diabetic's therapy of activity, diet, medication, and hygiene pointing to a more positive prognosis for those with diabetes mellitus. There is little information on the sexual aspects of the diabetic and his or her partner. Perhaps this is due to diabetics and health care professionals focusing most of their concern on learning to control the disease. The majority of diabetics that the writer has worked with have not reported any sexual changes, nor have they voiced any expectation to experience any. Often myths are circulated concerning possible side effects (including sexual changes) that result from certain diseases. This does not appear to be true for diabetes mellitus. It is, therefore, quite important for nurses to be knowledgeable of the types of sexual changes that can directly result from diabetes mellitus.

For example, diabetics and their partners who are interested in having children have a need for information concerning potential problems the diabetic may have with reproduction. Diabetic women should be aware they are more prone to complications during pregnancy and at delivery than nondiabetics. If women are knowledgeable of these potential dangers and if they seek good antepartum health care they will be less likely to experience serious problems as a result of their diabetes.

In some instances the diabetic male may experience retrograde ejaculation (ejaculation into the bladder), which would necessitate the utilization of artificial insemination if he and his partner desired a child. There have been no documented problems with fertility for the diabetic female.

The potential problems of male impotence and female orgasmic dysfunction for the diabetic have been identified. However, it is believed they should not be overemphasized with patients and their partners, unless there are symptoms present or unanswered questions voiced. The rationale behind this is that sometimes individuals who have a preconceived idea that they will develop a sexual problem will in time actually begin to experience it. It is extremely important that the male or female diabetic who presents with these problems be thoroughly assessed, and if the symptoms are pathophysiological in nature that the patient receive confirmation of this. It is vital to determine the etiology of the sexual problem before the correct therapy can be started.

Changes and Fears Regarding Sexual Functioning Experienced by Patients and Partners after the Onset of Diabetes Mellitus

Initially people with diabetes mellitus do not experience pathophysiological sexual dysfunction with the exception of those whose sexual difficulty leads to the diagnosis of diabetes mellitus. Twenty to 30 per cent of diabetic males are impotent, and by the time the male reaches 50 to 60 years of age there is a 50 per cent chance of impotence (AASECT, 1979). Usually the change occurs gradually over a period of six months to two years and generally the impotence occurs within 10 years after the disease is present (AASECT, 1979). The impotence is believed to be a "result of impaired transfer of the nervous impulse which leads to penile artery dilatation" (Jones, 1978). This problem with the autonomic nervous system seems to override the hypothesized hormonal relationship to impotence in diabetes mellitus. Ellenburg (1971) studied plasma testosterone levels of 45 impotent diabetics and found all measurements within normal range. He supports the theory that impotence is primarily due to neuropathic changes caused by the disease process of diabetes mellitus. The decreased vascularity to tissues that occurs in most diabetics should also be considered a factor leading to impotence.

Although female diabetics have not been studied in as much detail as males, some sexual dysfunction experienced more by diabetic females than by nondiabetic females has been identified. Diabetic females experienced a significantly greater incidence of secondary orgasmic dysfunction than a matched group of nondiabetic females (AASECT, 1979). Kolodny (1971) defined this orgasmic dysfunction as "where impaired sexual response is felt to be due to an organic basis and when the women had been orgasmic previously." In this study, 35 per cent of 125 diabetic females were nonorgasmic as compared with 6 per cent of a group of 100 nondiabetic women. This manifestation in diabetic women is thought to be evident from six months to one year after the onset of diabetes mellitus. Ellenburg (1977) studied female diabetics further with the purpose of assessing their sexuality in general. He found that such complications of diabetes mellitus as blindness, nephropathy, peripheral vascular disease, and angina had no measurable effect on the woman's sexual performance. He prefaced these findings with a limitation of his descriptive study, which is that the data were obtained strictly from the responses of the participants and did not include any objective measurements. His conclusions regarding his opinion on the diabetic male/ female differences in changed sexual function were most interesting. He stated that the difference in severity of sexual dysfunction experienced by diabetic males and females may revolve upon the male sex drive being primarily physical, whereas the female sex drive has a greater psychological basis. He felt that this biological consideration may partially account for the greater sexual changes experienced by some male diabetics.

It is most significant to realize that not all diabetic males encounter impotence nor do all diabetic females experience decreased orgasmic response. Most diabetics do not have a physiologically induced change in their libido. However, it would be reasonable to believe that diabetics who experience frequent periods of glucose-insulin imbalance may be fatigued and have a decreased sexual desire.

Nursing Interventions with the Diabetic Patient and His or Her Partner

The nurse should assist patients in finding any underlying causes for their sexual difficulty. In this way, appropriate counseling or therapy can be instituted. Often diabetics who have advanced disease may have little desire for sexual self-gratification. They may be more interested in trying to fulfill their partner's needs. The nurse can help by facilitating opportunities for the patient and partner to discuss their needs and possibly foster improved patient-partner communication.

The nurse can help the adolescent patient to realize that he or she is "not so different from the others" by having individual or group therapy sessions, or both. The nurse may also utilize the adolescent diabetic's family to aid in supporting their child through the more difficult teen years. Often the family will need to be counseled regarding methods of helping their son or daughter or brother or sister to establish self-dependence, to cope with body image changes due to the diabetes, and to develop a healthy self-image. All of these components may indirectly or directly produce problems in coping with the adolescent's emerging and developing sexuality.

The nurse can discuss with patients and their partners methods to decrease fatigue and improve physical appearance and ways to balance insulin and food intake in order to maintain control of diabetes and a generalized level of wellness; and, if appropriate, can explain the pathophysiology responsible for the sexual dysfunction. In some instances patients or partners may request information on educational resources for diabetics. It may be beneficial to review these pamphlets and/or audiovisual aids with the patient and partner rather than to just distribute them or refer the patient to them. Often patients will have questions regarding some of the general inferences they have drawn about sexuality that may need clarification from the nurse. The pamphlets can also serve as a reference point for the patient and may assist him or her in verbalizing questions to the nurse.

The nurse may counsel diabetics and their partners if there is a physical or psychological problem concerning sexual functioning. If a diabetic woman is experiencing orgasmic dysfunction, this problem needs to be discussed first with respect to how the woman feels about this, and then with respect to how the woman's partner feels about it. After this initial discussion, alternative methods of sexual pleasure should be discussed.

Often it is the impotent male's desire to satisfy his partner that causes him the most frustration. In this situation, the patient may benefit from a penile implant. The inflatable penile prosthesis, although more expensive and more prone to mechanical problems than the semirigid prosthesis, does have the capability of being controlled by the wearer. There is a squeeze bulb on the scrotum which the patient can utilize when he wants an erection. Some of the semirigid prostheses, such as the Small-Carrion implant, have the disadvantage of being rigid at all times. Patients should be told to expect some discomfort at the penis initially. A thorough discussion is necessary prior to the surgery. The patient should realize that if there was no ejaculation prior to the operation, there will be none postoperatively. If no genitourinary problem exists, the patient may be a good candidate for the inflatable penile prosthesis or the semirigid penile prosthesis. Usually patients are able to resume sexual activities four weeks postoperatively.

Nurses do need to raise the consciousness of their patients to afford them a greater ability to identify their sexual needs. Suppressing one's needs is usually more destructive than admitting them. The nurse can be very helpful in helping the individual and partner to identify internal coping mechanisms and also in acquainting them with external resources.

Renal Disease

This section focuses on the person whose diagnosis is end stage renal disease (ESRD). This includes any individual with irreversible kidney disease requiring dialysis or a kidney transplant in order to maintain life.

Lancaster (1979) stated that in the United States alone there are approximately 38,000 patients receiving maintenance dialysis and/or who are preparing for kidney transplantation. He anticipated an increase in patients requiring dialysis in the future and suggested that by 1980 there could be 10,000 to 20,000 more patients undergoing dialysis.

The primary medical problem of many dialysis patients may not have been renal disease. The original primary disease or the treatments given for this disease may have temporarily or permanently damaged the kidneys of these patients. This section deals with areas of concern regarding sexuality resulting from the loss of renal function.

Patient/Partner Knowledge of Renal Disease Necessitating Hemodialysis or Transplant

The loss of renal function, or uremia, causes the patient to retain nitrogenous substances in the blood system. This uremic syndrome results in nausea, vomiting, anorexia, jaundice, weight loss, headache, fatigue, dry, irritating skin, hypertension, tachycardia, very scanty to no urine output, and, if not treated, coma and eventually death. It is certainly understandable why uremic patients feel uncomfortable, irritable, and lethargic. Since the renal disease process is usually slow in progressing, these individuals may experience minor changes in their sexual response and/or functioning prior to being diagnosed. Depending on the etiology of the renal dysfunction (i.e., congenital, trauma-induced, side effect of medical treatment, acquired disease, infection), renal patients will react in a variety of ways to the diagnosis of irreversible renal dysfunction. Since the majority of these individuals will experience hemodialysis rather than kidney transplant, the acknowledgment of the ESRD diagnosis and its ramifications will be a turning point for most individuals and their families. Those who are potential candidates for kidney transplant will undergo periodic dialysis until a suitable donor can be located, and this can be a very long process.

For those who have been chronically debilitated by their disease process, it may be a relief to utilize dialysis, but for most people it is rather difficult to accept the fact that their lives will be temporarily or permanently dependent on a machine. This dependency may induce various feelings regarding one's self-concept, gender identity, and body image. Factors such as age, occupation, presence of supportive family/friends, overall physical health, potential for kidney transplant in the future, and financial situation, to list a few, will greatly affect one's sexuality and ability to adjust to dialysis.

Reichsman and Levy (1972) have studied hemodialysis patients and have identified three stages through which individuals pass during the course of their maintenance therapy. Knowledge of these stages can assist the nurse in assessing his or her patients' adaptation to dialysis and ability to cope. The first stage begins about three weeks after onset of treatment and is called the honeymoon phase. It usually lasts from six weeks to six months and is characterized by improved physical health and feelings of joy and hope. Approximately three to 12 months after onset of therapy and following the honeymoon phase, the second phase called the period of disenchantment and discouragement begins. At this time the individual usually feels hopeless and dejected. Frequently it occurs as a result of experiencing a stressful event such as planning for returning to work, moving to another location, or being unable to perform some type of activity at which the individual was successful before dialysis. The final stage is the period of long-term adaptation and, according to the individual's ability to utilize his or her external and internal resources, usually indicates an acceptance of one's new life and of the dialysis therapy.

It is important to appreciate the intense adjustment that the dialysis patient and his or her partner must go through. It is this emotional adjustment that can greatly affect one's feelings about resuming sexual intercourse and even feeling "good" about oneself. Most patients experience a temporary decrease in sexual excitement and performance as a result of this process of adjustment. In all likelihood, being aware of what to expect psychologically and physically will be helpful to both the patient and partner.

For instance, most uremic females will be amenorrheic; however, their menstrual periods usually will return after dialysis has begun. Patients who are aware of this will not feel that they are hemorrhaging when their period reappears. It is also important for these patients to realize that they may become pregnant now that their menstrual cycle has returned. Both male and female dialysis patients usually have no dialysis related difficulty with fertility. It should be explained to young men who are on dialysis or who receive transplants during puberty that they may become impotent (Levy, 1974).

The pathological vascular and neurological changes that occur with renal disease and that may physiologically impair sexual functioning are usually reversed once dialysis or transplant corrects the renal problem. It is really a combination of psychological and physical factors that may cause sexual problems. Levy and associates (1974) studied 345 men and 174 women who had had a renal transplant or were on dialysis. These researchers sent a questionnaire directly to the patients' homes and asked them to report about their sexual functioning prior to developing uremia, after developing uremia but prior to therapy, and at present. Fifty-six per cent of the respondents were on home dialysis, 21 per cent went to dialysis more than once a week, 6 per cent went once a week, and 17 per cent had received transplants. Their findings reflected no difference in frequency of sexual intercourse between males and females in the three types of hemodialysis regimens. However, males reported a significant decrease in frequency of sex from before they were uremic to the present. Females did not experience this decrease in sexual activity but rather remained the same. It is of interest that frequency of dialysis does not seem to affect sexual activity. More research is needed in the area of changes in sexual functioning following transplantation and during dialysis to confirm these results and to obtain new information.

Changes and Fears Regarding Sexual Functioning Experience by the Patient Requiring Hemodialysis or Transplant and His or Her Partner

Most researchers (Lancaster, 1979; Anger, 1975; Hekelman and Ostendarp, 1979; Levy, 1974; and others) cited renal patient reports of a deterioration in sexual activity. The main change regarding sexual functioning experience by dialysis patients seems to relate to the psychological adjustment to being dependent on a machine. There could be some physiological problem with erection or sexual arousal due to vascular or neuropathic damage from the disease causing the renal failure; however, the dialysis treatment is not responsible for any physical detrimental effect. For the posttransplant patient there also are no negative physiological changes to expect. Usually after a kidney transplant the patient's sexual functioning is restored to the prerenal disease status.

Most patients who receive dialysis treatments will gradually become stronger and less fatigued. This strength, in itself, can help to increase the patient's sexual response. Partners of these patients need to be aware that the individual may experience emotional changes due to the treatments and that the previously mentioned fatigue will not disappear immediately. Even though impotence or other sexual dysfunctions are not considered an effect of the therapy, patients should still be questioned about this in case they are experiencing problems.

Dialysis patients can experience many fears regarding their sexual functioning. Some patients have expressed fears such as "The machine will remove hormones which are necessary for good sex"; "I do not feel like a real man any longer since my penis doesn't work properly"; "I'm afraid the machine is not working correctly and the poisons are building up in me. I really don't want to give them to my wife, so I don't want to have sexual intercourse any more." All of these fears are real to the patient and/or partner who perceives them to be founded on fact but are due to a lack of knowledge of anatomy, physiology, and/or the mechanics of the machine.

It is common for male and female patients to masturbate during dialysis treatments. The activity may help them to feel more confident in themselves, may help them to forget their problems, or may be a means to communicate their need for sex. This latter reason is usually manifested by very overt behavior and should be identified by the nurse. The patients should be confronted and asked about it, thus affording an opportunity for the patient to feel that he or she can openly talk about their sexual needs.

Renal transplant patients can resume sexual relations from four to six weeks after surgery as long as there are no complications. Patients should be aware that there are no limitations regarding positioning or frequency of intercourse. They should be given instructions regarding the identification of symptoms that may indicate a kidney infection.

Although one might imagine the transplant patient to adjust better than the dialysis patient, this is not always true. For example:

Miss Unger, a 28-year-old with severe cystic kidneys, has been receiving hemodialysis therapy for the last three years. She teaches elementary school, lives with her parents, and goes out frequently with her fiance and friends. She is well adjusted to her dialysis and is hopeful the "right" kidney donor will eventually be located.

Finally she is notified that the proper donor has been found, and surgery is scheduled for that same week. After the transplant Miss Unger does very well physically and experiences no rejection or com-plications. However, she returns to her home with great fear and apprehension. Her parents and fiance recognize the changes exhibited by her and insist that she return to the hospital for follow-up. Miss Unger relates her primary fears that she could get a kidney infection from her husband-to-be; that she would be unable to have a child; and that she could not trust the new kidney to work properly. After much discussion she admits that she is scared of not having her dialysis treatments but equally scared of having to resume them if this kidney fails.

This is one example of a patient's experiences and serves to illustrate the importance of giving accurate information regarding sexual functioning to post-transplant patients and also of treating each patient as an individual.

Nursing Intervention with the Patient Who Requires Hemodialysis or Transplant and His or Her Partner

Perhaps the most important area of patient teaching regarding sexuality that the nurse can perform for dialysis patients is explaining the basic anatomy and physiology of the kidneys and their relationship to the reproductive system. Second to this would be thorough instructions and opportunities for return demonstrations by the patient and/or partner of the working of the dialysis machine. Many patients have dialysis at home and in order for the patient to feel in control of the situation and less dependent on the machine he or she needs to understand how the machine works.

If the patient is experiencing sexual dysfunction and has questions about positioning, frequency of sexual activities, drug effects, or other problems, the nurse should be able to answer them or obtain an answer from another resource.

Sometimes dialysis patients and transplant patients benefit from meeting other people with the same condition. Hickman (1977) conducted twice a week seminar discussion periods about sexual adjustment for all adult home dialysis patients and their partners. Her objectives for the program were 1) to create an environment of openness, acceptance, and support; 2) to identify common concerns relating to human sexuality; and 3) to identify the effects on sexual functioning of dialysis and the drugs commonly used in renal disease. The patients participating in the discussions found them very helpful. Others have had group meetings for patients at dialysis centers while they were being dialyzed. Nurses can utilize these meetings as informal teaching sessions and as support group get togethers. Periodically the groups could meet to discuss their needs; usually, however, a structured meeting has been found most effective.

Many authors have stressed the importance of including the partner of the patient in all teaching and counseling sessions. In order to best evaluate a sexual problem, it is necesary for the nurse to have as much information as possible, and this would include the partner's opinions. Sometimes with home dialysis patients, a visit by the nurse into the home is needed in order to accurately assess the patient's situation. A patient who complains of not having interest in sexual activities or of inability to perform with his or her partner may be unaware that the presence of the dialysis machine in the bedroom may be affecting his or her sexuality. Perhaps the patient would feel more comfortable and confident and be more successful with sexual activities if he or she engaged in sexual actions only after dialysis treatments. It takes an objective and accurate observer, such as the nurse, to help patients and their partners to adjust or to make referrals to sex therapists. The nurse must realize that it is not only the individual who has recently started on dialysis who may need assistance in coping. Often it is those who have been experiencing dialysis for a while who need help or support in re-establishing their sexual activities.

The reader might review the next chapter on surgical conditions for some general nursing interventions regarding the return to sexual activity of the patient and partner following transplant surgery. Often the kidney donor is a relative of the patient, and the partner may feel excluded since he or she has not been able to donate a kidney to their loved one. The nurse can be helpful in this situation by educating the person regarding the body's reception capabilities, by listening to the person's ideas, and by attempting to ease any feelings of guilt that may be present. The nurse can introduce transplant patients and partners to others with similar situations and could start support groups.

As mentioned previously in this text, a person's sexuality is not only the person's physical sexual actions; it emanates from her or him in a variety of ways. Both the patient who is dependent upon a dialysis machine and his or her partner can benefit from the sensitivity and empathy of nurses to their position. The nurse must actively pursue his or her instincts regarding patients' or partners' needs.

CONCLUSION

Information that patients and their partners may be interested in having about the effects of illness on their sexuality has been discussed in relation to general medical conditions. Three examples of these conditions, cardiovascular disease, diabetes mellitus, and renal disease, have been specifically focused upon. Some of the fears and changes regarding sexual function anticipated and/or experienced by previous diabetic, cardiac, and dialysis and transplant patients have been discussed. It is hoped that this information will assist nurses in recognizing the sexual health care needs of medical patients and their partners. Implications for nurses in the areas of advocacy, education, and counseling have also been suggested.

SEXUALITY AND THE SPINAL CORD INJURED (SCI) PATIENT

by JANIE WEINBERG

INTRODUCTION

Paralyzed patients have difficult physical and psychological problems to face during and after their rehabilitation. Their physical losses may initially seem insurmountable. With time and rehabilitation, losses are seen more realistically, and patients begin to see themselves as people with capabilities, rather than as people who have suffered tremendous losses. Psychologically, SCI people must face their own beliefs and the beliefs of their families that sexual function has been completely lost (Singh, 1975). Since most spinal cord injuries occur in males from 15 to 30 years of age, viewing the sex life as over condemns most SCI people to lifelong celibacy (AASECT, 1979).

Some form of sexual expression is possible for and is the right of everyone, regardless of disability (Parkinson, 1980). While it is true that for most SCI patients intercourse either is not a possibility or will be greatly changed as the result of loss of sensation, the genitals are not the only body area that can be sexually excited. Certainly, intercourse is not the only means of sexual expression.

Sexuality is often one of the major concerns of SCI people. The person asking about sexuality deserves a careful appraisal of his or her potentials, and a thorough discussion of the possibilities available. A great deal of the success of education and counseling will depend on the character and personality of the spinal cord injured person prior to the injury (AASECT, 1979).

In attempts to integrate sexuality and sexual functioning into the lives of SCI patients, some counselors perpetuate the notion that the only satisfaction that physically disabled people can obtain from sexual relationships is the pleasure they receive from satisfying their partners. This is particularly evident in literature concerning sexuality and SCI women. Much is said about their ability to have "normal" intercourse. It is assumed that they take the passive role, disabled or able-bodied; the fact that they will no longer have genital sensation is often not addressed. SCI women are led to believe that their satisfaction must come solely from the pleasure their partners experience. While some individuals may gain tremendous satisfaction from pleasing their partners, instructing people that this is their *only* sexual pleasure would probably lead to a feeling of being left out. Generally, the SCI person would probably lose interest in sex. Receiving sexual pleasure is possible and necessary for all individuals. SCI people and their partners learn new ways to give and receive pleasure through their bodies and the bodies of their sexual partners. The goal of sexual counseling and sexual rehabilitation of SCI patients is pleasure for *both* partners. The greatest pleasure is found in making the most of what the individual has and not focusing on the functions that may be lacking (Source Book for the Disabled, 1979).

SPINAL CORD INJURY AND SEXUAL RESPONSE

Cervical spine injury is the most commonly encountered spinal cord injury. The functional problems encountered with these injuries are the most devastating. A complete severing of the cord (a complete lesion) results in quadriplegia-paralysis of the lower extremities and trunk, with varying degrees of paresis or paralysis of the upper extremities, depending on the level of the injury. Often level of injury is used as a descriptive phrase to indicate the level of functioning present in a given patient. While the level is a general base for describing and predicting function, it is not absolute, since cord damage may occur above or below the level of the injury. Because of this, two patients with the same injury level may demonstrate different capabilities (Singh, 1975). With this individual variability in mind, the reader is advised to review the chart included at the end of this section for a brief review of the functioning generally encountered in individuals with complete spinal cord lesions.

Male Sexual Response. Following SCI there is no change in the libidinal drive. That is, the sex drive remains intact. Because the main nerve routes to the external genitalia in both men and women occur at the S2-S4 level, practically all complete lesions will result in decreased sensory input in the genital regions. The man will not feel that he is being stimulated. This decreased sensory input seems to lead to a change in the arousal pattern of many men in which secondary erogenous zones develop.

Erection is generally possible for quadriplegics. The reflex arch is located at the L2 level and remains intact in the quadriplegic. People with injuries below the cervical levels generally do not experience reflexogenic erections from tactile stimulation. SCI men do not experience subjective feelings of sexual arousal from tactile stimulation or from the resulting erection. The caretaker should be aware that the reflex erection will occur following any stimulation of the inner thighs or the penis. Reflexogenic erections are common during catheterization and bathing and do not indicate sexual arousal. In fact, most men will be totally unaware of the erection (unless they happen to see the erection or the sometimes flustered activity of the caretaker). Should reflex erection occur and should the patient notice this, the nurse should assure him that this is common and may be a positive sign of some of the sexual options that he will have.

Many men report the presence of "phantom orgasm" or feelings of voluptuousness and sexual satisfaction subjectively similar to the sensation of orgasm, even though the stimulation of the new erogenous areas does not produce genital responses (AASECT, 1979; Marquette, 1981; Parkinson, 1980). The new orgasm is different, but is qualitatively reported to be as good as orgasm prior to the injury (Marquette, 1981).

Ejaculation rarely occurs in spinal cord injured man. Should the man ejaculate, it would usually be an uncoordinated ejaculation which is often retrograde (ejaculation into the bladder rather than out the urethra) (Marquette, 1981). Retrograde ejaculation seems to be most common in cases where the erection is reflex rather than psychogenic.

Female Sexual Response.   As in men, there is no change in the libidinal drive of SCI women. The decreased genital sensation may also change the arousal pattern of the woman leading to the development of secondary erogenous zones above the level of the injury. Reflex lubrication and engorgement of the genitalia occurs in many women who are quadriplegics. There may be a decreased amount of lubrication, requiring the use of a lubricant such as KY-jelly or some other form of lubricant. Vaseline should not be used, since it is not water soluble and tends to deteriorate rubber. This is especially important for SCI women, who will generally be using a catheter. If the catheter is indwelling, and if the couple decides to have intercourse with the device in place, additional lubrication may be needed. (The catheter will be taped, usually on the woman's thigh or hip.) Phantom orgasm or paraorgasm is also reported by spinal cord injured women. (Liberto, 1981).

Problems Encountered in Sexual Expression of SCI People.   Bowel and bladder incontinence, autonomic dysreflexia (hyperreflexia), and spasticity may be encountered during sexual excitement. None of these problems is insurmountable, but they should be discussed in order to prevent their occurrence whenever possible.

Autonomic dysreflexia is a pathological reflex condition that is characterized by exaggerated autonomic responses to stimuli. The spinal cord, no longer "connected" to the brain, continues to generate massive responses to stimuli which are no longer inhibited by the brain's higher control (Luckman, 1980; Task Force on Concerns of Physically Disabled Women, 1978). Symptoms of hyperreflexia include severe hypertension (as high as 300/160); severe throbbing headaches; profuse diaphoresis (sweating); flushing of the skin above the level of the injury; nasal stuffiness; blurred vision; nausea; and bradycardia (Luckman, 1980). Often a distended bladder or bowel will start the response. Sexual arousal during intercourse or masturbation may also cause hyperreflexia. Generally, once the source is eliminated, the symptoms subside (Luckman, 1980; Parkinson, 1980; Task Force on Concerns of Physically Disabled Women, 1978). If the symptoms do not disappear, medications such as hydralzine (Apresoline) may be necessary to decrease the blood pressure. If the bladder or bowel is emptied prior to sexual activity, the incidence of autonomic hyperreflexia is decreased.

In addition to preventing autonomic hyperreflexia, emptying the bowel and bladder prior to sexual activity decreases the risk of incontinence during sexual excitement. In some cases, following the return of reflex arcs (after spinal shock ends) reflexive emptying of the bladder may occur. If the bladder is empty when sexual activity begins, the risk of incontinence is reduced.

Some spinal cord injured people choose to have their indwelling catheter remain in place during sexual activity. For the man, the catheter can be doubled back over the erect penis and enclosed in a condom. The vagina can accommodate this enlarged penis should intercourse be desired. Some additional lubrication may be necessary. For women with indwelling catheters, the tube can be taped to the abdomen or the thigh during sexual activity (AASECT, 1979).

Spasticity may be another problem encountered by disabled people who wish to have sexual relationships. Spasms may be triggered by many stimuli, including anger, apprehension, crying, laughing, tickling, stroking, pinching, and emotionally upsetting or tense situations (Luckman, 1980). Should increased spasticity occur during lovemaking activities, the partner or the disabled person may be able to decrease the spasticity by exerting gentle pressure on the affected limb (Szasz, 1979). There are times, though, that this maneuver may not be successful. Partners should be informed of this and helped to develop a realistic attitude about the possibility of increased spasticity.

Disabled people operate with definite performance expectations, much as able bodied people do. If they dwell on their loss of ability, they tend to become depressed and further withdrawn from social situations (Diamond, 1974). In rehabilitation efforts, genital sex is usually not stressed for SCI patients. A great deal of supportive counseling and permission giving is necessary to help the SCI individual feel comfortable experimenting sexually. The only appropriate criteria for performance lie in the desires and ability of the couple or individual involved.

Sex cannot be as spontaneous for the disabled person as it can for the able bodied. The disabled person may need help getting into bed, getting undressed, removing or taping urinary apparatuses, and washing of genitals (Smith, 1975). Needing this help requires more planning prior to intercourse than is necessary for able bodied couples. Often, the sexual partner can incorporate into the sex play the activities necessary for sexual activity to take place.

FERTILITY AND CONTRACEPTION

Fertility in males who are SCI is severely compromised, with fertility rates generally between 1 and 10 per cent (AASECT, 1979; Eisenberg, 1976; Marquette, 1981; Melnyk, 1979; Parkinson, 1980). SCI men with incomplete and lower cord lesions are the most likely to be fertile. Four main reasons for this low fertility are:
1. Lack of erection or sustained erection and inability to ejaculate
2. Uncoordination of ejaculations causing retrograde ejaculation
3. Damage to the temperature regulation mechanism of the body leading to reduced sperm count.
4. Repeated urinary tract infections leading to scar tissue formation on the urethra

Women are much more likely to retain their fertility following SCI. After a period of amenorrhea of six months to one year, the woman's menstrual cycle and ovulation generally resume (AASECT, 1979; Melnyk, 1979; Murta, 1980; Parkinson, 1980).

Because of their fertility, part of the sexual rehabilitation that SCI women require is counseling on contraceptive methods, including how the woman's disability will affect her choice of methods and how pregnancy would affect her. Many SCI women can and do have children and are excellent parents. In addition to discussing her disability in terms of contraception, the role of her partner in contraception must also be discussed, since it can have an effect on the method chosen (Task Force on Concerns of Physically Disabled Women, 1978).

Birth control pills may be considered to be absolutely contraindicated because of the danger of thrombophlebitis. The SCI woman is at greater risk of this and will probably not be aware of the warning signs of thrombus formation such as severe leg, arm, or abdominal pains. She may also fail to notice reddened areas (Melnyk, 1979; Parkinson, 1980; Source Book for the Disabled, 1979; Task Force on Concerns of Physically Disabled Women, 1978).

Intrauterine devices (IUD) are sometimes thought to be the best choice for a SCI woman since the insertion is not painful, and since there is no requirement to do anything that may not be possible for the disabled woman. The difficulty with the IUD for SCI women is the fact that the woman will not be able to feel early signs of pelvic inflammatory disease (Melnyk, 1970, Parkinson, 1980; Source Book for the Disabled, 1979). Some signs that the woman *may* notice and can be taught to look for that may indicate difficulty with the IUD are: spotting, irregular periods, increased spasticity, fever, or increased or changed vaginal discharge (Task Force on Concerns of Physically Disabled Women, 1978).

Foam and condoms are a highly effective method of contraception. Their use in SCI women requires a manual dexterity that the woman may lack. If the partner is willing and able to apply the condom and insert the foam, this method can be successfully utilized. Women who have intercourse with their indwelling catheter in place may not find this to be a good method, however, since the catheter may tear the condom (Source Book for the Disabled, 1979).

The diaphragm presents some problems for the SCI woman. First, dexterity is required to insert the diaphragm. A willing partner could be taught to do this. The diaphragm may not remain in place because of weak pelvic muscles. Finally, if the woman empties her bladder by the Credé method (putting pressure on the abdomen to empty the bladder), the diaphragm may be dislodged (Source Book for the Disabled, 1979).

In discussing sexual activity with SCI women, the nurse should not stress contraception to the point that the patient feels that intercourse is her only option for sexual expression. Intercourse is only one method available to her.

Pelvic examination and Pap smears are still part of the normal health care of the SCI woman. The pelvic exam may be difficult to accomplish in the normal lithotomy position, since the woman will not be able to hold her legs in the stirrups. The stimulation of the exam may also cause spasms. If this occurs, the examiner must have a helper on each side of the patient to ensure that she does not fall from the table. A side-lying position in which the patient's upper foot is placed on the examiner's shoulder may be the best alternative for positioning for the pelvic exam (Task Force on Concerns of Physically Disabled Women, 1980).

Jim was an active, happy 17-year-old high school student when one year ago he was involved in a motorcycle accident that left him paralyzed from the upper chest down. His spinal cord was completely severed at the C-6 level. Jim was hospitalized for six months following the injury. Because his home is far away from the rehabilitation center, and because his parents felt that they could not be with him at the rehabilitation center, it was decided that Jim would receive the education for his return home from the physical therapy department at the local community hospital. Despite his C-6 level, Jim is now able to transfer from the wheelchair to the bed with the help of a transfer board. He uses an electric wheelchair, and can feed himself. He does need to have meat cut for him. Jim sleeps in a hospital bed. He is able to dress himself completely except for putting on his shoes and socks. Luckily, Jim's house is a ranch style house, requiring very few modifications for his new requirements. Jim has not returned to school to finish his final year of high school, although he reportedly would like to do this.

As the year has progressed, it has become more apparent to Jim and to his parents that he now needs the kind of rehabilitation that only professionals in the field can offer. It is decided that Jim will go to the rehabilitation center. His parents will visit as often as possible, and will keep in contact with him by telephone. The trip to the center is a difficult one for Jim, who fears that his dependency will not be accepted by the staff.

When Jim arrives at the rehabilitation center, he is greeted by Claudia, the nurse who will be his primary nurse for the duration of his stay. She takes a history, including sexual history, and finds that Jim was sexually active prior to his injury, but that his girl friend left him shortly after the accident. Jim states that he didn't blame her for wanting someone who could be a "real man" with her. Further discussion leads to Jim's statement that he feels he will never find a woman to love and to marry. He feels that this is no longer an option for him. He reports that he is most interested in going back to school so that he can begin to prepare for a career.

As time goes on, Jim begins to feel more confident of his abilities to get through school, but he seems to be more restless generally. Claudia, the nurse, finds that Jim is beginning to make subtle references to sex and past sexual behaviors. One day he asks her if she ever "made it" with a quadriplegic. Claudia responds by acknowledging that sex seems to be more important for Jim of late. She tells him that she would like to discuss his sexual potential with him, but that although she is most interested in him as a person, their relationship is and will remain a professional one. Claudia and Jim then begin some individual counseling dealing primarily with education about sexuality. In addition to the fact that Jim had received no sexual information following his injury, Claudia discovers that his knowledge of sexuality is severely limited. After Jim and Claudia have been discussing sexuality for some time, Claudia suggests that Jim sit in on one of the group sessions that the rehab unit has twice a week. Jim is at first reluctant but agrees. By the time Jim leaves the rehabilitation unit, he feels more confident in himself as an individual, and is beginning to view himself in terms of his capabilities, rather than his disabilities. He plans to actively seek out new friendships and is looking forward to trying out his newfound sexual knowledge.

DISCUSSING SEXUALITY WITH THE SPINAL CORD INJURED PERSON

Studies have shown that the degree of sexual adjustment and functioning of adults with SCI is directly related to their success in vocational training and employment (Berkman, 1978; Conine, 1979). By meeting the individual's needs to discuss sexual concerns, the nurse contributes greatly to the reestablishment or the establishment of general feelings of self-worth in the SCI patient (Diamond, 1975). If SCI individuals feel that they are sexually inadequate, they may feel even more alienated from society and more likely to see themselves as members of a deviant subculture (Smith, 1975).

Despite studies emphasizing the importance of sexual counseling and guidance, many SCI patients receive little or no sexual counseling during or after their rehabilitation. The health team is generally focused on getting the patient back in society in a job functioning as independently as possible (Diamond, 1974). Often, they have not thought of the importance of sexuality. The patient may have feelings that any interest or effort that does not focus directly on the disability and the rehabilitation should be considered minor.

Anxiety on the part of the professionals dealing with the SCI patient is another explanation for the lack of sexual information given to SCI patients.

The professionals may avoid the topic or convey to the patient that the topic is unacceptable. Some patients are not viewed as potentially sexual by the professionals working to rehabilitate them (Bardach, 1978).

Some patients may sense the discomfort of the staff about sexuality. They may turn to a person who is not a professional or who is not knowledgeable in the field with their questioning. For example, the SCI patient who has developed a rapport with one of the nursing assistants may very well ask the person sexual questions. Awareness of this has led to training programs for all people dealing with SCI patients.

In the case study, the role of the parents in the sexual education of the SCI adolescent arises. Often parents of disabled children avoid the topic of sexuality (Task Force on Concerns of Physically Disabled Women, 1978). Often the parents lack the information to give. In addition, they may wish to protect their child, fearing that he or she will be exploited sexually because of the disability. They may wish to spare the child the rejection they see as inevitable. In a wish to avoid the fact that no one will want to marry their child, the entire subject of sex may be avoided. Still other parents may assume that the child has learned or will learn sexual information related to the disability somewhere else, such as during hospitalization. Finally, the parent of the disabled teenager may find it difficult to see his or her child as a sexual person, much as parents of able-bodied children have this difficulty.

NURSING INTERVENTIONS IN SCI PATIENTS

Discussing sexuality and sexual functioning is generally more acceptable now than it has been in the past. Owing to medical and technical advances, more SCI people now survive than ever before. The need for sexual rehabilitation is generally recognized. Often nursing has taken on this role.

The question of when to initiate discussions and teaching about sexuality is a difficult one to answer. Certainly, when the injury is new enough that there is still concern for that patient's survival, sexuality will not be an appropriately discussed topic. Often, though, by the time the staff feels that the time is "right" the patient has already begun to think about sexual functioning (Bardach, 1978; Cole, 1975).

One indication that a patient is thinking about sexual activity and that the time may be "right" to discuss it may be when the patient makes a pass at or in other ways discusses sexuality with the nurse (Parkinson, 1980). As in other cases in which a patient may behave inappropriately sexually, the nurse must keep in mind that the patient needs to view himself or herself as a sexual person. The "acting out" may be an acknowledgement of the patient's need to be seen as a sexual person. Regardless of the motivation, reprimands are not appropriate. In Jim's case, Claudia correctly interpreted his advances as a signal that Jim was ready to discuss his future sexuality.

Not all patients will behave so blatantly when they wish to discuss sexuality. Indeed, some patients may never bring up the topic at all. If it is addressed, however, it is often the nurse who will be asked. This is easily understood when one considers the high degree of intimate contact that the nurse has already had with the SCI patient during routine care. If the patient perceives that the nurse is a caring and open individual, and if the care is of high quality, approaching the nurse is a natural thing for the patient to do.

Often patients will enter a rehabilitation center after they are no longer acutely ill. At this time they should be informed that sexual rehabilitation is a part of the overall rehabilitation program. The inclusion of sexual histories as part of the intake history reinforces this (Bardach, 1978; Luckman, 1980). By informing patients that their sexual concerns will be addressed, the nurses have indicated that sexuality is an acceptable topic, and that they are people with whom patients may discuss such topics. Even if the patients are not ready at that time to attend to their sexuality, the knowledge that the subject will be covered can be comforting (Szasz, 1979).

A fairly common practice in the past was to encourage the SCI patient to "try out" having sexual relations (on weekends home) with his or her partner once before counseling began. This was intended to encourage the patient to experiment with his or her remaining capabilities, and to help the professional determine the functional capacities of the patient. The negative effects of this approach far outweigh its benefits, however. Patients who do not have partners available to them at the time receive the message that they will have to be celibate. They also get the message that sex is a taboo subject with health professionals (Smith, 1975). While it is true that a realistic assessment of the sexual capabilities of a given patient is hard to determine before six weeks after the injury (when spinal shock has subsided), forcing the patient into a stressful situation without the knowledge and support of experts can do much to undermine the precarious confidence the patient may have developed.

THE ROLE OF THE NURSE IN SEXUAL REHABILITATION OF SCI PATIENTS

The following six areas define the role of nurses in sexual health care and rehabilitation of SCI patients (Cole, 1975A; Murta, 1981; Parkinson, 1980; Smith, 1975):

1. To assess the person's fears and feelings about sexuality
2. To encourage the person's efforts to establish human relationships that could lead to sexual relationships
3. To provide practical information to help people develop competence in human sexual expression
4. To facilitate expressions of feelings and concerns in a straightforward manner
5. To convey hope
6. To provide for individual or group counseling as appropriate

Assessing the Person's Fears and Feelings About Sexuality. The initial sexual history forms the basis of the nursing assessment of the person's feelings and fears about sexuality. In addition, the nurse will learn of past sexual activity and attitudes. Often discussion of losses the patient feels will aid the nurse in determining more specific sexual information as well as allow patients to discuss their concerns. Physical, occupational, recreational, and self-image losses should be discussed in addition to sexual losses. Nurses must take care not to project their own concerns or their own perceptions of losses onto patients. Learning what the patient views as losses is an integral part of planning for future teaching.

Discussions of activity and performance prior to and since the injury will provide nurses with additional information about the losses that the patient perceives. Generally, the nurse will also find out whether there is a partner in the picture and may be able to help the patient to assess the likelihood of the relationship's continuing.

The patients' future plans, including those regarding sexual activity, may not agree with the preconceived notions of nurses caring for patients. It is essential for nurses to learn what adjustments the patient feels will be necessary, as well as those that are viewed as more difficult than others.

Basically, for the nurse to assess patients' feelings about sexuality, assessments of their views of themselves and the injury is necessary. With a thorough assessment, the nurse can then begin to plan for the teaching and counseling that the patient will require.

Encouraging the Person's Efforts to Establish Human Relationships that Could Lead to Sexual Relationships.   Many disabled people when asked will report that they are anxious and willing to find sexual partners. On further examination, though, many tend to withdraw from social interactions when they could potentially meet sexual partners. Most often they fear the reactions of others to their disability and withdraw rather than face what they may see as inevitable rejection. Mobility may also be a problem in meeting new people. The SCI individual who does not have an electric wheelchair may have difficulty on slight inclines, for example. Given a relatively barrier-free design, however, the SCI individual with an electric wheelchair will have more independence and therefore more confidence in approaching potential social contacts (Smith, 1975).

Communication is a topic that will be discussed many times, both in the context of establishing relationships that may become sexual and in the context of learning to be recognized as a complete person who happens to be in a wheelchair. Since much of the body language previously utilized will not be possible for the SCI patient, discussion of the use of the face and areas that have function for nonverbal behavior will also be discussed. (Task Force on Concerns of Physically Disabled Women, 1978).

SCI patients must learn that they are still entitled to sexual relationships. While it is appropriate to avoid overemphasizing the importance of sexual functioning at the risk of underplaying the importance of sexuality as a whole, sexual function must be seen as a right of all people, regardless of their disabilities.

Assumptions about the patient's sexuality or sexual preferences are inappropriate and can be damaging to the patient's already tenuous self-esteem. Disabled people, like able bodied people, express their sexuality in different ways (Eisenberg, 1976; Task Force on Concerns of Physically Disabled Women, 1978).

Providing Practical Information to Help People Develop Competence in Human Sexual Expression.   The practical issues and information that the nurse will provide to the SCI patient necessitate that the nurse be comfortable with the area of sexuality. Because the variety of sexual outlets available for SCI patients is more limited than that available to able-bodied individuals, the entire range of sexual expression should be considered according to the capabilities and desires of the patient (Bardach, 1978). No practice that is acceptable to both partners should be overlooked. For example, even in cases where genital sensitivity is lacking, the anal area may retain feeling and be a potential source of sexual pleasure. Oral-genital sex is another sexual option that should be discussed (Source Book on the Disabled, 1979). The nurse's role in providing positive sanctions to sexual experimentation is essential (Smith, 1975).

An important and practical bit of information that may have to be learned by the patient as part of sexual rehabilitation is that the real goal of sexual activity is intimacy — a sense of being close to another human being (AA-SECT, 1979). Noncoital sexual activity can lead to much the same sexual pleasure as was experienced prior to the injury, especially when alternative erogenous zones have been discovered (Task Force on Concerns of Physically Disabled Women, 1980).

Nurses must be aware of the dominant societal attitude that assumes all disabled people are asexual. Patients must learn to be clear to potential partners that they can engage in sexual activity.

After the patient has recovered from spinal shock and the reflex arcs have returned, a realistic assessment of potential sexual function is possible. Following the physical exam, which will include neurological testing, the patient and the nurse should discuss the findings and their relevance for the future sex life of the patient. Genital sex is not usually stressed, since alternatives are generally more satisfying for both partners. The capabilities of genital sex as well as the mechanics required should be discussed.

When the patient is aware of the potentials for sexual expression available, the issue of competence in sexual relationships should be addressed. Partners should be told what feels good, what hurts, what is comfortable, what is pleasurable. Able-bodied people rarely understand how the body of the disabled person works and may need to discuss limitations and strengths. Generally, the disabled person should ask the partner what he or she needs to know about the disability. Waiting for the able-bodied partner to ask, or assuming that the partner knows, can lead to uncomfortable situations. It is the assertive responsibility of disabled people to explain their physical condition to their potential partners and to tell the partners what they can do or think they can do (Source Book for the Disabled, 1979). If potential partners are unwilling or unable to deal with the limitations of a sexual relationship with the disabled person, discussion of this type can determine this before the situation has progressed to the point when both partners will be frustrated and hurt by the lack of understanding.

Facilitation of Expressions of Feelings and Concerns. An important part of helping patients express their feelings is to talk about the issues they want to discuss (Parkinson, 1980). Often nurses lead the discussion to topics they feel are important rather than listening to the patient's concerns. Listening skills are essential in facilitating discussion.

Sometimes nurses will unconsciously make nontherapeutic statements that can be detrimental to the establishment of a trusting relationship. For example, telling a patient, "I admire your courage" or "I don't know how you manage so well, I could never do it," implies heroic qualities that may make the patient feel most uncomfortable (Task Force on Concerns of Physically Disabled Women, 1980). Saying something like "... but all of us have handicaps" is also insulting. Few people face the losses faced by those who are paralyzed. This statement devalues the difficulties faced by the patient and will tend to have a negative effect on future interactions.

Terminology is another important aspect in helping to form a trusting relationship. The term "handicapped" has a very negative connotation for most people. Disabilities are what people have. Handicaps are what other people attribute to disabled people (Parkinson, 1980). The words disabled, paraplegic, and quadriplegic should be used as adjectives rather than nouns. That is, it is better to call someone a quadriplegic man than a quadriplegic. By referring to him as a quadriplegic, the nurse is describing him as *only* a quadriplegic rather than as a man who happens to be quadriplegic.

The SCI person generally will experience the injury and resulting disability as a tremendous loss. The stages of grieving are likely to be encountered and should be accepted by the nurses involved. The anger and bargaining are part of the recovery process. It is not unusual to hear quadriplegic and paraplegic men state that they would rather have their sexual function back than be able to walk again. This is an example of bargaining that may be seen even after the acceptance of the loss has occurred.

Conveying Hope.   The situation for a SCI person in terms of sexuality and general function is not bleak. Without being overly optimistic, nurses can help the SCI person to learn that life will still offer pleasures and joys, despite their disability. Nurses' outlooks should be realistic, avoiding false hopes or overly pessimistic predictions (Sovensen, 1980).

Providing for Individual or Group Counseling.   Generally, the initial counseling that SCI patients receive regarding sexuality is individual. Some patients are too shy to benefit from group counseling, which has been found to be very beneficial for SCI patients, who hear that they are not alone. They are able to hear of the successes and failures of others and receive a great deal of support. Most people tend to receive the greatest benefit from group counseling if it is not begun until they have been injured from three to six months. An awareness of the nature and consequences of the injury, initiation of physical therapy, and the development of concrete rehabilitation goals may be necessary prerequisites for successful group participation (Bardach, 1978; Eisenberg, 1976; Melnyk, 1979). Individual counseling can and should begin as early in the rehabilitation process as possible.

SUMMARY

The role of the nurse in the sexual rehabilitation of SCI patients is a complex and demanding one. The six components discussed may need to be reviewed or repeated often as the patient progresses to acceptance and understanding of new possibilities of sexual expression. Nurses have the information necessary and can serve as teachers, counselors, and advocates to patients who are generally still viewed by the majority of our society as asexual.

References

AASECT: *Sex Education, Counseling, and Therapy for the Physically Handicapped.* Washington D.C., The American Association of Sex Educators, Counselors, and Therapists, 1979.

Anger, Diane: The Psychologic Stress of Chronic Renal Failure and Long-term Hemodialysis. *Nursing Clinics of North America,* 10:449–460, 1975.

Bardach, Joan L.: "Sexuality in the Disabled: Some Current Work: Clinical, Training, and Research Aspects." *Bulletin of the New York Academy of Medicine,* Vol. 54, No. 5, May, 1978.

Cole, C., Sevin, E., Whittley, J., and Young, S.: Brief Counseling During Cardiac Rehabilitation. *Heart and Lung,* 8:124–129, 1979.

Cole, Theodore M.: "Reaction of the Rehabilitation Team to Patients with Sexual Problems." *Archives of Physical Medicine and Rehabilitation,* Vol. 56, 1975a.

Cole, Theodore, M.: "Spinal Cord Injury Patients and Sexual Dysfunction." *Archives of Physical Medicine and Rehabilitation,* Vol. 56, 1975b.

Conine, Tali, Disher, Catherine, Gilmore, Susan, Fischer, Bette A. and Perry,:

"Physical Therapists' Knowledge of Sexuality of Adults with Spinal Cord Injury." *Physical Therapy*, Vol. 59, No. 4, April, 1979.

Cromwell, V., Huey, R., Korn, R., Weiss, J., and Woodley, R.: "Understanding the Needs of Your Coronary Bypass Patient." *Nursing 80, 10*:34–41, 1980.

Cummings, J.: "Hemodialysis — Feelings, Facts, Fantasies." *American Journal of Nursing, 70*:70–76, 1970.

D'Afflitti, Judith, and Swanson, Donna: "Group Sessions for the Wives of Home Hemodialysis Patients." *American Journal of Nursing, 75*:633–635, 1975.

De-Nour, A. K.: "Hemodialysis: Sexual Functioning." *Medical Aspects of Human Sexuality, 19*:229–235, 1978.

Diamond, Milton: "Sexuality and the Handicapped." *Rehabilitation Literature,* Vol. 35, 1974.

Eisenberg, M. G., and Rustad, L. C.: "Sex Education and Counseling Program on Spinal Cord Injury Service." *Archives of Physical Medicine and Rehabilitation,* Vol. 57, March, 1976.

Ellenberg, M.: "Impotence in Diabetes Mellitus: A Neurologic Rather Than an Endocrinologic Problem." *Medical Aspects of Human Sexuality, 1*:12–20, 1973.

Ellenberg, M.: "Impotence in Diabetes: The Neurologic Factor." *Annals of Internal Medicine, 75*:213–219, 1971.

Ellenberg, M.: "Sexual Aspects of the Female Diabetic." *The Mount Sinai Journal of Medicine, 44*:495–500, 1977.

Ellenberg, M.: "Sexual Function in Diabetic Patients." *Annals of Internal Medicine, 92*:331–333, 1980.

Ellenberg, M.: "Effect of Respiratory Difficulties on Sexual Function." *MA of HS.* April, 1980.

Furlow, W.: "Patient-Partner Satisfaction Levels with the Inflatable Penile Prosthesis." *Journal of American Medical Association, 243*:1714, 1980.

Green, R. (ed.): *Human Sexuality: A Health Practitioner's Test,* 2nd ed., Baltimore, The Williams & Wilkins Co., 1979.

Griffith, G. "Sexuality and the Cardiac Patient." *Heart and Lung, 2*:70–73, 1973.

Hekelman, Francine, and Ostendarp, Carol: *Nephrology Nursing: Perspectives of Care.* New York, McGraw-Hill Book Co., 1979.

Hellerstein, H., and Friedman, E.: "Sexual Activity and the Post-Coronary Patient." *Archives of Internal Medicine 125*:987–999, 1970.

Hott, Jacqueline: "Sex and the Heart Patient: A Nursing View." *Topics in Clinical Nursing, 1*:75–84, 1980.

Hickman, B.: "All about Sex...Despite Dialysis." *American Journal of Nursing, 77*:606–607, 1977.

Jones, Dorothy A., Dunbar Claire F., and Jirovec, Mary M.: *Medical-Surgical Nursing.* New York, McGraw-Hill Book Company, 1978.

Kinsman, Robert, Jones, Nelson, Matus, Irwin, and Schum, Robert: "Patient Variables Supporting Chronic Illness." *The Journal of Nervous and Mental Disease, 163*:159–165, 1976.

Kolodny, R.: "Sexual Dysfunction in Diabetic Females." *The Journal of the American Diabetes Association, 20*:557–559, 1971.

Kolodny, R., Masters, W., Johnson, V., and Biggs, M.: *Textbook of Human Sexuality for Nurses.* Boston, Little, Brown and Company, 1979.

Labitz, P.: "Sexual Concomitants of Disease and Illness." *Postgraduate Medicine, 58*:103–111, 1975.

Lancaster, Larry (ed.): *The Patient with End Stage Renal Disease.* New York, John Wiley & Sons, 1979.

Levy, Norman (ed.): *Living or Dying: Adaptation to Hemodialysis.* Springfield, Ill., C. C Thomas, 1974.

Levy, N.: "The Psychology and Care of the Maintenance Hemodialysis Patient." *Heart and Lung,* May/June, 1973, pp. 400–405.

Liberto, Lana: "Sexuality and the Spinal Cord Injured Female" Seminar in Human Sexuality (Unpublished). Thomas Jefferson University, May, 1981.

Littleton, V.: "The Surgical Patient's Sexuality." *Association of Operating Room Nurses' Journal, 26*:649–658, 1977.

Luckman, Joan, and Sorensen, Karen: *Medical-Surgical Nursing.* Philadelphia, W. B. Saunders Co., 1980.

MacRae, I., and Henderson, G.: "Sexuality and Irreversible Health Limitations." *Nursing Clinics of North America, 10*:587–597, 1975.

McLane, M., Krop, H., and Mehta, J.: "Psychosexual Adjustment and Counseling after Myocardial Infarction." *Annals of Internal Medicine, 92*:514–519, 1980.

Marquette, Carl: "Sexuality and the Spinal Cord Injured Male." Seminar in Human Sexuality (Unpublished). Thomas Jefferson University, May, 1981.

Melnyk, Roger, Montgomery, Robert, and Over, Ray: "Attitude Change Following a Sexual Counseling Program for Spinal Cord Injured Persons." *Archives of Physical Medicine and Rehabilitation,* Vol. 60, December, 1979.

Meyer, J., ed.: *Clinical Management of Sexual Disorders.* Baltimore, Williams & Wilkins Co., 1976.

Mims, F., and Swenson, M.: *Sexuality: A Nursing Perspective.* New York, McGraw-Hill Book Company, 1980.

Murta, Adelaide C.: "Sexuality and the Spinal Cord Injured." Unpublished manuscript, 1981.

Owens, J., et al.: "Cardiac Rehabilitation: A Patient Education Program." *Nursing Research, 27*:148–150, 1978.

Page, L.: "Advising Hypertensive Patients About Sex." *Medical Aspects of Human Sexuality,* Jan., 1975, pp. 103–104.

Papadopoulos, C., et al.: "Sexual Concerns and Needs of the Post-Coronary Patient's Wife." *Archives of Internal Medicine, 140*:38–41, 1980.

Parkinson, Margaret Helen, Bogle, Jane Elder: "Sexuality." *In* Luckman, Joan, and Sorensen, Karen: *Medical-Surgical Nursing.* Philadelphia, W. B. Saunders Co., 1980.

Parkinson, Margaret Helen, Bogle, Jane Elder: "The Psychology and Care of the Maintenance Hemodialysis Patient." *Heart and Lung, 2*:400–405, 1973.

Puksta, N.: "All About Sex After a Coronary." *American Journal of Nursing, 77*:602–605, 1977.

Reichsman, F., and Levy, N.: "Problems in Adaptation to Maintenance Hemodialysis: A Four Year Study of Twenty-Five Patients." *Archives of Internal Medicine, 130*:859–865, 1972.

Sacerdote, A., et al.: "Sexual Dysfunction in Diabetes Mellitus." *Annals of Internal Medicine, 93*, 147, July, 1980.

Santopietro, Mary: "Meeting the Emotional Needs of Hemodialysis Patients and their Spouses." *American Journal of Nursing, 75*:629–632, 1975.

Satterfield, Sharon: "Sexual Rehabilitation for the Post Coronary Patient." *Topics in Clinical Nursing, 1*:85–89, 1980.

Scalzi, C., and Dracup, K.: "Sexual Counseling of Coronary Patients." *Heart and Lung, 7*:840–845, 1978.

Sexton, Dorothy: *Chronic Obstructive Pulmonary Disease.* St. Louis, The C. V. Mosby Co., 1981.

Singh, Silas P., and Magner, Tom: "Sex and Self: The Spinal Cord Injured." *Rehabilitation Literature,* Vol. 36, No. 1m, 1975.

Small, D.: "A Patient Education Program." *American Journal of Nursing, 78*:889–891, 1978.

Smith, Jim, and Bullough, Bonnie: "Sexuality and the Severely Disabled Person." *American Journal of Nursing,* Vol. 75. No. 12, December, 1975.

Smith, Jim, and Bullough, Bonnie: *The Source Book for the Disabled.* London, Imprint Books Ltd., 1979.

Stein, R.: "The Effects of Exercise Training on Heart Rate During Coitus in the Post Myocardial Infarction Patient." *Circulation, 55*:738–740, 1977.

Stevens, Carolyn: *Special Needs of Long-Term Patients.* Philadelphia, J. B. Lippincott Co., 1974.

Stewart, W.: "Sexual Rehabilitation — a Gap in Provision for the Disabled." *Nursing Mirror,* Feb. 5, 1976, pp. 48–49.

Strauss, Anselm: *Chronic Illness and the Quality of Life.* St. Louis, C. V. Mosby Co., 1975.

Szasz, George: "Sexual Health Care Service to the Physically Handicapped." *AASECT Convention,* Washington, D.C., 1979.

Task Force on Concerns of Physically Disabled Women: *Toward Intimacy: Family Planning and Sexuality Concerns of Physically Disabled Women,* New York, Human Sciences Press, 1980.

Task Force on Concerns of Physically Disabled Women: *Within Reach: Providing Family Planning Services to Physically Disabled Women,* New York, Human Sciences Press, 1978.

Trieschmann, R.: "Coping with a Disability: A Sliding Scale of Goals." *Archives of Physical and Medical Rehabilitation, 55*:556–561, 1974.

Ueno, M.: "The So-called Coition Death." *Japanese Journal of Legal Medicine, 17*:330–340, 1963.

Vemireddi, N.: "Sexual Counseling for Chronically Disabled Patients." *Geriatrics,* July, 1978, pp. 65–69.

Watts, R. J.: "The Physiological Interrelationship Between Depression, Drugs, and Sexuality." *Nursing Forum, 77*:168–183, 1978.

Wood, R., and Rose, K.: "Penile Implants for Impotence." *American Journal of Nursing, 78*:234–238, 1978.

Woods, N. F.: *Human Sexuality in Health and Illness.* 2nd ed., St. Louis, The C. V. Mosby Co., 1979.

13

SURGICAL CONDITIONS

by SHEILA GROSSMAN

INTRODUCTION

The purpose of this chapter is to increase nurses' awareness of the importance of recognizing sexual health care needs of surgical patients and their partners. Nurses must utilize data concerning their patients' sexuality in developing patient care plans if holistic nursing is to be attained. There has been little in the nursing literature concerning the sexuality of surgical patients. This information must be incorporated into surgical-medical texts in the future.

Patient Responses to Surgery with Respect to Sexuality

People respond in different ways to surgery. Some will exhibit anger, having participated in surgery without success; others may express relief, since preoperative symptoms such as pain, polyuria, or headaches have been eliminated; and still others may feel indifferent, having undergone an elective surgery with no sequential side effects. Usually a person's response will be related to the reason surgery was required and the inherent threat. However, factors related to one's sexuality will also affect one's response, and need to be considered either preoperatively or postoperatively, or both. Nurses need to assess patients and their partners regarding the surgery: if it was perceived as mutilating; if it caused changes to the mind or body with regard to sexual functioning; and if there was a resultant loss of self-esteem. Body image encompasses one's perception not only of physical appearance but also of function, sensation, and mobility (McCloskey, 1976). An example cited by Littleton (1977) describes these concepts well:

A young woman experiences extensive oral surgery and then manifests severe depression due to a change in her sexual activity. She and her husband had considered kissing significant, and now, due to the surgery, were unable to resume this sexual expression.

Five problem areas related to sexuality have been identified which the physically handicapped may experience as a result of their situation (AA-SECT, 1975). Included are 1) impaired body image; 2) loss of self-esteem due to dependency on others; 3) difficulty with gender identity and gender role; 4) difficulty with decision-making and responsibility for sexual functioning; and 5) possibility of being the victim of sexual exploitation by others, including health care staff. These can be, in part or in entirety, experienced by patients recovering from surgery, and so can be areas of patient assessment postoperatively.

Effect of Surgery on Patients' Sexuality

The surgical patient may have little psychological energy to expend on sexual concerns. This appears to be especially true preoperatively and shortly after surgery. Caught up in the stress and excitement of the surgery, their partners may experience a similiar effect. However, often partners may not understand the patient's postoperative lethargy, desire to be alone, and unattractive appearance. This behavior may be perceived by the patient's partner as a rejection by the patient. In many situations the nurse can intervene by preparing the partner ahead of time concerning what to expect. A nurse and partner discussion of frequent manifestations exhibited by the ill may assist him or her in relating to the convalescing partner. If the nurse-patient relationship allows, the nurse might also share observations of the patient's behavior and physical appearance with the patient, who may be unaware of this change. Some people may be indifferent to the image they project to their partners, and so nursing intervention should be limited to making them aware of their appearance and to supporting the well partner, who may be feeling isolated.

In planning patient care, nurses need to consider their patients' developmental and chronological age, for surgery may cause acceleration or regression with regard to their sexual functioning. Nurses also need to be aware of the effect that the patient's surgery might have on sexual functioning; of drugs the patient may be taking that alter sexual response; and of the generalized effects that hospitalization can have on one's sexuality. If the patient's surgical intervention and/or related treatments produce changes in vision, hearing, balance, or speech, there is a detrimental effect on his or her sexuality (Littleton, 1977). For example, in caring for an adolescent who has undergone an orthopedic maneuver requiring continuous leg abduction, the nurse should consider the obvious effect this may have on the patient's developing sexuality. Nurses also need to consider the sexual health care needs of patients who undergo the numerous routine surgeries, such as cholecystectomy, hernia repair, and appendectomy, that may not necessitate such an obvious exposure.

All patients have the right to receive information regarding the effect of their surgical procedure on their sexual functioning. Some examples of what to tell a patient follow: 1) most postoperative patients are in a weakened state; 2) resumption of physical activity is gradual and restrictions of activity are enforced; 3) coitus may be difficult or painful initially (after selected procedures); 4) most postoperative patients feel dependent; and 5) depression is very common. Some surgical patients are very concerned about the damage and odor from their wound and also about the extent of scarring that will exist when the surgical incision heals. These fears can affect a person's self-concept and, in turn, sexuality. Prior to discharge, each patient should be told exactly when sexual activity can resume. If relevant, information regarding the integrity of the stitches should also be communicated to prevent possible fears of reopening the incisions. Many people will assume, if nothing is said about resuming their sexual activities, that they should avoid any physical sexual expression. Others may not have questions or concerns regarding sexual activity and limitations until they are at home, where there will be no one to give them this information. To avoid these problems, nurses should give straightforward, non-opinionated information to each of their patients prior to their discharge.

Nursing Interventions with Surgical Problems: The Nurse as a Patient Advocate, Educator, and Counselor

As an advocate for the patient, the nurse can assist in preoperative teaching and in fully informing the patient about the surgery. Preoperatively, the nurse can explain the anatomy and physiology involved in the surgical procedure. Postoperatively, he or she can be instrumental in discussing alternative methods of sexual expression that the patient and partner can engage in until their more accustomed sexual relations can be resumed. As a counselor, the nurse can support the patient and his or her partner by encouraging verbalization and the sharing of coping methods that have been successful for others. The nurse can also introduce the patient and/or partner to a qualified sex therapist if the need arises. Obviously, nurses must be aware of their own attitudes regarding sexual expression, and must not impose them on their patients. It is important to realize that all patients will adjust to the manifestations of their surgeries and that this adjustment will be closely related to their presurgery sex lives.

COMMON, SELECTED SURGICAL PROCEDURES WITH SEXUAL IMPLICATIONS

The remainder of this chapter focuses on common selected surgical procedures, including hysterectomy, prostatectomy, ostomy, and mastectomy. Each procedure will be discussed in terms of the following: 1) patient/partner knowledge of the surgery; 2) changes and fears regarding sexual function experienced by patients and their partners; and 3) the role of the nurse as a patient advocate, educator, and counselor in working with these patients.

Hysterectomy

Gynecological surgery may be ominous to the woman involved and to her partner. Perhaps surgery in the pelvic and genital-rectal areas commands such suspicious respect because of the general lack of awareness or ignorance of what it entails. Current American societal beliefs seem to focus somewhat less on the child-bearing and child-rearing functions of the woman. However, many ethnic groups still have deep-rooted beliefs in the procreative functions as the major role of the female. Also predominant in our society is the strong emphasis on portraying women as sexy, youthful, and attractive. For many couples, reproductive capability is extremely significant. This section deals with these issues with regard to the most common gynecological surgery, the removal of the uterus.

Patient/Partner Knowledge of the Surgery

Physicians, with follow-up reinforcement by the nurse, are responsible for explaining the full ramifications of hysterectomy. In some instances, the woman and her partner may participate in selecting the procedure. For example, in the case of uterine cancer the actual surgery can be less extensive if radiation and/or chemotherapy is used in conjunction with the surgery. This, of course, will depend on the site of the tumor and/or the extent of the metastasis.

Hysterectomy, either vaginal or abdominal, is the removal of the uterus. If the ovaries are removed, the procedure is hysterectomy with oophorectomy. If the woman is being operated on for reasons other than malignancy, she and her partner may have more doubts about the rationale for removing the uterus than will a woman with a cancerous uterus.

Often women will fear that more radical surgery is imminent for them. It is the responsibility of the nurse to insure that the patients and their partners are fully knowledgeable of what organs are to be removed. In addition, both partners need to understand how the surgery will affect their sexual functioning. The importance of full knowledge of the surgery is most significant in avoiding unnecessary stress. For example, a woman may think (possibly because of religious beliefs or ignorance) that since she no longer has a womb she can no longer participate in sexual intercourse. Often people do not know the function of the uterus, and therefore believe that without it intercourse is not possible. Of course, it is the vagina that is necessary for intercourse to occur. This remains intact after the hysterectomy.

There are no significant physiological side effects of sexual functioning as a result of a hysterectomy except the possibility of a slightly shortened vagina if malignancy was involved. Premenopausal women who have their ovaries removed will begin menopause as a result of their surgery, whereas those having just the uterus removed will not. Psychosexual changes may be experienced by either the woman or her partner, or both. Fears of becoming asexual, of being incapable of performing sexually, of being unable to satisfy one's partner, and of becoming more masculine have been experienced.

Changes and Fears Regarding Sexual Function Experienced by Hysterectomy Patients and Their Partners

Women who have experienced vaginal bleeding, abdominal pain, dyspareunia, and/or dysmenorrhea will probably be greatly relieved and may have greater sexual response as a result of the relief of symptoms. Many women do not experience any of the above mentioned symptoms but find they have a cancer following a routine Pap smear. It is perhaps more difficult for these women to adjust to losing their uterus, since they have no pre-existing symptoms and little time to psychologically prepare for surgery.

The removal of the possibility of pregnancy may have either a positive or a negative effect on sexual response. For some, the end of the need for contraception can be of positive value to sexual expression. For others, the inability to become pregnant may serve as a constant reminder of the loss of fertility.

Although many women may be more fearful of the loss of sexual response and femininity after a hysterectomy with oophorectomy, there is no physiological basis for this. Removal of both ovaries stimulates the onset of menopause but does not affect one's femininity, sex drive, or sex enjoyment, because it is the adrenal glands and not the ovaries that produce the androgens, which are the primary libidinal influence (Coope, 1975). Post-oophorectomy women may experience a decrease in vaginal lubrication. Artificial water-soluble lubrications (e.g., KY jelly) or supplemental estrogen therapy can easily remedy this situation.

In one study, in which women were well informed about the nature of their operations, the incidence of sexual dysfunction was less. Approximately 37 per cent experienced decreased sexual function, whereas 34 per cent actually increased sexual function. The remaining 29 per cent detected no change (Dinnerstein, 1977).

Women and their partners should be advised against sexual intercourse for four to six weeks after surgery. This is especially relevant if a vaginal hysterectomy was performed. This prohibition of coitus is done to promote adequate time for tissue healing to occur and to prevent the possibility of infection or hemorrhage.

Nursing Interventions with the Hysterectomy Patient and Her Partner

Nurses as patient advocates have the same role with hysterectomy patients and their partners as they do with any surgical patient. This vital function is to insure that the patient is adequately informed of the consequences of surgery.

The nurse can explain the reasons for avoiding sexual intercourse for four to six weeks after surgery. He or she can discuss alternative methods of sexual expression for the patient to practice for this time interval. A description of the anatomy and physiology of the female reproductive system may be necessary for some women. For women who have undergone oophorectomy, various suggestions can be made for coping with the symptoms of menopause. All posthysterectomy women should be reminded of the importance of and reasons for having a Pap smear performed on a routine basis.

Sometimes nurses limit sexual counseling to women who have undergone radical gynecological procedures, such as pelvic exenteration, vaginectomy, or vulvectomy. Nurses should not overlook the posthysterectomy patient and her partner. Male partners of women who have had malignancies may believe that they will contract cancer, and thus may hesitate to resume sexual intercourse. This is a good illustration of the need for nurses to discuss the ramifications of the hysterectomy with both the patient and her partner. Sometimes problems unrelated to the surgery may arise. The nurse can hold further discussions with the couple or refer them to a counseling program.

If the couple are of child-bearing age and desire to have children, the nurse can advise them about appropriate resources. The woman may feel particularly depressed about her loss of reproductive capacity and will need the nurse's assistance. In some cases the nurse might introduce the woman to a support group so that she may share her feelings with others who are experiencing similiar losses.

Kreuger et al. (1979) studied 108 posthysterectomy women's knowledge of sex functioning, sex attitudes, and sex behavior. More than 75 per cent stated that doctors supplied the majority of their information to them. Half of the participants felt that nurses should provide more information concerning sexual adjustment after the surgery. The researchers recommended more nurse awareness concerning the necessity for discussion of the sexual problems experienced by some posthysterectomy women. Nurses and physicians need to work together to educate and counsel posthysterectomy women and their partners in a manner that individualizes the adjustment of each patient or couple.

Prostatectomy

There is an increased incidence of prostate hyperplasia (excessive build-up of tissue) with increased age. The American Cancer Society lists the prostate as the most common site of cancer in men. Thus, prostatectomy is becoming more necessary as a surgical intervention.

Patient/Partner Knowledge of the Surgery

There are a variety of types of prostatectomies, of which transurethral, suprapubic, retropubic, and radical perineal resection are the most common. The lay and professional literature is ambiguous and in some instances seems to magnify the extent of potential sexual problems that may result from prostatectomy. Investigators (DeBacher et al., 1977) studied the sexual activities, including frequency, desire, and quality of intercourse, of three sample groups of 100 men each. One hundred men had undergone a prostatectomy, 100 had some other type of urological procedure performed, and the remaining 100 men had experienced some type of general surgery. The results concluded that prostatectomy in itself is no more likely to affect sexual functioning than is nephrectomy or gastrectomy (DeBacher et al., 1977).

Impotence usually follows the radical perineal resection procedure, which is frequently used in cases of malignancy. This physiological impotence results from the severing of perineal nerves. If a man undergoing one of the other procedures has a belief that the surgery will cause impotence, it is not unlikely for this to occur. This psychologically produced impotence can be treated and is reversible. Often good preoperative discussion regarding all aspects of the surgery can greatly reduce the individual's fear of impotence. If physiological reasons will lead to impotence, the individual should be made aware of this and not be led to believe the impotence can be reversed.

The common postprostatectomy side effects of bleeding, bladder spasms, dysuria, and occasional incontinence need to be explained to the patient prior to surgery. All of these symptoms can have relevance to one's masculinity. It is not uncommon for patients to awaken postoperatively and grasp out for the involved area only to find a catheter or drain connected to the penis or the incision site. This can produce fear, anxiety, and confusion in the patient regarding his self-wholeness, and therefore should also be accurately discussed preoperatively.

With some prostatectomy procedures, the patient experiences a change in the subjective feeling of ejaculation. In some cases the man may produce less or no ejaculate. This is due to retrograde ejaculation into the bladder, which is harmless and does not decrease sexual sensations. The patient and his partner should be made aware of this change prior to his discharge. Some patients have found this absence of ejaculate very alarming. Their fears alone can lead them to sexual dysfunction.

Changes and Fears Regarding Sexual Function Experienced by Prostatectomy Patients and Their Partners

It is necessary to emphasize that sexual function following prostatectomy will be similar to preprostatectomy function for most patients, unless radical perineal resection is utilized. Those who have had malignancy may fear recurrence, and this will likely decrease their interest in sex. This preoccupation with the unknown may be more detrimental than a tangible physical loss.

Men who had experienced severe urinary discomforts preoperatively may enjoy sexual activity more, having alleviated embarrassing symptoms, such as urinary frequency or hematuria. They may require reassurance and support from their partners in readjusting to their sexual actions. Partners may need added assurance that engaging in sexual intercourse will not hurt the operative site.

The impotent patient does have sexual options. Alternative methods of sexual expression that do not necessitate the use of a penis with erectile capacity should be discussed with both patient and partner. Some people may need permission to practice these other methods of sexual gratification. The nurse can have an important part in this by encouraging patient-partner verbalization and by sharing knowledge of successful methods that other patients have reported in adjusting to this change in sexual functioning.

Some men are good candidates for an inflatable erectile prosthetic implant or for insertion of a bilateral silicone prosthesis along the shaft of the penis. One study (American Medical Systems, Inc., 1978) reported success in restoring sexual function in all 59 postprostatectomy patients receiving inflatable penile prostheses. However, even though physical restoration of the sexual function is achieved, most men and their partners experience some anxiety in adjusting to this. Further study is necessary to provide clarification on the psychosexual ramifications of men and their partners using penile prostheses.

It is important for men to avoid penile stimulation or sexual intercourse for a short period of time, commonly cited as two to four weeks postprostatectomy, in order to prevent hemorrhage or infection.

Nursing Interventions with the Prostatectomy Patient and His Partner

Because there has been so much misinformation disseminated concerning prostatectomy, many choose to suffer unnecessarily rather than to seek medical assistance. The nurse can be instrumental in recommending to men with prostate hyperplasia that they have the disorder corrected. Nurses must be aware of the side effects of prostatectomy so that they can explain them to their patients. The functions of the prostate gland, its anatomical relationship to the rest of the body, and the role that the gland plays in the male's sexual response should be discussed. In some cases it would be advisable for the nurse to teach either the patient or the partner, or both, the testicular examination procedure. This would be especially important for the individual who has had cancer or has a family history of cancer.

As a counselor, the nurse can offer special support, for he or she has probably spent more time with the patient than any other member of the health care team. Hopefully, the nurse-patient relationship will bring about open communication between nurse, patient, and partner. The person with psychologically induced impotence can benefit greatly from continuous support and sincere commitment from the nurse. The nurse may need to refer the patient to a sex counselor or psychologist. The patient's partner must also be encouraged to participate in the counseling.

Although many prostatectomy patients and their partners will not experience any postoperative changes in sexual function, there are a variety of psychosocial and biophysical aspects the nurse should consider in implementing holistic nursing care. Evaluate the following and determine the correct nursing actions:

Mr. Carew, 55 years old, is one day post-transurethral resection. A diagnosis of cancer was made one week prior to his admission and he has now been told that the entire cancer has been removed. His father died of prostate cancer at the age of 65.

He is quiet and asks his nurse to leave him alone since he wants to think over the last week's events. Upon leaving the room, the nurse reminds Mr. Carew to use the call button to reach her if he should need anything or desire to talk.

An hour later, Mrs. Carew comes out of her husband's room crying, and says to the nurse, "He's so sad, he thinks he'll always have that horrible odor; he won't, will he? It has something to do with the cancer, doesn't it? I wonder if we'll ever be like we were before all of this—he should never have had this operation. . . . "

The nurse should first attempt to communicate with Mrs. Carew by answering her questions; then the nurse should discuss the postprostatectomy convalescent period with both Mr. and Mrs. Carew. Both also need to be reinforced by being assured of Mr. Carew's positive prognosis. It is possible that Mr. Carew may need one-to-one counseling concerning his father's death from prostate cancer. The nurse should also check the dressing and catheter site, for the odor is probably due to wound drainage or urine, and could be easily remedied. A dressing change schedule should be instituted and the collected urine should be more frequently emptied. The cause of the odor should be explained to Mr. and Mrs. Carew to make them aware that this is a normal finding following prostatectomy.

Ostomies: Colostomy, Ileostomy, and Urinary Diversions

One hundred and twenty thousand people have ostomies performed on them each year in the United States alone (Wilpizeki, 1981). Few people require ostomies for congenital defects; the majority of ostomy operations are necessitated by disease processes that require removal of part or all of an organ. The term "ostomate" refers to anyone having a stoma. The terms "colostomate," "ileostomate," and "urostomate" will be used when the specific surgery is being discussed. Some individuals will require only a temporary ostomy, while others will need a permanent stoma. Many people and their families will be faced with a diagnosis of cancer, which may further detract from their sense of well-being. The purpose of this section is to increase awareness of sexual perspectives that relate to the colostomate, ileostomate, and patient with a urinary diversion apparatus.

Patient/Partner Knowledge of the Surgery

The majority of people who have undergone ostomy surgery for cancer will be more concerned with survival than with their sexuality. Individuals with ulcerative colitis may focus more on relief of their discomfort and embarrassing symptoms than on possible postoperative effects on their sexual functioning. Nevertheless, a complete, detailed description of the surgical procedure should be explained to the individual and his or her partner.

It is possible in some instances for a person to elect palliative, alternative therapies or less radical procedures rather than to experience a perceived mutilating surgery that may prevent them from being "themselves" ever again. People should have the opportunity to participate in their surgical treatment plan. For example, a pre-colostomy patient may strongly desire to have input in the placement of his or her stoma. This patient participation should be encouraged, for most individuals will adjust more easily if they are a part of the decision-making process that causes the change.

Certainly there should be no surprises postoperatively. Pre-ostomates need to be told if their entire colon and rectum will be removed. Ostomates-to-be should be aware if they will have one or more stomas. People with urinary problems need to know whether the diversion of urine will be internal or external. For example, ureteroenterostomy allows for excretion of urine via the anus, whereas the ileal conduit utilizes a portion of the ileum and attaches ends of the ureters to it, which then allows excretion via an external ileal stoma. The main pre-surgery focus of most ostomates seems to be on changes in body image, with loss of control of self-elimination and with lowered self-esteem. Concern for actual sexual functioning appears to follow surgery when the individual is recovering and planning to return to a regular life style and to the activities of daily living.

In the literature are found some general sexual function altering side effects of these procedures. The method of Dr. Weinstein, as given in the journal *Medical Aspects of Human Sexuality* (1978), explains two common procedures for treatment of rectal cancer. Anterior resection is used for patients who have only partial malignant involvement of the rectum. This surgery certainly has implications affecting one's sexuality with regard to lowered self-esteem and may cause a temporary change in one's sexual activities. For example, the person who enjoys oral-anal sex or anal intercourse may be temporarily drastically affected by his or her surgery. However, there are no permanent physiological side effects that alter sexual function as a result of this procedure. The person having more extensive rectal malignancy will need the abdominoperineal procedure, which necessitates removal of both the rectum and the anus and requires a permanent colostomy. The majority of men having this surgery become impotent because the perineal portion of the procedure irreversibly damages the pudendal nerves. Women who have this procedure can enjoy a normal sex life, however, because the anatomical placement of the female's pudendal nerves differs greatly from that of the male's and the nerves are therefore unaffected by the procedure. Most patients who need a colostomy will suffer from inflammatory bowel disease or an obstruction of the bowel. Many will receive a diagnosis of cancer as the cause of their gastrointestinal difficulties.

Most female colostomates will not have physiological changes involving sexual function. Although male colostomates often become partially or totally impotent as a result of nerve damage, male ileostomates tend to suffer from diseases other than cancer, and usually the procedure does not result in nerve damage (AASECT, 1979).

A urostomy usually has no physiological effect on a woman's sexual functioning. Depending on the procedure utilized, men may experience problems in attaining or maintaining erections, absence of ejaculate, and/or decreased sperm count (AASECT, 1979). Often male urostomates fear impotence if they are unable to excrete urine via the penis.

The patient and partner should be told not only of the physical changes but also of the body image and function changes they will experience. It is important that the patient's partner or some significant other be available throughout the stages of the surgical procedure and be part of the physician-patient-nurse relationship.

Changes and Fears Regarding Sexual Function Experienced by Ostomy Patients and Their Partners

The presence of a stoma will tend to impair the return to sexual functioning of many ostomates and their partners. Many patients have fears that their ostomy devices will leak and also that escaping odors will repulse their partners. Many partners of ostomates have expressed their fear of harming the stoma by close physical contact.

Fear of recurrence of malignancy bothers some individuals so much that they are unable to resume sexual functioning. Others consider their ostomy to be a punishment and refrain from resuming sexual activities for fear of additional problems. Often partners of ostomates will blame the stoma for any sexual problems that develop, and will be unable to identify the real stresses affecting their sexual functioning.

In the female colostomate, or the woman who has had her rectum removed, it is common for some dyspareunia to occur until the perineal wound has completely healed. She should be told to expect this beforehand.

It has been mentioned previously that physiological impotence in men as a result of certain ostomy procedures will greatly alter sexual functioning. It is believed, however, that if patients and partners are included in the decision-making process prior to surgery and are advised of the prognosis, they will be more likely to adjust to the irreversible changes. Another important consideration regarding ostomates' adjustment to changes is the nature of the ostomy. Is it temporary or permanent? Evaluate the following situation and determine how Mr. Spier may have reacted if the physician and nurses had been more truthful from the beginning.

Mr. Spier, 45 years old, is married and enjoys an active sex life. He has never been hospitalized prior to this. His chief complaint is diarrhea with periods of constipation, inability to tolerate his regular diet, and some minor abdominal discomfort. He has had numerous tests, including barium enemas and gastrointestinal x-rays, and his diagnosis is bowel obstruction.

Mr. Spier's physician tells him that his surgery will include a temporary ostomy. Mr. Spier asks, "How long will I need the opening?" The physician replies, "No more than four weeks." Surgery goes well with no complications and Mr. Spier gradually regains his normal level of health. The nurses care for his stoma and change the bags accordingly. They feel there is no need to teach Mr. Spier or his wife, since it is only a temporary situation.

After three weeks, the physician decides to discharge Mr. Spier with the colostomy and tells him he wants Mr. Spier to care for the stoma at home. He explains to his patient that he will follow him through the surgical clinic so he can assess the appropriate time for removal of the external stoma. As time passes, Mr. Spier feels he has been tricked, and thinks that he will never have the additional surgery. He wishes he had not gone along with the original surgery. He spends most of his time feeling sorry for himself. He has lost trust in his wife, physician, and everyone who cared for him during his hospitalization. Mrs. Spier has found her husband intolerable to live with and so just ignores him.

Analysis.   Mr. Spier should have been told initially that his colostomy would probably be temporary but that it would require a long time (approximately eight weeks) before his colon was sufficiently healed to reverse the procedure. He should have participated in his own stoma care and bag changes from the beginning. Mr. and Mrs. Spier have experienced a drastic and possibly irreparable deterioration in their communication. The idea of engaging in sexual activities has probably been far from his thoughts. Everything has been put at a standstill for the Spiers until the reverse surgical procedure is performed. This is an example of how sexual function can be disrupted as an indirect result of the surgery. The next section, on nursing interventions, discusses some actions that the nurse can implement with ostomates and their partners.

Nursing Interventions with Ostomy Patients and Their Partners

As a patient advocate, the nurse can be helpful with patients who are experiencing permanent ostomies by reinforcing information that physicians and/or other nurses have shared with the patient. They can act as a sounding board for both the patient and his or her partner regarding all aspects of the surgery. Often the fears of either the patient or the partner will not be shared with anyone but the nurse, as a result of fear of embarrassment and feelings of not wanting to appear stupid to the physician, or for many other reasons. The nurse, who is available over the longest period of time, is the person with whom the patient and partner usually become closest.

The staff nurse can sometimes act as an intermediary between the patient and the ostomy nurse specialist. Even though the ostomy nurse works more closely with the patient in caring for his or her stoma and bag, he or she may not have the information the staff nurses have collected during their numerous interactions with the patient.

The nurse who is caring for ostomy patients must be interested and motivated toward health teaching. The subject of this chapter is sexual health care only, but there is a wealth of information that can be shared with patients to help them return to a normal life. Much of this information refers to self-control of elimination and prevention of skin breakdown, which indirectly effects the sexual image.

One of the most important aspects of teaching the ostomate and his or her partner is to allow both an opportunity to view the stoma and the drainage. The stoma and bag should not be covered. If the patient and partner can become accustomed to the sight of the stoma and its excretions, adjustment to what the surgery represents can be easier for both.

Many ostomates' partners need to be told that bodily contact cannot harm a stoma. Suggestions of positions for sexual intercourse would perhaps be helpful. If the ostomate can avoid the bottom position, the appliance and stoma may be less in the way. Side-to-side positions might be a good way to begin when both partners feel inhibited, for there will be less emphasis on the stoma or the appliance.

For the ileostomate, a drainage bag or pouch will be necessary at all times, for there is a constant liquid excretion from the small intestine. A routine should be established that would allow emptying of the bag prior to sexual activity. This would prevent any spilling or leaking. If odor is a problem, deodorants can be obtained for the appliance. A method of assessing the appliance for adherence to the stoma should be developed so that it can be checked prior to sexual activity. If controlled bowel function is present, the colostomate may not need to wear a drainage bag. Again, this patient should be taught to regulate himself or herself so that sexual activity can take place at an appropriate time.

The nurse must take a pre-surgery sexual assessment of the ostomate in order to plan counseling postoperatively. The nurse's goal is to form and maintain an objective, empathetic relationship with the patient and partner from the preoperative stage to the patient's discharge. Often patients appear to adjust very well, as do their partners, until they return or attempt to return to their presurgery life style. Each ostomate should have a designated health care professional to contact once he or she returns home. The United Ostomy Association, Inc., Dept. N81, 2001 Beverly Blvd., Los Angeles, Calif. 90057, provides ostomates with free literature that may answer questions or serve as guidelines for the patient. If the client or partner has difficulty adjusting to his or her new style of living, the nurse may need to set up formal counseling meetings on a routine, scheduled basis to assist them in coping with their changes. Sometimes it is necessary for the nurse to refer the person(s) to a sex counselor, psychiatric nurse specialist, or psychologist for assistance.

MASTECTOMY

"At the present rate, one out of every 14 (7%) American women will develop breast cancer at some time in her life" (U.S. Department of Health, Education and Welfare, 1979). Many women are predisposed to breast cancer and have a fear of losing a breast many years prior to actually developing the cancer. More and more women and their partners are having to adjust to living with a mastectomy. Men rarely are afflicted with cancer of the breast, and therefore this section will focus on the woman and her partner with regard to their sexuality.

Text continued on page 300

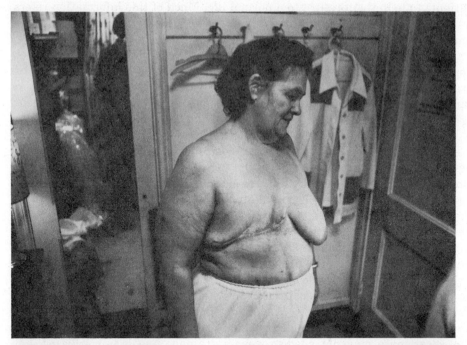

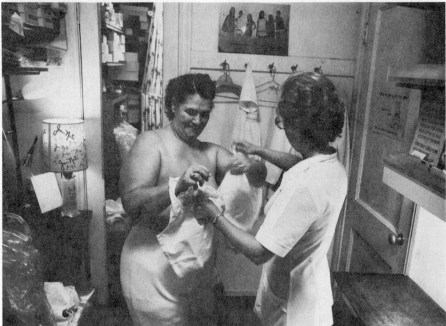

"When I first went back to work, I felt everyone knew that I had something done, whether they did know or not. Everyone was looking at me, watching me to see how things fit. I just knew that everyone else knew."

"Three months
For the feeling
That I could again be comfortable.
And know that I look normal
And know that I look all right.
And that people
Don't know"

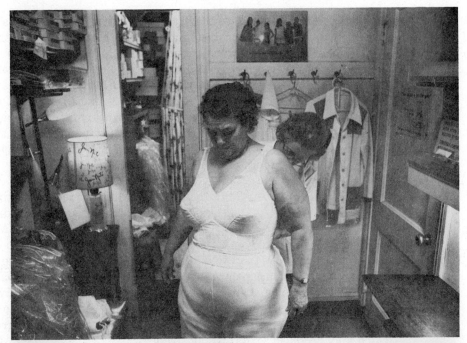

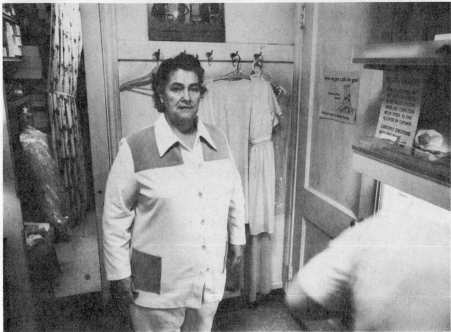

[My husband] "states he cannot sleep with me yet as he is afraid that in thrashing, he would hurt me physically. He is still unable to look at my surgery. I'm not pushing this part, as I feel less of a woman; I also feel a great loss, an embarrassment . . . I don't understand this feeling. Sometimes a feeling of not being whole. I know this sounds foolish, but it is real to me."

These photographs were taken by Mark L. Rosenberg, M.D., and appear in his book *Patients: The Experience of Illness* (Saunders Press, 1980).

Patient/Partner Knowledge of the Surgery

There are a variety of mastectomy procedures available, such as the radical mastectomy, the simple mastectomy, and the lumpectomy. There has been much controversy as to the therapeutic effect of removing a portion of the breast as compared with removing the entire breast. It is the responsibility of the physician to describe and the nurse to reinforce information on the various procedures, along with the alternatives and/or adjuvant nonsurgical procedures available so that the woman and her partner can participate in the decision-making process. In most cases, it is advantageous to the patient's sense of well-being and maintenance of self-control if he or she shares in the determination of the action that will lead to the loss of a body part and/or function. Thomas and Yates (1977) advise a premastectomy consultation which includes the above and also the possibilities of reconstructing a breast. It is imperative that the patient be given all information regarding possible risks and realistic outcomes of the procedure she is to undergo. Many people involved with a mastectomy are more concerned with change in body image and loss of femininity than in actual or potential changes in sexual function.

There is no relationship between mastectomy and the acceleration or deceleration of menopause. However, if the woman is also receiving chemotherapy, an artificial menopause may occur. For the woman receiving radiation therapy before and/or after mastectomy, there is usually great fatigue, which may decrease sexual responsiveness.

With the exception of loss of the ability to breast-feed, the side effects of mastectomy related to sexual function are psychosocial and psychosexual in nature. Very little is known about these side effects or, of most significance, about the effect the mastectomy has on the woman's sexual behavior and that of her partner (Frank, 1978).

Changes and Fears Regarding Sexual Function Experienced by Mastectomy Patients and Their Partners

Our society gives much attention to the female breast and considers it a source of much pride and pleasure. Depending on the extent of the surgery, women will experience many difficulties related to losing one or both of their breasts. Frank identified the following as some areas of sexual concern for the woman who experiences breast surgery: fears of loss of femininity; changes in behavior related to sexual activity such as resumption of sexual intercourse after discharge from the hospital, viewing of the scars by the woman and her partner, wearing a bra or prosthesis during sexual interactions, hurting the incision area, and resumption of behaviors related to the breast, such as manual and oral stimulation (Frank, 1977).

Abt, McGurrin, and Heintz (1978) studied 47 postmastectomy women with regard to their perceived changes in sexual self-image, sexual attitudes, and sexual behavior. Their findings supported Frank's (1977). In addition, women reported the desire to undress privately, not in full view of their partners.

There are several biologic, psychologic, and social factors that influence the responses of the woman and her partner to the loss of a breast. The biologic factors include 1) the fact that the breast is a prominent, easily visible organ, and when excised it leaves a very apparent anatomical void; 2) preoperative breast size; 3) age; 4) pain or discomfort at the operative site

(Woods, 1975). Psychologic variables are 1) the woman's assigned value to her breasts; 2) the woman's preoperative body image; 3) the woman's perception of her partner's reaction; and 4) the value of breast stimulation in sexual expression (Woods, 1975). The quality of the preoperative sexual relations, the actual reaction of the male partner, and the occupational role of the woman are social factors (Woods, 1975). All of these contribute to the postmastectomy woman's adaptation or maladaptation to the loss of her breast.

Self-acceptance seems to be stressed less than acceptance by the patient's partner. One might conclude a definite need for the partner to participate in all aspects of the surgical experience in order to increase the woman's opinion of her partner's acceptance of her. Perhaps then the chief concern of the woman's acceptance of herself can be dealt with, since the woman's strongest support (her partner) will be perceived as willing to accept the woman without a breast.

Nursing Interventions with the Mastectomy Patient and Her Partner

As an advocate with mastectomy patients, the nurse needs to empathize with her patients throughout the entire experience. The nurse is probably the person who will spend the most time with the woman and will hopefully establish a special involvement with her. The nurse who cares for the premastectomy patient may best identify the woman's reactions postoperatively. Woods (1975) suggests taking a thorough sexual history prior to the surgery to ascertain the woman's response to the loss of her breast. With this information and the other cues the nurse observes during interactions with the patient and her partner, an individualized method of helping the patient to adapt successfully to her breast loss can be developed and implemented.

The nurse can have a strong influence on increasing the woman's awareness of the need for routine self-examination of the unaffected breast. Classes can be set up with individuals or groups wherein the need, technique, and rationale can be taught. It is recommended that each learner give a return demonstration to the nurse-teacher at the end of the class.

Preoperative and postoperative teaching by the nurse concerning the importance of various exercises is imperative for uncomplicated recovery. There is a high potential for the arm on the affected side to swell postoperatively. There also may be some tenderness in the incisional area. Therefore, alternative positions for sexual intercourse might be suggested to allow the arm the utmost flexibility. Sexual activity can resume immediately after discharge.

The nurse can also teach the patient proper techniques in changing the dressing. The literature and experience indicate that it is important to have the woman and her partner participate in the dressing change prior to discharge. In this way, the woman will not have to fear her partner's viewing the operative area when she returns home.

Various support groups such as ENCORE and Reach-to-Recovery can be a good resource for the mastectomy patient if planned at an appropriate time. If the woman expresses interest, the nurse can educate her about the various prostheses and reconstructive procedures.

In a study of approximately 50 women who had experienced a mastectomy, the majority of women did not feel adequately prepared for either their surgery or the postoperative experience (Woods and Earp, 1978). Other researchers (Abt, McGurrin, and Heintz, 1978) described similar findings with one-half of their sample (N = 47), suggesting that the single most significant help they could have utilized would have been counseling, especially preoperative. Perhaps with the current emphasis on sexual awareness and the emerging, expanded role of the nurse, this void cited by mastectomy patients can be prevented. Nurses are in a most opportune position to counsel these women and their partners. If the nurse caring for a mastectomy patient reviews the section on changes and fears regarding sexual function experienced by mastectomy patients and their partners, it will assist him or her in knowing the appropriate areas for counseling.

References

Abt, V., McGurrin, M., and Heintz, L.: "The Impact of Mastectomy on Sexual Self-Image, Attitudes, and Behavior." *Journal of Sex Education and Therapy, 4*:43–46, 1978.

American Association of Sex Educators, Counselors and Therapists. *Sex Education, Counseling, and Therapy for the Physically Handicapped.* Washington, D.C., The American Association of Sex Educators, Counselors, and Therapists, 1979.

American Medical Systems, Inc.: "A Summary of Clinical Experience to Date With the AMS Inflatable Penile Prosthesis". Minnesota, American Medical Systems, Inc., 1978.

Bouchard-Kurtz, R., and Owens-Speese, N.: *Nursing Care of the Cancer Patient.* 4th ed., St. Louis, The C. V. Mosby Co., 1981.

Carter, S. K.: "What You Can Do for Your Patient with Breast Cancer." *Medical Times, 106*:50–57, 1978.

Coope, J.: "Post-Hysterectomy Symptoms." *Nursing Times, 71*:1284–1286, 1975.

DeBacher, E., Lauverigns, A., and Willem, C.: "Sexual Behavior after Prostatectomy." *European Urology, 3*:295–298, 1977.

Dinnerstein, L., Wood, C., and Burrows, G.: "Sexual Response Following Hysterectomy and Oophorectomy." *Obstetrics and Gynecology, 49*:92–96, 1977.

Dulcey, Martino: "Addressing Breast Cancer's Assault on Female Sexuality." *Topics in Clinical Nursing, 1*:61–68, 1980.

Frank, Deborah: "You Don't Have to Be an Expert to Give Sexual Counselling to a Mastectomy Patient." *Nursing 81, 11*:64–67, 1981.

Frank, D., Dornbush, R., Webster, S., and Kolodney, R.: "Mastectomy and Sexual Behavior: A Pilot Study." *Sexuality and Disability, 1*:16–26, 1978.

Gallagher, K.: "Body Image Changes in the Patient with a Colostomy." *Nursing Clinics of North America, 7*:669–676, 1972.

Golub, S.: "When Your Patient's Problem Involves Sex." *RN,* March 1975, pp. 27–33.

Guendeman, B. J.: "The Impact of Surgery on Body Image." *Nursing Clinics of North America, 10*:635–643, 1975.

Jones, D., Dunbar, C., and Jeiovec, M.: *Medical-Surgical Nursing—a Conceptual Approach.* New York, McGraw-Hill Book Co., 1978.

Kentsmith, D., and Eaton, M.: *Treating Sexual Problems in Medical Practice.* New York, Aklo Publishing Inc., 1979.

Kolodney, R., Masters, W., Johnson, V., and Biggs, M.: *Textbook of Human Sexuality for Nurses.* Boston, Little, Brown and Co., 1979.

Krizinofske, M. T.: "Symposium on the Patient with Long-Term Illness, Human Sexuality and Nursing Practice." *Nursing Clinics of North America, 8*:673–681, 1973.

Kroz, R.: "Becoming Comfortable with Sexual Assessment." *American Journal of Nursing, 78*:1036–1038, 1978.

Krueger, J., Hassell, J., Gaggins, D., Ishimatu, T., Pablico, M., and Tuttle, E.: "Relationship Between Nurse Counseling and Sexual Adjustment with Hysterectomy. *Nursing Research, 28*:145–150, 1979.

Lamanshe, J.: "Helping the Ileostomy Patient to Help Himself." *Nursing 77,* January 1977, pp. 34–39.

Littleton, V.: "The Surgical Patient's Sexuality." *Association of Operating Room Nurses' Journal, 26*:649–658, 1977.

Marino, Lisa: *Cancer Nursing*. St. Louis, The C. V. Mosby Co., 1981.

McCloskey, J.: "How to Make the Most of Body Image Theory in Nursing Practice." *Nursing 76*, May 1976, pp. 68–72.

Mims, F., and Swenson, M.: *Sexuality: A Nursing Perspective*. New York, McGraw-Hill Book Co., 1980.

Phipps, W., Long, B., and Woods, N.: *Medical-Surgical Nursing Concepts and Clinical Practice*. St. Louis, The C. V. Mosby Company, 1979.

Robusto, Nancy: "Advising Patients on Sex After Surgery." *AORN Journal*. *32*:55–61, 1980.

Ryan, C., and Ryan, K.: *A Private Battle*. New York, Simon and Schuster, 1979.

"Sex after Ileostomy and Colostomy." *Medical Aspects of Human Sexuality*. January 1975, pp. 107–108.

"Sexual Function After Surgery for Rectal Cancer." *Medical Aspects of Human Sexuality*. September 1978, pp. 53–54.

"Sexual Rehabilitation of Gynecologic Cancer Patients." *Medical Aspects of Human Sexuality*. February 1978, pp. 51–52.

Shipes, E., and Lehr, S.: *Sexual Counselling for Ostomates*. Springfield, Ill., C. C Thomas, 1980.

Thomas, S., and Yates, M.: "Breast Reconstruction After Mastectomy." *American Journal of Nursing*, 77:1438–1442, 1977.

Tully, J.: "Breast Cancer—Helping the Mastectomy Patient Live Life Fully." *Nursing 78, 8*:18–25, 1978.

U.S. Department of Health, Education, and Welfare Staff. *The breast cancer digest: a guide to medical care, emotional support, educational programs, and resources*. Maryland: National Cancer Institute, Public Health Service National Institutes of Health, December 1979.

von Eschenbach, A., and Rodriguez, D. (eds.): *Sexual Rehabilitation of the Urologic Cancer Patient*. Boston, G. K. Hall Medical Publishers, 1981.

Vredeval, D., Derdiarian, A., Sarna, L., Friel, M., and Shiplacoff, J.: *Concepts of Oncology Nursing*. New Jersey, Prentice-Hall, Inc., 1981.

Wabrek, A., and Wabrek, C.: "Mastectomy: Sexual Implications." *Primary Care, 3*:803–810, 1976.

Watson, P., Wood, R., Wechsler, N., and Christensen, L.: "Comprehensive Care of the Ileostomy Patient." *Nursing Clinics of North America, 77*:427–444, 1976.

Wilpizeski, Marcia: "Helping the Ostomate Return to Normal Life. *Nursing 81, 11*:62–66, 1981.

Winker, W.: "Confronting One's Changed Image: Choosing the Prosthesis and Clothing. What a Mastectomy Patient Needs to Know About Buying a Prosthesis and Clothing." *American Journal of Nursing, 77*:1433–1436, 1977.

Wood, R., and Rose, K.: "Penile Implants for Impotence." *American Journal of Nursing,* 78:234–238, 1978.

Woods, N.: "Facts and Opinion—Influences on Sexual Adaptation to Mastectomy." *Journal of Obstetrics, Gynecologic, and Neonatal Nursing*, May/June 1975, 33–37.

Woods, N.: *Human Sexuality in Health and Illness*. 2nd ed., St. Louis, The C. V. Mosby Co., 1979.

Woods, N., and Earp, J.: "Women with Cured Breast Cancer—a Study of Mastectomy Patients in North Carolina." *Nursing Research, 27*:279–285, 1978.

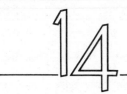

SEXUALLY TRANSMITTED DISEASES

INTRODUCTION

Sexually transmitted diseases (STDs) have long been a part of the history of civilization. Today, despite tremendous advances in the diagnosis and treatment of sexually transmitted diseases, the incidence continues to rise. The most drastic increases are in the 15- to 19-year-old group (Felman, 1978). Explanations for the continuation and increasing incidence of sexually transmitted diseases are complex. The following components help explain some of the reasons for the tenacity of sexually transmitted diseases: moral aspects, social factors, and medical factors.

Tremendous negative bias exists about sexually transmitted diseases. The term "venereal disease" has a highly negative connotation to most people. Because of this, most health care professionals who deal with STDs have begun to use the less emotionally charged term "sexually transmitted disease" rather than "venereal disease." Although people from all social classes and all professions can and do contract STDs, the prevalent view of the individual who has a STD is one who is dirty, sexually promiscuous, and generally of low moral character. To seek treatment may be seen as admitting to falling into this stereotypical role. The individual with a sexually transmitted disease may suffer great guilt and loss of self-esteem as a result of moralistic attitudes toward STDs, particularly gonorrhea and syphilis (Fong, 1977). It has been suggested that the legal requirement for use of names in reporting these diseases may be a significant factor in the failure of people to report the disease and in inadequate contact tracing (LeBourdois, 1975). It has been proposed that codes be used to protect the identity of the individuals. This reluctance to be identified surely is due in part to the negative feelings our society holds in regard to STDs.

Social factors also affect the incidence of STDs. In our culture, sex is everywhere—in advertisements, television, newspapers, magazines, radio, in all areas. People are constantly bombarded with sex and sexual innuendo from the mass media. This, combined with mobility and increased leisure time, may contribute to a relaxation of previous restrictions on sexual behavior. The negative social stigma that was attached to nonmarital sexual activity does not seem to be as rigid today (Donald, 1979).

Perhaps the greatest barrier to the eradication of STDs is a medical one— the increasing incidence of asymptomatic disease. As a rule, most individuals do not seek preventive care in terms of STDs. By and large, people seek medical care for two reasons: if they are experiencing symptoms of a disease; or if they have learned that they were exposed to a disease. Unless individuals are educated toward primary prevention and periodic prophylactic evaluation for STDs, a significant portion of the population may suffer from these diseases and unknowingly spread them.

An additional medical problem that has deterred the treatment of STDs is the tendency of the organisms, over time, to develop immunities to the treatment. The most common example of this is in the newer penicillin-resistant strains of gonococci. The organisms have begun to produce an enzyme that actually breaks down the penicillin, thereby rendering it ineffective in treatment.

The last medical problem to be discussed that has led to reductions in prevention of the spread of STDs is the advent of some of the more effective and popular methods of contraception. Neither the birth control pills nor the intrauterine devices offer any protection from STDs. In fact, the pill may actually enhance a woman's chances of contracting gonorrhea if she is exposed while taking the pill. As the diaphragm and foam and condoms gain in popularity once again, their STD barriers may be seen as a definite advantage.

Although strict disease orientation has been avoided throughout this text, the subject material of this chapter does necessitate more of a medical approach. For the reader's convenience, charts have been provided at the end of the chapter summarizing diagnostic tests, treatments, and follow-up recommendations for the common STDs. Each disease will be covered in the text of the chapter in terms of symptoms, incubation periods, complications of untreated disease, and patient instructions. The increasing incidence of pelvic inflammatory disease (PID), sexually transmitted enteric disease, and hepatitis will also be discussed for their epidemiological importance. The final section of the chapter will be devoted to nursing implications for dealing with patients with STDs. Instead of the case study approach, values clarification exercises for education about STD's have been included.

SPECIFIC DISEASES

Nongonococcal Urethritis (NGU)

Nongonococcal urethritis is perhaps the most commonly sexually transmitted disease among men in the United States (McCormack, 1978; Tenenbaum, 1980). For those individuals who experience symptoms, the most commonly encountered ones include dysuria (pain on urination) and a scanty or moderate mucopurulent urethral discharge, which is clear or white in color. The urethral discharge may be observed after penile stripping during examination, or on awakening after a long period without urination (Felman, 1979a). In addition, the patient may complain of urinary frequency and meatal or urethral irritation or itching. The incubation period for NGU is from one to three weeks. Sometimes the disease is not discovered until treatment for gonococcal urethritis has been found to be ineffective (Felman, 1979a; Jupa, 1979).

The two most commonly encountered organisms for NGU are *Chlamydia trachomatis* and *Ureaplasma urealyticum* (Holmes, 1978; Rein, 1981; Sparling, 1979). These organisms have been found to be responsible for other diseases as well. For example, 31 per cent of women who were found to be *Chlamydia* positive although asymptomatic, were found to have hypertrophic erosion of the cervix. Of these women, 46 per cent had mucopurulent endocervical discharge on examination (Sparling, 1979). A full 50 per cent of women who were found to have positive *Chlamydia* cultures from the cervix were asymptomatic and showed no signs of disease on examination. Salpingitis, infection in the tubes, may also be caused by *Chlamydia*. Because of the incidence of these disorders in asymptomatic females, it is recommended that all partners be treated for the disease (Felman, 1979a; Jupa, 1979). In the case of NGU, most female contacts of heterosexual males with NGU and most male contacts of homosexual men with NGU are asymptomatic. On examination of the partner, proctitis may be found in males, or cervicitis in females (Felman, 1979a). Regardless of the sex or number of partners, all contacts should be treated at the same time, when possible, to avoid later reinfection and the Ping-Pong effect often encountered in treatment of STDs.

Complications of untreated NGU include proctitis in males who practice anal intercourse with an infected partner and epididymitis. For women, the most commonly encountered complications of untreated NGU are hypertrophic erosion of the cervix and/or salpingitis. Salpingitis may eventually lead to pelvic inflammatory disease (Felman, 1979a).

When instructing patients with STDs that require treatment of more than one application of some medication, careful explanation of the importance of finishing the medication is necessary. In symptomatic patients, the symptoms will often disappear after several days of treatment. When the patient no longer experiences the symptoms, he or she may falsely conclude that the infection is "cured" and that the medication may be discontinued. This is both common and dangerous. Although the symptoms have disappeared, the infection is usually not cleared up until the whole course of the medication is followed.

All attempts to treat partners simultaneously should be made in order to prevent Ping-Pong type reinfection at a later date. The health care professional must guard against assumptions about the clients' sexual partners and habits. Informing clients of the possibility of reinfection from partners and the need for simultaneous treatment, while giving them the opportunity to maintain their self-esteem, encourages them to inform their partners, regardless of their sexual orientations and practices.

Gonococcal Urethritis

Gonococcal urethritis is the classic cause of purulent urethritis in men, which is its major symptom (Jupa, 1979). There is a two to five day incubation period for the disease. Often dysuria will accompany the discharge. If the disease is untreated, the discharge may last for two months.

Penicillin has traditionally been the treatment of choice for gonococcal urethritis. Recently, the advent of penicillin-resistant strains of gonococci has led to more vigorous treatment. The penicillin-resistant strains actually break down penicillin, rendering it ineffective, and may also show an increased resistance to tetracycline, which has long been an alternative choice in the treatment of gonococcus (Jupa, 1979). If penicillin is ineffective, or if the organisms have been found to be the penicillin-resistant type, alternative methods outlined at the end of the chapter are followed.

If gonococcal urethritis is left untreated, the patient may develop local abscesses, epididymitis, seminal vesiculitis, and/or urethral strictures. These possible complications are serious and are particularly frustrating for workers in the field of STDs, since the infection itself is asymptomatic in 20 to 50 per cent of the contacts of males with the urethral infection (Sparling, 1979). It has been determined that approximately 30 per cent of homosexual males exposed to gonococcal urethritis will contract the disease. Of these, about one-third will be asymptomatic. In addition, there seems to be a higher incidence of transmission of gonococcal infection to women. Women who contract the disease also tend to be asymptomatic.

In instructing clients about care and follow-up treatment, completion of the medication course (if tetracycline is given) must be stressed. All contacts should be checked and treated when necessary. Clients should also be instructed to return for a follow-up culture seven to 14 days after the treatment is completed. This is particularly important in ruling out the penicillin-resistant strains and in preventing further spread of the disease (McCormack, 1978).

Gonorrhea

Gonorrhea is caused by a gram-negative bacteria called *Neisseria gonorrhoeae*. The disease may be totally asymptomatic in both males and females (Hatcher, 1979). Traditionally, it was thought that males were more likely than females to experience symptoms of the disease. However, the asymptomatic rate for males has been increasing recently. Individuals in the 15- to 19-year-old group are now responsible for 25 per cent of all reported cases of gonorrhea (Felman, 1978).

In males who are suffering from symptoms, the most commonly encountered complaints include dysuria with frequency and urgency of urination and penile discharge, which may at first be scant and then become a heavier, yellowish-green discharge. The client may complain of irritation and swelling of the urethra and testicular pain. If untreated, the symptoms in the male usually disappear within six weeks.

Symptomatic females will usually complain of symptoms from two days to three weeks after exposure. The complaints may include a creamy yellow vaginal discharge that may coexist with some other form of vaginitis, inflammation, increased discharge from the cervix, and reddened urethra, vaginal introitus, rectum, Bartholin's glands, and/or Skene's glands. The urethra and Skene's glands, when milked, may evidence a purulent discharge. Pain during intercourse and urination may also be present. Both males and females have been found to have gonococcal pharyngitis.

If gonorrhea is left untreated in women, permanent sterility due to salpingitis may occur, leading to pelvic inflammatory disease (PID) and scarring of the tubes. Pelvic inflammatory disease will be discussed in greater depth later in the chapter. In all cases of suspected PID, appendicitis must be ruled out. Other potential complications from untreated gonorrhea include arthritis, endocarditis, gonococcal septicemia, hepatitis, and meningitis (Holmes, 1978).

Newborns of mothers infected with gonorrhea may suffer from a disease called ophthalmia neonatorum. In this condition, the newborn's eyes become the site of gonococcal infection as a result of exposure in the mother's vagina during delivery. If untreated, blindness may follow. In order to prevent this, hospitals are now required by law to prophylactically treat for this condition by the instillation of either silver nitrate drops or penicillin drops into the eyes of all newborns. The silver nitrate is very irritating to the mucous membranes of the eyes and causes the swelling and reddened eyes often seen in newborns.

The most effective method of diagnosis of gonorrhea is culture on modified Thayer-Martin media. In the past, the urethra in the male and the cervix in the female were the primary sites for obtaining specimens for culture. However, it has been found that taking cultures from the urethra, cervix, throat, and anus will significantly increase the yield of positive results (Crespo, 1978; Donald, 1979). Increase in the incidence of oral coitus (both fellatio and cunnilingus) have led to the increased incidence of pharyngeal gonorrhea. Similarly, the increase in anal intercourse with both males and females has led to an increase in anal gonorrhea. These two locations are potentially primary sites of infection and must not be overlooked because of the ignorance or embarrassment of the health care worker (Donald, 1979). Infections at these sites are frequently asymptomatic (Sparling, 1979).

In instructing heterosexual clients about gonorrhea and the treatment for the disease, discussion of contraception is appropriate. There is some thought that the IUD (intrauterine device) may enhance a woman's susceptibility to gonorrhea (Felman, 1979a; Jupa, 1979). In addition, women taking birth control pills have been found to be more susceptible to gonococcal infection than those not taking the pill (Felman, 1979a; Hatcher, 1979). These facts may significantly affect the client's choice of contraception.

All clients who have been treated for gonorrhea should be evaluated by post-treatment cultures from seven to 14 days after treatment. In cases where cure has not been attained, the practitioner will usually suspect a penicillin-resistant gonococcus and will treat accordingly (McCormack, 1978).

Treatment of contacts is of utmost importance and must be stressed. For heterosexual clients, use of a condom for intercourse should be advised until negative cultures of both the clients and the contacts have been obtained. Couples who engage in anal intercourse should also be advised to use condoms until cultures are negative. In addition, oral-genital sex is to be discontinued until negative cultures are obtained. Patients who understand that oral sex provides another method of spreading the disease will be more likely to follow the instructions than clients who are not informed as to why such a prohibition may be given them. Finally, clients should be alerted to the possibility of side effects of the medication, such as diarrhea from tetracycline or ampicillin, or in women, the development of a concurrent yeast infection secondary to the use of antibiotics (Hatcher, 1979).

Genital Herpes Virus

Genital herpes is a viral infection related to the herpes simplex organism that is marked by latency periods and repeated recurrent localized lesions, for which the body does not usually form an immunity (McNab, 1979). The virus is similar to the virus causing fever blisters on the mouths of susceptible individuals. It was thought that herpes simplex Type I was responsible for fever blisters, while Type II was responsible for genital herpes. However, research has indicated that both types of the virus are implicated in the genital disease. Type I seems to be much more common in patients experiencing their first infection, while Type II is usually isolated from patients with recurrent infections (Sparling, 1979).

Symptoms of primary infections usually appear from two to 20 days after exposure. The most commonly encountered incubation period is six days. Symptoms usually begin as a minor itching or rash in the genital area. Blister-like lesions may then form, break open, and ulcerate. These lesions may cause extreme itching and intense pain, especially during intercourse. The external lesions usually last from three to 10 days. In addition to the lesions, the infected individual may experience pain on urination, swollen and tender lymph nodes, fever, general malaise, and pain radiating into the legs. In some cases where lesions may be present in the urethra, the individual may be unable to void because of the pain. In these cases, catheterization may be necessary. The most common infection sites in the male are the glans and shaft of the penis, the urethra, the scrotum, the inner thighs, and the anal area. In women the most common sites are the labia, within the vagina and/or cervix, and the anal area (Jupa, 1979; McNab, 1979; Tenenbaum, 1980).

The primary herpes infection is usually the most severe that the individual will suffer in terms of number of lesions, intensity and duration of pain, duration of virus shedding, and total duration of the lesions (Sparling, 1979). It is also during the primary infection that the individual is most likely to develop a concurrent infection. This is particularly true in women, who often develop a severe monilial infection as a result of the scratching. Any coexisting infections must be treated. It has been estimated by the Venereal Disease Control Center that the average patient experiences from four to five recurrences in the first year and two or three in subsequent years (McNab, 1979). The recurrences usually are less severe and last about two weeks. Some individuals report that they experience stress-related recurrences. For example, nervous tension, emotional upset, general fatigue, poor diet, and the onset of menstruation or ovulation have been reported as precipitating factors of recurrent infections.

Genital herpes is very contagious during the symptomatic phase when the lesions are present both in primary and recurrent infections (Hatcher, 1979; McNab, 1979). Patients should be advised to avoid intercourse or to use condoms from the time the lesions appear until about two weeks after they are healed (McNab, 1979; Sparling, 1979). Contact of any mucous membrane with the lesions may result in spread of the disease.

Complications of herpes include neuralgia, urinary retention, aseptic meningitis, zoster-like illness, anal canal infection, and infection of the neonate. Infection of the neonate is highly life threatening and will be discussed further (Sparling, 1979).

The woman who develops an acute case of herpes while pregnant is three times more likely to suffer from a spontaneous abortion or premature labor than the pregnant woman who does not have the infection. Prior to the birth of the child, the infection may spread through the placenta. If the child is born before the maternal antibodies are transferred across the placenta, the neonate may suffer severe systemic infection. Fifty per cent of the neonates who are exposed to the disease during the birth process will contract the disease. Of these neonates, 75 to 100 per cent of those infected in organs other than the skin will suffer either brain damage or death (McNab, 1979). Because of the potential hazards to the newborn, the management of pregnant women who have active herpetic lesions at the end of pregnancy requires delivery by cesarean to avoid contact with the lesions. In some cases, to be certain that no lesions in the vaginal canal have been missed on exam, the physician and the client may decide on cesarean delivery even when no active lesions are visible.

Another condition that has been linked with herpes is cervical cancer. It has been found that women who had cervical and uterine infections of herpes are eight times more likely to have cancer of the cervix than are noninfected women. It has been postulated that herpes infection in women may be an etiological factor in later development of cancer of the cervix. A direct cause-and-effect relationship between herpes and cervical cancer has not been proved (Donald, 1979; Holmes, 1978; McNab, 1979; Sparling, 1979). The possibility that such a link exists does require explanation to the patient, who should also be advised to seek at least yearly Pap smears to determine the presence of cervical dysplasia or cancer. (Some physicians still recommend Pap smears every six months for women who have had herpes.)

Perhaps the most frustrating aspect of herpes virus is the fact that at present there is no known treatment for the disease other than symptomatic treatment for pain. In the past, red dye was applied to the lesions, followed by photoactivation of the dye. This treatment was found to be ineffective. In addition, it was found that photoactivation with red dye was associated with sarcoma formation in experimental animals. The treatment has been largely eliminated (Jupa, 1979). Other treatments have been tried but none have been successful. "Until an effective, safe treatment is found, there is no justification for the use of ineffective and potentially toxic remedies (Holmes, 1979).

Syphilis

Syphilis is a systemic disease caused by the motile spirochete *Treponema pallidum*. It has been cited as the major health threat to homosexual males with multiple sex partners (Henderson, 1977). More than 50 per cent of the cases in males occur in homosexual or bisexual individuals (Holmes, 1978). Syphilis must be ruled out in any case of genital lesions, unexplained papulosquamous skin rash, or anal lesions (Holmes, 1978). To control the spread of the disease, greater attention must be given to providing competent and compassionate health services for the homosexual population.

Syphilis is generally divided into three stages, the primary, secondary, and the tertiary stages. Because of differences in diagnosis and treatment during these stages of the disease, each will be discussed separately here.

Primary Stage.   Syphilis is the classic cause of the venereally transmitted genital ulcer, although genital herpes now occurs with far greater frequency than syphilis (Jupa, 1979). The ulcer generally appears as a single lesion and is painless. It may appear from 10 to 90 days after exposure to the disease. Usually, the incubation period is about 21 days. If left untreated, the ulcer will usually heal in two to six weeks. Many patients are unaware of the primary lesion and therefore do not seek treatment.

The VDRL blood test is generally not very effective in the diagnosis of in the early primary stage of the disease. It becomes more effective at about seven weeks after the start of the primary stage (Jupa, 1979). The more specific test, the FTA-ABS, is not helpful early in the primary stage, since it does not distinguish between recent and prior infections; that is, an individual who has been treated for syphilis may still test positive on an FTA-ABS at this stage.

Secondary Stage. If untreated, some individuals with primary syphilis may remain without any clinical manifestations after the lesion disappears. Others will develop a generalized maculopapular rash, which usually involves the palms of the hands and the soles of the feet. Lesions that may resemble chancres may appear on mucous membranes.

The secondary stage of syphilis usually lasts from six weeks to six months after the chancre formation. In addition to the rash, the individual in this stage may experience hair loss. During the secondary stage of syphilis, a positive VDRL will be obtained in the vast majority of cases.

Tertiary Stage. The late or latent stage of syphilis follows the secondary stage, and may last from 10 to 20 years. As with the secondary stage, some individuals may not develop further symptoms, although the disease will still be present. During the early phase of the third stage, the individual is still contagious. After about two years, the individual no longer seems to be contagious to others.

About one-third of the individuals with tertiary syphilis will demonstrate severe symptoms, which result from invasion of the bacteria into the organs. Particularly affected are the brain and the heart. Complications include heart disease, brain damage, and blindness (Hatcher, 1979; Jupa, 1979).

Testing for Syphilis

The incidence of false positives in testing for syphilis is not uncommon and must be considered in cases of positive VDRLs. False positive results may be obtained in collagen vascular diseases, in heroin addicts, and in a wide variety of acute infections including hepatitis, measles, chickenpox, and mononucleosis.

The pregnant woman who is infected with syphilis is a special case. During pregnancy, after about 16 to 18 weeks of gestation, the spirochete can usually cross the placenta of an infected woman. Children with congenital syphilis may be born dead or profoundly retarded. To prevent this, the condition of congenital syphilis has been largely eliminated by routine VDRL tests and recommendation for early treatment for all pregnant women.

It is generally recommended that sexual contacts of individuals with proven syphilis be treated without waiting for serology or the development of symptoms (Jupa, 1979). Obviously, the benefits of this aggressive stance must be weighed in individual cases. Following treatment, the patient is usually asked to return for repeat VDRL tests 30 days after initial treatment. Then the patient is asked to return every three months for one year. As can be imagined, this follow-up is often impossible to ensure and makes up one of the major problems in the eradication of syphilis. If treated in the first stages, before organ damage has occurred, the effects of the disease are usually completely reversible. However, if organ damage has occurred, treatment will usually result in the prevention of further damage only.

Vaginitis

The next three diseases to be discussed have been traditionally placed together under the catch-all phrase of "vaginitis." It has been demonstrated that these diseases are also found in the male, but it is in the female that the symptoms are most marked, and it is the female who will usually initiate health care.

In the past, it has not been unusual for practitioners to prescribe so-called "all-purpose" vaginal creams for the treatment of vaginal symptoms. This is a poor practice that is unnecessary in the light of the ease with which these diseases are diagnosed (Holmes, 1978). All the practitioner needs are a microscope, glass slides, normal saline, 10 per cent potassium hydroxide, and the ability to recognize the infections by a microscopic examination. In the vast majority of cases, all-purpose creams will not cure the infection and may only mask the symptoms. The patient may become very frustrated with the ineffective treatment and may discontinue care before the disease is cured, thereby leading to increased spread of sexually transmitted diseases. With appropriate diagnosis and care, the patient should be relieved of symptoms and free of disease in a very short time. In addition, contacts may be treated, thus eliminating the source for spread of further infection.

Trichomoniasis

It has been estimated that trichomoniasis is twice as commonly found in the United States as gonorrhea or herpes. The disease is caused by a protozoan found in both men and women. In one study, one in five women were found to have trichomoniasis without any symptoms (McNab, 1979). Forty per cent of women with gonorrhea will on examination be found to also have trichomoniasis (Donald, 1979). Both diseases must be diagnosed and treated. Treatment for gonorrhea will not cure trichomoniasis, nor will treatment for trichomoniasis cure gonorrhea.

The most commonly encountered symptom of trichomoniasis is a thin, watery, foamy discharge of greenish or yellowish liquid that has a foul odor. In addition, the patient may complain of itching, burning of the vagina, pain on intercourse, and pain on urination (Jupa, 1979; McNab, 1979). The disease is transmitted by contact with the discharge during sexual activity. The sexual mode is not the only method of transmission, however. The organism requires a warm, moist environment, and can survive on towels and wash-cloths, and in bathtubs, and other moist places. Patients should be cautioned not to borrow or lend towels and washcloths.

If left untreated, trichomoniasis may lead to cystitis. It has also been implicated in the development of pelvic inflammatory disease. Treatment of this disease was the cause of great controversy in the late 1970s, when it was discovered that metronidazole (Flagyl) caused sarcoma formation in experimental animals. The toxicity studies demonstrated that these sarcomas formed only following long-term use of the drug. Because of this, the Food and Drug Administration did not withdraw the drug from use (Holmes, 1978; Hatcher, 1979). Some practitioners have changed their treatment regimens to allow a shorter exposure to the drug and thus minimize the dangers to the client.

In instructing the client about the treatment of the disease, all clients should be warned of the Antabuse effect of metronidazole. Individuals taking the drug have been found to suffer mild to severe nausea and vomiting when they ingested alcohol while taking the medication. It is recommended that patients be advised to avoid alcohol (including beer and wine) during treatment and for at least one day after the completion of treatment.

Partners should also be treated for trichomoniasis. Although males are usually asymptomatic, they can contribute to recurrences of the infection. Flagyl is not recommended more frequently than every six to eight weeks. If, during a recheck, a client is found to have the disease, alternative treatment should be provided (Hatcher, 1979). Clients should be advised to use condoms for intercourse (either vaginal or rectal) and to avoid oral-genital sex for the course of the treatment.

Moniliasis (Candidiasis)

Moniliasis, or yeast vaginitis, is caused by the fungus *Candida albicans,* which normally exists in the anus and vagina. The symptoms occur as a result of an overgrowth of this fungus. Symptoms include thick, curdlike chunks of white, cottage-cheese–like vaginal discharge and intolerable vaginal and vulvar itching (McNab, 1979). Clients may also complain of pain on intercourse and burning on urination following intercourse.

Yeast infections may occur when any change of the normal acidity of the vagina occurs. Contributing factors to such changes include pregnancy, emotional upsets, and the use of "feminine hygiene" sprays and products, antibiotics, and birth control pills high in progestins. In cases of recurrent yeast infections, diabetes mellitus should be ruled out, since the normal elevation in blood sugar seems to make women more prone to yeast infections. During pregnancy many women are more prone to develop yeast infections (Holmes, 1978). Recently, fecal contamination of the vagina and sexual contact with an infected partner have been added to the list of potential causes of monilial infections (McNab, 1979).

In terms of sexual transmission, some studies have found an increased prevalence of penile colonization of *Candida* in the sexual partners of women diagnosed with moniliasis. In some cases, the male partner may have penile candidal dermatitis, while in others the men are asymptomatic (Holmes, 1978). Still other men with candidal infection may be diagnosed as suffering from nonspecific urethritis. Regardless of the sex of the partner, *Candida albicans,* the organism responsible for the disease, seems to have an affinity for the mucous membranes, particularly of the mouth (Poindexter, 1977). This, in combination with the increased incidences of oral sexual activities, can be seen as a potentially great source of the spread of the disease. In fact, White (1979) reported a high degree of correlation between oral sex and recurrent monilial infections in women.

When both the patient and his or her partner are to be treated, they both should be treated at the same time. Intercourse and oral sex should be avoided until the medication has been finished. The patient may find that the symptoms disappear very soon after the beginning of treatment. Because of this, many patients choose to discontinue the treatment as soon as the symptoms are relieved. Such short-term treatment for the infection will prove to be ineffective. Patients should be instructed to complete the medication.

Prevention of moniliasis is possible and should be discussed with patients. For example, the use of cotton underwear rather than nylon can help prevent the infection by allowing air flow to the perineum. Clients should be educated about douching and feminine hygiene products. The vagina is a self-cleaning organ that requires no additional use of products that can and do contribute to an overgrowth of yeast.

In cases where monilial infections seem to recur with some pattern, such as just before or just after menstruation, some women are advised to douche with a weak acid or weak Betadine solution. Using one tablespoon of vinegar with one quart of warm water will in some cases alter the vaginal acidity sufficiently to avoid the overgrowth of the organism. Care must be taken to avoid too much of a change in the acidity, since this can cause the infection to begin. Douching should be encouraged for women only when there is a medical purpose for it (Hatcher, 1979).

Nonspecific Vaginitis

The organisms responsible for the symptoms associated with nonspecific vaginitis have not been completely determined. The organism that is thought to be responsible for a large proportion of the infections is *Hemophilus vaginalis*. The symptoms of this infection include a minimal, watery gray vaginal discharge, which may be similar in appearance to that seen in trichomoniasis. The patient may complain of vaginal itching, pain on intercourse, and burning after intercourse or urination (Hatcher, 1979; Jupa, 1979).

Since no single organism has been implicated as the etiology of nonspecific vaginitis, no exhaustive list of specific causes can be formulated. Some of the causes associated with nonspecific vaginitis are the use of feminine hygiene products; the wearing of tight, dirty clothing; contamination of the vagina with fecal material; and poor lubrication of the vagina during intercourse.

When teaching patients appropriate self-care, it should be stressed that both partners should be treated; that the client should avoid sexual contact during the course of treatment; and that the woman and her partner should complete any medication prescribed, even if the symptoms should subside (Hatcher, 1979).

Condylomata Acuminata (Venereal Warts)

Venereal warts are dry, fungating, wartlike growths on the vulva, vagina, cervix, and penis (Hatcher, 1979). The warts are caused by a virus similar to those that cause common skin warts on other parts of the body. The incubation period for venereal warts usually is about three weeks to three months after exposure. Approximately 60 to 70 per cent of those who are exposed will contract the virus.

In diagnosing the disease, syphilis must be ruled out. As a rule, the lesions cause severe itching, while those of secondary syphilis do not. The itching and scratching may lead to secondary infections due to skin irritation.

Recently, genital warts have tended to respond less readily to podophyllin than they had in the past (Donald, 1979). If this is the case, removal of the warts through electrocautery or cryosurgery may be required. Partners must be treated, ideally at the same time, to avoid reinfection.

Infestations

The most commonly encountered sexually transmitted forms of parasitic infestations are *Pediculus pubis* and *Sarcoptes scabiei,* or crabs and scabies.

Crabs may be found on the skin and/or hair. The mites are usually seen as small black spots on the skin. Closer examination will reveal the crab-shaped mites. The symptoms for pediculosis may include severe itching. The scratching may lead to a secondary skin infection. Diagnosis is usually made on visual examination. In addition to the sexual mode of transmission, pediculosis may be spread by wearing the clothing of an infected person, by sleeping in bedding infected with the mites, and even by sitting on toilet seats used by infected individuals.

Treatment instructions to the patient require that he or she understands that the eggs mature in two to 14 days. To be sure that the mites are killed, treatment may be repeated two to three weeks after the initial treatment. Partners of infected individuals should also be treated. Bed linens and contaminated clothing should be laundered and dried in a clothes dryer. Mattresses can be treated with a lindane (Kwell) spray or a bug bomb.

The symptoms of *Sarcoptes scabiei* dermatitis usually differ from those of pediculosis in that the itching associated with scabies is particularly severe at night. The scabies mite penetrates into the upper skin of the infected individual. On examination, burrows may be noted in the superficial skin layer. Inflammatory skin changes also occur.

Partners should be treated with Kwell. Patients should be informed that the itching may continue for several days or even months after treatment, because of the allergic response to the mite that some people experience. Should this occur, the use of antihistamines is advised (Poindexter, 1977).

NEW EPIDEMIOLOGICAL INFORMATION ON SEXUALLY TRANSMITTED DISEASES

Pelvic Inflammatory Disease

In many cases of untreated or improperly treated STDs, pelvic inflammatory disease (PID) has been stated as a possible complication. The incidence of PID has risen dramatically in recent years. While most practitioners were taught that PID arose primarily from gonorrhea, it is now recognized that the syndrome known as PID can arise from any number of conditions, some of which are unrelated to STDs.

The major symptoms of PID include abdominal, pelvic, back, and leg pain. Clients may complain of fever or chills, prolonged menstrual bleeding, bleeding after intercourse, or pain on intercourse (Hatcher, 1979). If untreated, a major effect of PID is scarring of the tubes, leading to sterility. Tubo-ovarian cysts may form and rupture, possibly leading to peritonitis and sepsis (Hatcher, 1979; Jupa, 1979).

Ectopic pregnancy (pregnancy that occurs outside of the uterus), ovarian cyst, neoplasm, and endometriosis must all be ruled out in the diagnosis of PID (Hatcher, 1979). Treatment of all partners is essential, as is abstaining from sexual activity for at least one week. Most patients are placed on bedrest during the acute phase of PID.

Given the rising incidence of STDs in our society, it has been postulated that a concurrent increase in the complications of untreated STDs will also be noted. The two most easily observed complications of PID are sterility and ectopic pregnancy. In studies performed to determine the incidence of these conditions, Urquhart (1979) has determined that indeed these increases are found. Nonsurgical sterility among 27 million married women of reproductive age was found to have doubled between 1973 and 1976. This increase is statistically significant, and has been attributed to the increased rate of PID. The number of ectopic pregnancies was also found to have doubled between 1971 and 1977 (Urquhart, 1979).

This marked increase in PID and its consequences is of great epidemiological importance to everyone in our society. Untreated or improperly treated STDs may be significantly contributing to the increasing sterility of women in the child-bearing years in our culture. Prevention of the diseases and their spread becomes more urgent in the light of the potential long-term effects such diseases can have on our culture.

Enteric Diseases

Enteric diseases are those diseases traditionally associated with the ingestion of contaminated food or water (Felman, 1979b). Recently, however, it has been demonstrated that these diseases may in fact be sexually transmitted. Anolingus (mouth to anus contact) and fellatio of a fecally contaminated penis have been found to provide excellent mechanisms for the spread of common enteric pathogens (Sparling, 1979). For example, shigellosis has been found to have anolingus as a major mode of transmission. The incubation period for the disease is usually from one to seven days. Symptoms may range from severe abdominal cramping and diarrhea to no symptoms at all. In patients exhibiting symptoms, physicians have been perplexed in determining an adequate diagnosis unless the patient reported a recent history of foreign travel. It is essential, in the light of the sexual mode of transmission of these diseases, that health care professionals become aware of sexual transmission as a potential cause for these diseases in order to hasten appropriate treatment.

Hepatitis B, formerly called viral hepatitis, has also been found to be sexually transmissible. Any sexual practice that involves exposure to infectious saliva, semen, urine, vaginal secretions, or menstrual blood may lead to infection (Felman, 1979b).

Incidence rates for all of the aforementioned enteric pathogens and hepatitis seem to be greater in homosexual populations than in heterosexual ones, although anal intercourse and anolingus are practiced by both homosexual and heterosexual couples. Nonjudgmental care in a setting that will insure the patient's privacy is essential in treating homosexuals for sexually transmitted diseases. Homosexuals often will avoid care or will wait until symptoms are severe before seeking care because of fear of harsh treatment in today's health care delivery system. In order to adequately deal with the ever-increasing incidence of STDs in our society, care for all clients, particularly homosexual clients, must be closely examined and modified.

NURSING IMPLICATIONS

Management of Patients with STDs

It is the nurse's responsibility to give all patients understanding, reassurance, and nonjudgmental treatment. In addition, nurses have the responsibility as patient advocates and educators to educate their clients, both in the treatment of diseases and in future prevention of disease.

Sexually transmitted diseases cause patients as well as health care professionals to explore their moral values and beliefs. It is undeniable that the increasing incidence of sexual activity with more than one partner has contributed to the spread of STDs. Nurses must deal with the fact that people are having sexual relationships with more partners today than in the past. Nurses are responsible for examining their own feelings about this behavior in order to appropriately deal with clients who report such activities. Nurses who are unable to put aside their feelings about sexually transmitted diseases should consider the values clarification exercises to be discussed later in this chapter. If the exercises do not help, and nurses feel unable to give the quality of care necessary for patients who have STDs, perhaps these nurses should not work with these patients. As always, the nurse has the responsibility to be aware of appropriate referral sources for clients that can be relied upon to give nonjudgmental, quality care.

In many cases, the instructions the patient receives about treatment of STDs will be similar, regardless of the disease. It is appropriate and necessary that the nurse be sure that the client is informed of and understands these instructions. Fully informing clients will make them more motivated to take part in care and to follow directions. This is particularly important in cases that will require follow-up visits. While many patients, both symptomatic and asymptomatic, may visit a health care facility for treatment once, many do not return for follow-up visits. The major effort toward follow-up care must be made at the first (and sometimes only) visit. One technique found to be helpful in encouraging patients to return for follow-up testing and treatment is maintenance of a strict appointment schedule in order to minimize waiting time (Kahl, 1977). Assisting patients in taking part in their care is essential for their cooperation.

In most cases of STDs, all partners must be treated. Some clinicians will provide prescriptions for partners at the time of the client's first visit in order that the partners be treated simultaneously. While concurrent treatment is desirable, the ethics of providing patient treatment without proper examination is questionable. The clinician must be aware that more than one partner may be involved. All will need treatment. Careful case-finding is essential.

The use of condoms for the duration of the treatment and for some time following the treatment is usually encouraged for heterosexual patients. Some facilities supply condoms to both male and female patients for this purpose. Condoms do offer some protection against the spread of some STDs. The health care professional must guard against assuming that clients are involved in heterosexual relationships. The provision of condoms alone does not meet the protection needs for all types of sexual activity. Diseases that are transmitted by oral-genital sex are not prevented by the use of condoms. Teaching must be specific and must consider all potential modes of sexual expression utilized by a given client.

A common error made by many clients is stopping the medication before the required time. For most clients, symptomatic relief is quite rapid. The client who feels that the medication is no longer necessary may stop the treatment. This practice is to be avoided, since it may lead to inadequate treatment of the disease, which may later recur and spread, perhaps in an asymptomatic state.

Female clients who are taking antibiotics for the treatment of STDs should be warned about the possibility that they will develop monilial infections as a result of the alteration of the acidity of the vagina caused by these antibiotics. If this has occurred in the past, prophylactic treatment may be advised. If not, the women should be advised of the potential symptoms and instructed to return for treatment should a yeast infection occur.

Patients taking tetracycline for treatment of an STD should be advised to avoid milk and milk products for two hours before and two hours after taking the medication, since milk has been found to inhibit the absorption of tetracycline (Hatcher, 1979). Tetracycline should not be utilized in pregnant women for the treatment of any infection because discoloration of tooth enamel (in permanent teeth) may occur in the fetus.

Most patients are advised to avoid sexual activity while they are suffering from the symptoms of STDs. Often, they are told primarily to avoid intercourse. Such information does not give the client sufficient data. The mode of spread of the infection must be discussed, so that the client knows precisely how the disease can be contagious to others. The avoidance of intercourse alone will not offer sufficient protection for many of the STDs.

A final suggestion, and a very important one, is the avoidance by health care professionals of the term "venereal disease." "VD" has come to be an emotion-laden term, which often connotes "badness" to many people. In addition, it is no longer a precise term for the diseases that occur today. Instead, the term used in this chapter, "sexually transmitted diseases," should be used. This term does not carry with it the negative implications of venereal disease, and is therefore less threatening to the clients.

The Nurse as Educator

Education about STDs should focus on prevention, early diagnosis, and early treatment. One aim of education about STDs is to foster positive attitudes about the diseases in order to prevent infection and to promote early treatment. Decreasing embarrassment may be the most important factor in teaching about sexually transmitted diseases (Breckon, 1978; McNab, 1979; Niemiec, 1978). In order to foster more positive attitudes about STDs, teaching becomes of the utmost importance. The teacher must be able to present facts honestly, accurately, and objectively. Regardless of the information transmitted, the teacher who has strong moral objections to sexual activity outside of marriage, for example, will not be able to help foster a positive attitude about the incidence, prevention, and treatment of STDs. The teacher may be the most important factor in the quality of the education on STDs received by students and patients of all ages (Breckon, 1978).

In educating people about STDs, all students must understand that these diseases are not "dirty" or shameful. Such attitudes will only contribute to the reluctance to seek appropriate and early diagnosis if STD is suspected (McNab, 1979). Many students lack basic sexual health care knowledge, which should be supplied during the education about STDs. For example, most women do not know that some vaginal discharge is normal. Teaching the difference between normal vaginal discharge and discharges associated with infection is usually required in early STD education.

Prevention of STDs is the primary aim of education. Some preventive measures that may be covered include (McNab, 1979):

1. Use of contraceptives that can decrease the spread of STDs (condoms and some foams, diaphragms, and jelly)
2. Avoiding contacts with persons known to be infected
3. Use of soap and water after sexual contact (hands, genitals, mouth)
4. Voiding by the male after intercourse

5. Avoiding the sharing of washcloths or towels with others
6. Cleaning toilet seats
7. Regular checkups

Although these preventive measures may seem very basic to the educator, they must be discussed. As part of the discussion, some specific diseases and their spread can be easily included. The first preventive measure listed, the use of contraceptives that can decrease the spread of STDs, has been receiving more and more attention of late. The knowledge that a form of contraception can offer some protection against STDs, combined with the increasing fears about the more effective methods of contraception (notably the birth control pill and the IUD), may lead more people to choose methods such as the diaphragm and spermicidal jellies or contraceptive foam and condoms that, when combined, will offer high contraceptive effectiveness as well as protection against the spread of STDs.

Early diagnosis is the next goal in the education process. Students should be informed about the most common infections and their signs and symptoms. The high incidence of asymptomatic disease should be stressed, in order to encourage students to seek treatment if informed that they have been contacts. In addition, periodic check-ups that include testing for STDs in all individuals who could have been exposed to these infections should be encouraged.

Resources should be discussed, including their positive and negative aspects. For example, most students have the option of visiting a family physician or gynecologist. While this will ensure individual care, the expense of such treatment and the potential embarrassment of the patient may combine to make the private physician an unacceptable alternative.

Clinics that have treatment of STDs as their primary role offer the potential patient another alternative. In discussing clinics, local clinics—including hours, locations, and fees, if any—should be discussed. If there are particular clinics the teacher would recommend, this too should be covered. The toll free National Operation Venus Helpline telephone number (800-523-1885) should be distributed along with the telephone numbers of local STD clinics.

Specialized STD clinics, while maintaining the anonymity of the clients, sometimes require long waiting periods, which may be unacceptable to clients who do not have the time to wait for care. In addition, some clinics are limited, because of financial restraints, to diagnosis and treatment of gonorrhea and syphilis only. For treatment of other STDs, the clients would have to seek care elsewhere. The nurse who is teaching about the STD clinics must have the information concerning the type of care available in the local clinics, to appropriately inform the class (McNab, 1979).

Another potential source of sexual health care for STDs are the women's health care centers. There are a few of these centers currently in existence. An obvious shortcoming of these clinics is that they exclude men. Generally, though, women who are fortunate enough to seek treatment in such centers find compassionate and comprehensive care.

While many educators now agree that teaching about STDs is necessary, controversy still surrounds the issue of when and in what setting such teaching should occur. It has been suggested by Breckon (1978) that STD education should be given at least once in the junior high school and once in the senior high. However, because of the increase in the incidence rates in young teenagers in many communities, there seems to be a push, at least in some areas, to include STD education in the upper elementary school. Rather than having a separate unit on STDs, as has been done in the past in most cases, it is suggested that the unit be included as part of a unit on communicable disease. By doing this, the sexual aspects of transmission of these communicable diseases are discussed naturally, in the same manner used to discuss, for example, the transmission of chickenpox (Breckon, 1978). By including this material in such a way as to minimize the emotional impact, it is hoped that the students will be assisted in forming nonjudgmental attitudes about STDs and their treatment.

As noted earlier, in the discussion of gonorrhea, the teenage group is the section of the population in which STDs have seen the greatest increases. However, a large number of teenagers either ignore the symptoms of STDs or delay seeking treatment for the diseases (Niemiec, 1978). It appears that the severity of the symptoms and the teenager's perceptions of the symptoms are the key factors in the decision of whether or when to seek care. When the adolescent decides to seek care for a suspected STD, friends are usually the major source of information about the availability and acceptability of health care. This fact must be considered in education aimed at teenagers. The information about where to seek care must be easily available to the teenagers, such as on bulletin boards and the school newspaper, so that the teenagers themselves can help to spread the information.

Education about STDs involves not only the lay public but health care professionals as well. For many in the health care fields, the moralistic attitudes and misinformation found among the general public about STDs are also a problem. Virtually all health care workers are in settings in which they will encounter individuals with STDs. All practitioners must face and analyze their feelings about STDs and the people who contact them, in order to recognize their biases and strive to give the best quality care possible. The following exercises are values clarification exercises that have been proposed to help students get in touch with their feelings about STDs (Breckon, 1978). They are presented here as a valuable tool in the education of health care professionals. These simple exercises could become a part of any continuing education program involving nurses. They are, of course, of value to a basic education program as well.

The first exercise is called *Who's Who in Sexually Transmitted Disease*. The purpose of this exercise is to deal with the myth that only certain types of people contract STDs. Students are presented with randomly selected groups of famous people and instructed to rank the list in the order of probability that the individuals might have had a sexually transmitted disease. After each student ranks the famous people, discussion follows regarding the criterion utilized by the students to determine the order of the rankings.

Closely related to the first exercise is the *STD Top Ten*. In this exercise, famous and infamous people who are known to have had STDs are presented. In the discussion that follows the presentation of the list of names, attempts are made to analyze the feelings toward people who have had STDs. For example, the following list contains the names of ten famous people who are known to have suffered from STDs (Wallechinsky, 1977). Examine the list, and your feelings about these people. Pay particular attention to your feelings about the kind of person you tend to associate with being more likely to contract an STD. All health care professionals have biases. Our goal throughout is to recognize these in order to give the best care possible, given our own limitations.

1. Christopher Columbus
2. Peter the Great, Czar of Russia
3. Florence Nightingale
4. Henry VIII

5. Benjamin Franklin
6. Ludwig von Beethoven
7. Al Capone

8. Wild Bill Hickok
9. Friedrich Nietzsche
10. Paul Gaugin

Role play is another useful tool in values clarification about STDs. The nurse can be placed in the role of the patient, partner, etc., in order to experience STDs from another view. Role play has been useful in many other threatening situations, and can be of great value here.

Similar to role play is the exercise entitled *What Would You Do If?* In this game, the student is placed in a situation in which he or she must more personally examine feelings about STDs. The individual is given a situation or situations to consider. For example, the student may be asked to complete the statement, "What would you do if your 14-year-old brother (or sister) tells you he (or she) might have an STD?" Another example would be, "What would you do if you saw your favorite teacher coming out of an STD clinic?" These types of situations can be made appropriate to any age level student to help examine feelings. The students need not have to actually state what they felt they would do. Thinking about the situation and an open class discussion are often sufficient to achieve the desired goals of this experience.

Finally, a commonly used technique of teaching that may be utilized in many learning situations is the use of *Popular Myths* as a basis for discussion. Using this teaching method, each student is asked to discuss three myths that he or she has heard in the past. Discussion focuses on whether or not the myth is accurate. In addition, efforts are made to determine the source of the myth. Some of the more commonly-held ideas about STDs are incorrect, although based on some accurate information. Finally, the myths are discussed in terms of the effect they may have on efforts to control STDs. An obvious example of a myth that has been demonstrated to be false is the notion that only dirty people contract sexually transmitted diseases. However, the persistence of this belief is a major obstacle in controlling STDs, since many people deny symptoms rather than admit that they too are "dirty."

CONCLUSION

STDs have been a part of our past, and, if the present is any indication, will continue to be an important part of our future. As sexual mores change, attitudes toward STDs must also change. More people in our society are having sexual relationships with more partners than ever before. The increased potential for contact with STDs is a reality. As with many diseases, the strongest chance for the reduction of the disease lies in primary prevention. Periodic medical evaluations for STDs, so that asymptomatic as well as symptomatic infections can be detected, must become a part of the health-seeking behavior of all people in our society. Such medical evaluations must be carried out in the most matter of fact way, much as the Pap smear for women is carried out. The nurse is the appropriate person to transmit accepting attitudes, to educate clients, and to work as a patient advocate in ensuring quality care for all clients wishing to be seen for STD treatment check-ups. The nurse must work toward changing the negative attitudes toward STDs if the public is going to be able to benefit from the new advances in the treatment of STDs.

Text continued on page 327

Table 14–1.

Infection	Diagnosis	Treatment	Follow-up
Nongonococcal urethritis	Presence of significant urethritis after ruling out gonococcal infection	Tetracycline 500 mg orally four times a day for seven days	
		If recurs — 250 mg tetracycline orally four times a day for 30 days	
		or	
		Tetracycline 500 mg orally four times a day for seven days	
		then	
		Tetracycline 250 mg orally four times a day for 14 days	
		or	
		(for tetracycline allergy) Erythromycin 500 mg orally four times a day for seven days	
		then	
		Erythromycin 250 mg orally four times a day for 14 days	
		Treat partners simultaneously	

Adapted from Jupa, 1979; Felman, 1979a.

Table 14–2

Infection	Diagnosis	Treatment	Follow-up
Gonococcal urethritis	Gram stain of discharge — 85% diagnosis	4.8 million units penicillin injection with 1.0 gm probenicid orally	7–14 days after treatment repeat culture completed
	Culture on Thayer-Martin media	*or* Ampicillin 3.5 gm orally with 1.0 gm probenicid	
		or Amoxicillin 3.0 gm po with 1.0 gm probenicid	
		or (for penicillin allergy) Tetracycline 500 mg orally 4 times a day for 4 days	
		or Spectinomycin 2 gm injection	
Gonococcal urethritis with penicillin resistance		Spectinomycin 2 gm intramuscularly	
		or Cefazolin 2 gm intramuscularly with 1.0 gm probenicid orally	
		Check contacts	

Adapted from McCormack, 1978; Jupa, 1979.

Table 14–3

Infection	Diagnosis	Treatment	Follow-up
Gonorrhea	Gram stain Thayer-Martin culture — urethral, cervical, oral, anal	4.8 million units aqueous procaine penicillin intramuscularly with 1.0 gm of probenicid orally	Repeat culture 7–14 days after treatment is completed
		or (penicillin allergic nonpregnant) Tetracycline 500 mg orally 4 times a day for 4 days	Treat partners
		or Spectinomycin 2 gm intramuscularly	
		or (pregnant penicillin allergic patients) Cephalexin 500 mg orally 4 times a day for 7–14 days Erythromycin 500 mg late	
Gonorrhea with resistant strains	Ineffective treatment	Spectinomycin 2 gm intramuscularly	
Disseminated gonococcal infection		Aqueous crystalline penicillin G, 10 million units per day intravenously for 2–3 days	
		then Ampicillin 500 mg orally 4 times a day for 10 days	

Adapted from Hatcher, 1979; Crespo, 1978; Donald, 1979; Sparling, 1979; and McCormack, 1978.

Table 14–4

Infection	Diagnosis	Treatment	Follow-up
Herpes genitalis	Tzanck test (demonstration of multinucleated giant cells in base of lesion)	Symptomatic only	Pap smear every 6 months to 1 year
	Culture		
	FA (rapid immunofluorescent test)		
	Pap smear		

Adapted from McNab, 1979; Sparling, 1979.

Table 14–5

Infection	Diagnosis	Treatment	Follow-up
Trichomoniasis	Wet mount with normal saline to see organisms under microscope	Metronidazole (Flagyl) 2 gm orally for patient and partners	
		or	
	Pap smear	Flagyl 250 mg orally once a day for 10 days (patient and partners)	
		or	
		Flagyl 500 mg orally twice a day for 5 days (patient and partners)	
Candidiasis (yeast, monilia)	Microscopic exam with 10% potassium hydroxide for visual diagnosis	Nystatin vaginal suppository twice a day for 14 days	
	Culture	Monistat vaginal cream once a day before bed for 7 days	
Hemophilus vaginalis	Microscopic exam	Ampicillin or tetracycline 500 mg orally 4 times a day for 5 days	
		Nitrofurazone (Furacin) suppositories daily for 14 days	

Adapted from Holmes, 1978; Jupa, 1979; McNab, 1979; and Hatcher, 1979.

Table 14–6

Infection	Diagnosis	Treatment	Follow-up
Condylomata acuminata		Local application of podophyllin	May require repeated treatments
		Cautery	May need to have partners treated
		Cryosurgery	
Pubic lice	Lice or eggs seen in pubic hair	Lindane shampoo, lotion or cream	Repeat treatment 24–48 hours
			Repeat treatment 14 days

Adapted from Donald, 1979; Hatcher, 1979.

Table 14–7

Infection	Diagnosis	Treatment	Follow-up
Syphilis (primary, secondary, and early latent stages)	FTA-ABS	Benzathine penicillin G 2.4 million units intramuscularly *or*	Treat partners
	VDRL (late in stage only)	Aqueous procaine penicillin G 600,000 to 1.2 million units daily for 10 days *or* (penicillin allergic patients) Erythromycin 500 mg po 4 times daily for 15 days *or* Tetracycline HCl 500 mg po 4 times daily for 15 days	
Late latent or tertiary stages	STS (2nd and 3rd stages)	Aqueous procaine penicillin G 600,000 to 1.2 million units intramuscularly daily for 15 days *or* Benzathine penicillin G 2.4 million units intramuscularly every 7 days (three times: 7.2 million units total) *or* (penicillin allergic patients) Tetracycline HCl or erythromycin (for 30 days)	
Congenital, asymptomatic normal CNS		Benzathine penicillin G 50,000 units per kg intramuscularly, one time	
Congenital, symptomatic abnormal CNS		Aqueous procaine penicillin G 50,000 units per kg intramuscularly once daily for at least 10 days *or* Aqueous crystalline penicillin G 50,000 units per kg intramuscularly or intravenously daily in two divided doses for at least 10 days	

Adapted from Crespo, 1978; Jupa, 1979.

References

Breckon, Don and Sweeney, Don: "Use of Values Clarification Methods in Venereal Disease Education." *The Journal of School Health, 48*:3, 1978.

Crespo, Jorge and Rytel, Michael: "Venereal Diseases." *American Family Physician, 18*:2, 1978.

Donald, W. H.: "The Changing Pattern of Sexually Transmitted Diseases in Adolescents." *Practitioner, 222*:1329, 1979.

Felman, Yehudi and Nikitas, James: "Nongonococcal Urethritis." *New York State Journal of Medicine, 79*:6, 1979a.

Felman, Yehudi and Ricciardi, Nicholas: "Sexually Transmitted Enteric Diseases." *Bulletin of the New York Academy of Medicine, 55*:6, 1979b.

Felman, Y. M.: "A Plea for the Condom, Especially for Teenagers." *The Journal of the American Medical Association, 241*:23, 1979c.

Fong, R.: "Talking to Patients in Special Clinics." *Nursing Times, 72*:42, 1977.

Hatcher, Robert A., Stewart, Gary K., Stewart, Felicia, Stratton, Pamela and Wright, Angela: *Contraceptive Technology 1978—1979. (9th ed.),* New York, Irvington Publishers, 1979.

Henderson, Ralph H.: "Improving Sexually Transmitted Disease Health Services for Gays." *Sexually Transmitted Diseases, 4*:2, 1977.

Holmes, King K., and Martin, David: "Sexually Transmitted Diseases: Advances in Management." *Postgraduate Medicine, 64*:3, 1978.

Jupa, James: "Venereal Diseases." *Primary Care, 6*:1, 1979.

Kahl, I.: "A Potential Defaulter." *Nursing Times, 74*:37, 1977.

LeBourdois, Eleanor: "VD Apathy Among Doctors." *Dimensions of Health Service, 55*:2, 1978.

McCormack, William M.: "Common Sexually Transmitted Diseases and Their Treatment." *Bulletin of the New York Academy of Medicine, 54*:2, 1978.

McNab, Warren L.: "The 'Other' Venereal Diseases: Herpes Simplex, Trichomoniasis, and Candidiasis." *The Journal of School Health, 49*:2, 1979.

Niemiec, Marjean Austin, and Chen, Shu-Pi: "Seeking Clinic Care for Venereal Disease: A Study of Teenagers." *The Journal of School Health, 48*:1, 1978.

Poindexter, Hildrus A.: "Sexually Transmitted Disease." *Journal of the National Medical Association, 69*:8, 1977.

Rein, Michael F.: "Recent Developments in Sexually Transmitted Chlamydial Infections," *Medical Times, 109*(3), March, 1981.

Sparling, P. Frederick: "Current Problems in Sexually Transmitted Diseases." *Advances in Internal Medicine, 24*:203, 1979.

Tenenbaum, Marvin J.: "Grand Rounds: Sexually Transmitted Diseases," *Virginia Medical, 107*(4), April, 1980.

Urquhart, John: "Effect of the Venereal Disease Epidemic on the Incidence of Ectopic Pregnancy—Implications for the Evaluation of Contraceptives." *Contraception, 19*:5, 1979.

Wallechinsky, David, Wallace, Irving, and Wallace, Amy: *The People's Almanac Presents the Book of Lists.* New York, William Morrow and Co., Inc., 1977.

White, W., and Spencer-Phillips, R. J.: "Recurrent Vaginitis and Oral Sex." *Lancet,* vol. 1 (8116): 621, 1979.

INDEX

Note: Page numbers in *italics* refer to illustrations; page numbers followed by (t) refer to tables.